theclinics.com

EMERGENCY MEDICINE CLINICS OF NORTH AMERICA

Pain and Sedation Management in the 21st Century Emergency Department

GUEST EDITORS
John G. McManus Jr., MD, FACEP and
Benjamin Harrison, MD, FACEP

May 2005 • Volume 23 • Number 2

SAUNDERS
An Imprint of Elsevier, Inc.
PHILADELPHIA LONDON TORONTO MONTREAL SYDNEY TOKYO

W.B. SAUNDERS COMPANY
A Division of Elsevier Inc.

1600 John F. Kennedy Boulevard, Suite 1800 • Philadelphia, Pennsylvania 19103-2899

http://www.theclinics.com

EMERGENCY MEDICINE CLINICS OF NORTH AMERICA
May 2005
Editor: Karen Sorensen

Volume 23, Number 2
ISSN 0733-8627
ISBN 1-4160-2711-4

Emergency Medicine Clinics of North America (ISSN 0733-8627) is published quarterly by W.B. Saunders Company. Corporate and Editorial Offices: 1600 John F. Kennedy Boulevard, Suite 1800, Philadelphia, PA 19103-2899. Accounting and Circulation Offices: 6277 Sea Harbor Drive, Orlando, FL 32887-4800. Periodicals postage paid at Orlando, FL 32862, and additional mailing offices. Subscription prices are $170.00 per year (US individuals), $263.00 per year (US institutions), $225.00 per year (international individuals), $312.00 per year (international institutions), $205.00 per year (Canadian individuals), and $312.00 per year (Canadian institutions). International air speed delivery is included in all *Clinics'* subscription prices. All prices are subject to change without notice. POSTMASTER: Send address changes to *Emergency Medicine Clinics of North America*, W.B. Saunders Company, Periodicals Fulfillment, Orlando, FL 32887-4800. **Customer Service: 1-800-654-2452 (US). From outside of the US, call 1-407-345-4000. E-mail: hhspcs@harcourt.com.**

Emergency Medicine Clinics of North America is covered in *Index Medicus, Current Contents/Clinical Medicine, EMBASE/Excerpta Medica, BIOSIS, SciSearch, CINAHL, ISI/BIOMED,* and *Research Alert.*

Printed in the United States of America.

GUEST EDITORS

JOHN G. MCMANUS, JR, MD, FACEP, Lieutenant Colonel, United States Army; Research Physician Combat Casualty Care, United States Army Institute of Surgical Research, Fort Sam Houston, Texas; Adjunct Assistant Professor, Department of Military and Emergency Medicine, Uniformed Services University of the Health Sciences; Medical Director, Emergency Medical Services, Fort Sam Houston, Texas; Adjunct Assistant Professor, Department of Emergency Medicine, Oregon Health and Science University, Portland, Oregon

BENJAMIN HARRISON, MD, FACEP, Department of Emergency Medicine, Madigan Army Medical Center, Tacoma, Washington

CONTRIBUTORS

ELIZABETH L. BAHN, MD, Resident in Emergency Medicine, Department of Emergency Medicine, Madigan Army Medical Center/University of Washington Emergency Medicine Residency, Fort Lewis, Washington

ERIK D. BARTON, MD, Associate Professor, Division of Emergency Medicine, University of Utah School of Medicine, Salt Lake City, Utah

BEVERLY H. BAUMAN MD, Assistant Professor, Department of Emergency Medicine; Adjunct Assistant Professor, Department of Pediatrics; Chief, Pediatric Emergency Services, Doernbecher Emergency Department, Oregon Health & Sciences University, Portland, Oregon

ROBERT B. BLANKENSHIP, MD, Assistant Residency Director, Emergency Medicine Residency Program, Department of Emergency Medicine, Madigan Army Medical Center, Fort Lewis, Washington

CHAD S. CRYSTAL, MD, Staff Physician, Emergency Medicine Residency Program, Department of Emergency Medicine, Darnall Army Community Hospital, Fort Hood, Texas

JIM CZARNIK, MD, Major, United States Army; Emergency Medicine Physician, Staff Physician, WOMACK Medical Center, Fort Bragg, North Carolina

JAMES N. DILLARD, MD, DC, CAc, FAAPM&R, Assistant Clinical Professor, Columbia University College of Physicians and Surgeons; Medical Director, Rosenthal Center for Complementary and Alternative Medicine Under National Institutes of Health NCCAM Center Grant to Columbia University College of Physicians and Surgeons; Medical Director, Complementary and Alternative Medicine, Oxford Health Plans, New York, New York

JAMES DUCHARME, MDCM, FRCP, DABEM, Professor of Emergency Medicine, Department of Emergency Medicine, Dalhousie University; Clinical Director, Department of Emergency Medicine, Atlantic Health Sciences Corporation, Saint John, New Brunswick, Canada

WALTER ALLEN FINK, Jr, DO, FAAEM, FACEP, Major, United States Army; United States Army Clinical Instructor, Madigan Army Medical Center; Residency in Emergency Medicine, University of Washington-Madigan Army Medical Center, Tacoma, Washington

DAVID E. FOSNOCHT, MD, Associate Professor, Division of Emergency Medicine, University of Utah School of Medicine, Salt Lake City, Utah

GEORGE R. HANSEN, MD, Department of Emergency Medicine, Sierra Vista Regional Medical Center, San Luis Obispo, California

BENJAMIN HARRISON, MD, FACEP, Department of Emergency Medicine, Madigan Army Medical Center, Tacoma, Washington

STEVE HENDRIX, CRNA, Lieutenant Colonel, United States Army; Certified Registered Nurse, Anesthetist, Eisenhower Army Medical Center, Fort Gordon, Georgia

KURTIS R. HOLT, MD, FACEP, Associate Program Director, Department of Emergency Medicine, Madigan Army Medical Center/University of Washington Emergency Medicine Residency, Fort Lewis, Washington

GRANT D. INNES, MD, FRCP(C), Chairman, Department of Emergency Medicine, Providence Health Care and St. Paul's Hospital; Clinical Professor, Departments of Surgery and Emergency Medicine, University of British Columbia, Vancouver, British Columbia, Canada

TROY JOHNSON, MD, Major, United States Army; Emergency Medicine Physician, Assistant Professor, Uniformed Services University of Health Sciences, Bethesda, Maryland

SHARON KNAPP, MS, FNP, NP-C, Clinical Instructor, Department of Emergency Medicine, Oregon Health and Sciences University, Portland, Oregon; American Academy of Nurse Practicioners

LINDA L. LAWRENCE, MD, FACEP, Lieutenant Colonel, United States Air Force; MC Associate Professor, Department of Military & Emergency Medicine, Uniformed Services University of the Health Sciences, Bethesda, Maryland

PHILLIP LEVY, MD, Assistant Professor, Department of Emergency Medicine, Wayne State University, Detroit Receiving Hospital, Detroit, Michigan

DEREK R. LINKLATER, MD, Assistant Clinical Professor of Emergency Medicine, College of Medicine, Texas A & M University, College Station, Texas; Assistant Program Director, Emergency Medicine Residency Program, Darnall Army Community Hospital, Fort Hood, Texas

JOHN G. MCMANUS, JR, MD, FACEP, Lieutenant Colonel, United States Army; Research Physician Combat Casualty Care, United States Army Institute of Surgical Research, Fort Sam Houston, Texas; Adjunct Assistant Professor, Department of Military and

Emergency Medicine, Uniformed Services University of the Health Sciences; Medical Director, Emergency Medical Services, Fort Sam Houston, Texas; Adjunct Assistant Professor, Department of Emergency Medicine, Oregon Health and Science University, Portland, Oregon

MICHAEL A. MILLER, MD, Program Director, Medical Toxicologist, Department of Emergency Medicine, Darnall Army Community Hospital, Fort Hood, Texas

MANISH M. PATEL, MD, MSc, Assistant Professor, School of Medicine, Department of Emergency Medicine, Emory University, Atlanta, Georgia

LAURIE PEMBERTON, DO, Director of Pre-hospital Care and Teaching Faculty, Emergency Medicine Residency Program, Darnall Army Community Hospital, Fort Hood, Texas

CHRISTOPHER F. RICHARDS, MD, Associate Professor, Chief, Acute Clinical Care, Center for Policy and Research in Emergency Medicine, Department of Emergency Medicine, Oregon Health and Science University, Portland, Oregon

DONALD R. SALLEE, JR, MD, FAAEM, Commander, United States Navy; Director, Emergency Medical Services, Naval Medical Center, San Diego, California

JON STRELTZER, MD, Professor, Department of Psychiatry, University of Hawaii, Honolulu, Hawaii

ERIC R. SWANSON, MD, MS, Associate Professor, Division of Emergency Medicine, University of Utah School of Medicine, Salt Lake City, Utah

STEVE TAYLOR, DO, Resident, Emergency Medicine Residency Program, Madigan Army Medical Center-University of Washington, Tacoma, Washington

KNOX H. TODD, MD, MPH, Director, Pain and Emergency Medicine Institute, Beth Israel Medical Center, New York, New York

IAN S. WEDMORE, MD, FACEP, Lieutenant Colonel, United States Army; Emergency Medicine Physician, Deputy Chief, Department of Emergency Medicine, Clinical Instructor, University of Washington School of Medicine, Seattle, Washington; Physician, United States Army, Madigan Army Medical Center, Fort Lewis, Washington

PETER J. ZED, BSc, BSc(Pharm), PharmD, Pharmacotherapeutic Specialist, Emergency Medicine CSU Pharmaceutical Sciences, Vancouver General Hospital; Clinical Assistant Professor, Faculty of Pharmaceutical Sciences, University of British Columbia; Associate Member, Department of Surgery, Division of Emergency Medicine, University of British Columbia, Vancouver, British Columbia, Canada

WESLEY ZEGER, DO, Attending Faculty, Department of Emergency Medicine, University of Nebraska Medical Center, Omaha, Nebraska

CONTENTS

This article discusses the anatomy and physiology of pain sensations, concentrating on mechanism of acute pain. Limited discussion is offered regarding the modulation of pain sensations, as well as a brief overview of visceral pain.

This article provides a practical review of pain measures and assessment procedures most appropriate for emergency care researchers and providers. It reviews pain measures currently in use and suggests additional measures that could profitably be employed in the emergency department practice setting. The choice or preference for specific tools is based on the feasibility and ease of their use, or the likelihood that they can be standardized or disseminated between departments. There will always be a need for new tools with which to understand our patients' experience and inform our clinical decision-making. This field is ripe for input from our specialty.

A culture of suspicion, diverse and often difficult patient populations, and challenging clinical environments combine to present formidable barriers for effective pain management in the emergency

By operational we mean the austere deployed military setting, to include both noncombat and combat operations. The authors combined experience with wartime trauma pain management consists of experience in Operation "Just Cause" (Panama Invasion), Operation "Desert Storm" (Persian Gulf War), Operation "Uphold Democracy" (Haiti liberation), Operation "Enduring Freedom" (Afghanistan conflict), and Operation "Iraqi Freedom" (Iraq conflict).

GOAL *STATEMENT*

The goal of Emergency Medicine Clinics of North America is to keep practicing physicians up to date with current clinical practice in emergency medicine by providing timely articles reviewing the state of the art in patient care.

ACCREDITATION

The Emergency Medicine Clinics of North America is planned and implemented in accordance with the Essential Areas and Policies of the Accreditation Council for Continuing Medical Education (ACCME) through the joint sponsorship of the University Of Virginia School Of Medicine and Elsevier. The University Of Virginia School of Medicine is accredited by the ACCME to provide continuing medical education for physicians.

The University of Virginia School of Medicine designates this educational activity for a maximum of 60 category 1 credits per year, 15 category 1 credits per issue, toward the AMA Physician's Recognition Award. Each physician should claim only those credits that he/she actually spent in the activity.

The American Medical Association has determined that physicians not licensed in the US who participate in this CME activity are eligible for AMA PRA category 1 credit.

Category 1 credit can be earned by reading the text material, taking the CME examination online at http://www.theclinics.com/home/cme, and completing the evaluation. After taking the test, you will be required to review any and all incorrect answers. Following completion of the test and evaluation, your credit will be awarded and you may print your certificate.

FACULTY DISCLOSURE

As a provider accredited by the Accreditation Council for Continuing Medical Education (ACCME), the Office of Continuing Medical Education of the University of Virginia School of Medicine must ensure balance, independence, objectivity, and scientific rigor in all its individually sponsored or jointly sponsored educational activities. All authors/editors participating in a sponsored activity are expected to disclose to the readers any significant financial interest or other relationship (1) with the manufacturer(s) of any commercial product(s) and/or provider(s) of commercial services discussed in an educational presentation and (2) with any commercial supporters of the activity (significant financial interest or other relationship can include such things as grants or research support, employee, consultant, stock holder, member of speakers bureau, etc.) The intent of this disclosure is not to prevent authors/editors with a significant financial or other relationship from writing an article, but rather to provide readers with information on which they can make their own judgments. It remains for the readers to determine whether the author's/editor's interest or relationships may influence the article with regard to exposition or conclusion.

The authors/editors listed below have identified no professional or financial affiliations related to their presentation: Elizabeth L. Bahn, MD, PS; Erik D. Barton, MD, MS; Beverly Bauman, MD, FAAP, FACEP; Robert B. Blankenship, MD, MAJ, USA, MC; Chad S. Crystal, ND; Jim Czarnik, MD; James N. Dillard, MD, DC, CAc, FAAPM James Ducharme, MDCM, FRCP, DABEM; Walter Allen Fink, Jr., DO, FAAEM; David E. Fosnocht, MD; George R. Hansen, MD; Benjamin Harrison, MD, FACEP; Steven Hendrix, RN; Kurtis R. Holt, MD, FACEP; Grant D. Innes, MD, FRCPC; Troy R. Johnson, MD; Linda L. Lawrence, MD, FACEP; Phillip D. Levy, MD, MPH; Derek R. Linklater, MD; John G. McManus, MD, FACEP; Michael A. Miller, MD, LTC, USA; LCDR Manish M. Patel, MD MSc; Laurie Pemberton, DO; Christopher F. Richards, MD; Donald R. Sallee, Jr., MD, FAAEM; Karen Sorensen, Acquisitions Editor; Jon Streltzer, MD; Eric R. Swanson, MD; Steven Taylor, DO; Knox H. Todd, MD, MPH, FACEP; Ian S. Wedmore, MD, FACEP; Peter J. Zed, BSc, BSc (Pharm), PharmD; and, Wesley G. Zeger, DO.

Disclosure of discussion of non-FDA approved uses for pharmaceutical products and/or medical devices: The University of Virginia School of Medicine, as an ACCME provider, requires that all authors/editors identify and disclose any "off label" uses for pharmaceutical products and/or for medical devices. The University of Virginia School of Medicine recommends that each reader fully review all the available data on new products or procedures prior to instituting them with patients.

All authors/editors who provided disclosures have indicated that they will not be discussing off-label uses except:
Jim Czarnik, MD, Steven Hendrix, RN, and Ian S. Wedmore, MD, FACEP discuss use of fentanyl lozenges for acute traumatic pain control and the use of low dose ketamine for pain control.
Troy R. Johnson, MD discusses the use of Trans-mucosal Fentanyl Citrate (OTFC) for acute pain management. This is currently FDA approved for break through cancer pain. The article also discusses several studies using this preparation.
Beverly Bauman, MD, FAAP, FACEP will discuss the following drugs: Codeine: Safe dosage of acetaminophen and codeine phosphate oral solution USP has not been established in children below the age of 3 years; Hydropmorphone: Safety and effectiveness in children have not been established; Oxycodone: Safety and effectiveness in pediatric patients have not been established; Morphine: No information is available regarding the use of Astramorph/PF in patients under the age of 18; Hydrocodone: Safety and effectiveness in the pediatric population below the age of two years have not been established; Fentanyl: should not be administered to children (under 12 years of age) or patients under 18 years of age who weigh less than 50 kg (110 lbs) except in an authorized investigational research setting; Lorazepam The administration of lorazepam intravenously to patients younger than 18 years of age has not been; Methohexital The safety and effectiveness of methohexital sodium in children less than 1 month of age have not been established, 2001); Propofol: Safety and effectiveness of propofol injection has not been established for use in intensive care unit sedation or for monitored anesthesia care (MAC) sedation in pediatric patients; Etomidate The manufacturer indicates that ETOMIDATE should not be used in children less than 10-years-old because of lack of sufficient data. In children older than 10 years, the usual dose is 0.3 milligram/kilogram (range, 0.2 to 0.6 milligram/kilogram), which is the same as for adults; Ethyl Chloride -does not have FDA approval for pediatric use.
Wesley G. Zeger, DO will discuss the use of metoclopramide, prochlorperazin, and chlorpromazine for treatment of migraine headaches.

The following author has not provided disclosure or off-label information.
Sharon Knapp, MS, FNP, NP-C

TO ENROLL

To enroll in the Emergency Medicine Clinics of North America Continuing Medical Education program, call customer service at 1-800-654-2452 or visit us online at www.theclinics.com/home/cme. The CME program is available to subscribers for an additional fee of $165.00.

FORTHCOMING ISSUES

August 2005

Endocrine and Metabolic Emergencies
Mary Jo Wagner, MD, FACEP, and
Kathleen Cowling, DO, FACEP, *Guest Editors*

November 2005

Emergency Cardiology: Challenges, Controversies, and Advances
William Brady, MD, Wyatt W. Decker, MD, and
Amal Mattu, MD, *Guest Editors*

February 2006

The ECG in Emergency Medicine
Richard Harrigan, MD, William Brady, MD, and
Ted C. Chan, MD, *Guest Editors*

RECENT ISSUES

February 2005

International Emergency Medicine
L. Kristian Arnold, MD, FACEP, and Jeffrey Smith, MD, MPH, *Guest Editors*

November 2004

Unsuspected Killers in Emergency Medicine
Amal Mattu, MD, Deepi G. Goyal, MD, and
Andrew S. Ulrich, MD, *Guest Editors*

August 2004

Ultrasound in Emergency Medicine
Carlo L. Rosen, MD, and Richard E. Wolfe, MD
Guest Editors

EMERGENCY
MEDICINE
CLINICS OF
NORTH AMERICA

ELSEVIER
SAUNDERS

Emerg Med Clin N Am 23 (2005) xv–xvi

Preface

Pain and Sedation Management In the 21st Century Emergency Department

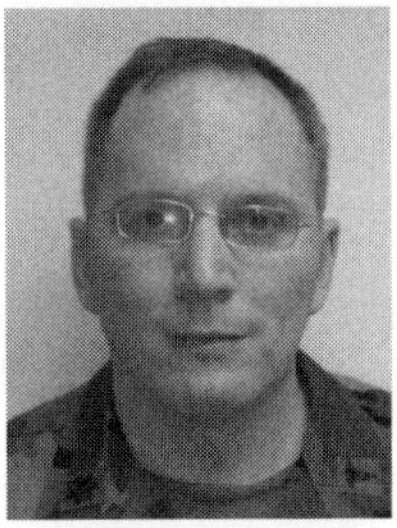

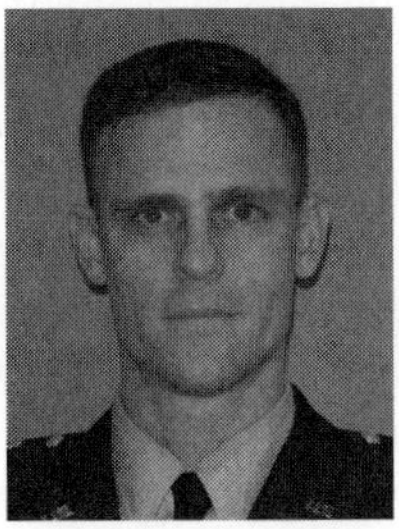

John G. McManus, Jr, MD, FACEP   Benjamin Harrison, MD, FACEP
Guest Editors

Pain is the most common reason patients seek care in emergency departments (ED), with as much as 70% of patients having pain as part of their presenting complaint. Emergency physicians treat many patients with many etiologies and levels of pain. The volume and severity of pain-related problems make pain management a core skill in emergency medicine, yet there is ongoing evidence that pain is inadequately treated in the ED. For more than a decade we have identified that pain is undertreated in emergency medicine. Wilson coined the term "oligoanalgesia" in 1989 for inadequate use of methods to relieve pain.

So, how then do we (emergency care providers) improve on our pain management? First, fundamental changes in the attitudes of emergency providers regarding pain assessment and pain management are necessary to prevent such "oligoanalgesia" in the emergency environment. This change in attitude requires that providers recognize and treat pain as a true emergency. Changing the attitudes of emergency medical providers about pain assessment and management will require attention in several areas of research, education, and training. Next, a better understanding of the pathophysiology, measurement, and optimal therapies for pain must be learned and taught to all our providers. Also, patient needs and expectations for pain relief, as well as continued efforts at patient education regarding pain, will also improve our treatment of pain in the ED. Finally, providers must understand various future aspects of education, evaluation, and therapy that may allow us to optimize pain care.

0733-8627/05/$ - see front matter
doi:10.1016/j.emc.2004.12.019   *emed.theclinics.com*

The last 15 years have seen a substantial increase in ED research focused on pain and pain management. Continued research efforts and focused clinical application of these efforts are still required. Recognition by providers of the ethnic, cultural, and gender differences in the expression, reporting, and expectations for treatment of pain should also continue to be a priority in changing attitudes toward pain and pain control. These goals must be realistic within the chaotic and unpredictable environment that defines emergency medicine. Practical and time-sensitive approaches to pain and pain management will continue to be a challenge to enact and enforce in our EDs.

The consequences of "oligoanalgesia" in the ED are not insignificant. To improve our treatment of pain in the ED, a fundamental change in attitude toward pain and the control of pain is required. This is unlikely to occur until pain is adequately addressed and treated appropriately as a true emergency. This edition of *Emergency Medicine Clinics of North America* hopes to reinforce the importance of pain education, management, and treatment for our emergency medical patients.

John G. McManus, Jr, MD, FACEP
The Army Institute of Surgical Research
Brooke Army Medical Center
San Antonio, TX 78258, USA

Benjamin Harrison, MD, FACEP
Department of Emergency Medicine
Madigan Army Medical Center
Tacoma, WA 98431, USA

ELSEVIER
SAUNDERS

EMERGENCY
MEDICINE
CLINICS OF
NORTH AMERICA

Emerg Med Clin N Am 23 (2005) 277–284

The Pathophysiology of Acute Pain

Walter Allen Fink Jr, DO, FAAEM, FACEP

United States Army, Major, Department of Emergency Medicine, Madigan Army Medical Center-University of Washington, Tacoma, WA 98431, USA

The sensation of pain is a neural-biochemical phenomenon. When acute tissue damage occurs, neurochemical reactions at the site of injury activate the free nerve endings of special nerves called nociceptors. Nociceptors initiate an afferent nerve impulse that propagates through the peripheral nerve, enters the spinal cord, and synapses with higher order neurons. The impulse then traverses specific ascending spinal tracts, landing in cerebral centers for interpretation. Modulation of the afferent information can occur in many areas, including the periphery, spinal cord, midbrain, and cerebral cortex. Interpretation of the impulse yields a response signal, again traveling through specific descending spinal tracks and out through peripheral motor nerves. This process partially accounts for the delay in feeling a sensation of pain after experiencing an acute injury. Pain sensations can be categorized in many ways, based upon their speed in traveling in the nervous system (fast and slow pain), the length of time the pain has continued (acute or chronic pain), or the anatomical etiology of the sensations (somatic or visceral pain). This article discusses the anatomy and physiology of pain sensations, concentrating on acute pain mechanisms. Limited discussion is offered regarding the modulation of pain sensations, and there is a brief overview of visceral pain. Discussion of chronic pain pathophysiology is included in the article by Hansen on chronic pain elsewhere in this issue.

Pain receptors and peripheral nerve fibers

Nociceptors transduce noxious stimuli into a nerve impulse, and the feeling of physical pain is initiated with its activation. The cell bodies of nociceptors are located in the dorsal root ganglion of the spinal nerve at each level, or the trigeminal ganglion for the trigeminal nerve. This is typical for all peripheral nerves. Each cell body possesses two branches, one

E-mail address: Walter.fink@nw.amedd.army.mil

0733-8627/05/$ - see front matter
doi:10.1016/j.emc.2004.12.001 **emed.theclinics.com**

projecting to the periphery where its terminal is sensitive to noxious stimuli. The second branch projects to the spinal cord, where it synapses with higher-order central nervous system (CNS) neurons. Unlike the free nerve ending associated with sensation, nociceptors lack a specific encapsulated receptor. Instead, they broadly interweave with the local tissue, based upon anatomical location [1]. Nociceptors are found throughout the body, but are most extensively located in the integumen, periosteium, arterial walls, teeth, and joint surfaces, as well as the falx and tentorium of the cranial vault [2]. Pain receptors are less frequently found in other deep tissues of the body; however, tissue damage can initiate pain in these areas. Two broad categories of polymodal nociceptors are recognized. The C (chemical) polymodal receptors are the most common, and compose 80% of all peripheral nociceptors. A full range of mechanical, thermal, and chemical stimuli activate ploymodal C receptors [3]. The second type of nociceptors are the Aδ polymodal nociceptors. Less numerous than the polymodal C receptor, these receptors are activated primarily by thermal or mechanical stimuli [4].

Tissue damage causes the release of numerous chemicals, including leukotrienes, bradykinins, serotonin, histamine, potassium ions, acids, acetylcholine, thromboxanes, substance P, and platelet activating factor. Chemical pain receptors (polymodal C type) react to the release of these mediators to deliver the sensation of pain. These chemicals can be important factors in the development of ongoing pain after acute injury. Prostoglandins cannot directly activate receptors, but are involved as a local mediator or cofactor, enhancing the sensitivity of the free nerve ending. Mechanical and thermal receptors react to excessive mechanical stretch or temperature, activating both the polymodal Aδ and C nociceptors [2].

The speed of signal transmission of each type of polymodal peripheral nociceptors can be delineated by its unique anatomical characteristics. The polymodal C fibers are nonmylinated and transmit afferent pain sensation at a slower velocity than do the mylinated Aδ fibers. The faster-mylinated Aδ pain fibers deliver mechanical and thermal pain sensations at a velocity of 5 to 30 m/second, and have a neuronal diameter of 1 to 5 microns. Sensation that travels via the Aδ fibers can be initiated by cutting the skin with a knife, or by an electric shock, and is often described as "fast pain" sensation. These pain sensations are less common in the deep tissues of the body, because there are a decreased number of the Aδ fibers to those regions. Sensation that is ascribed to the polymodal C receptors begins a second or more after a painful encounter, and increases in intensity over seconds or minutes. The sensation has been referred to as "slow pain." The slow pain sensation travels via the nonmylinated C fibers with a velocity of 0.5 to 2 m/second, with the neurons having a diameter of less than 1.5 microns. The feeling ascribed to slow pain is a dull, throbbing, aching pain sensation, and it is associated with tissue destruction as well as deep visceral pain. This is also the sensation associated with chronic pain [3,5].

The dual system of the faster Aδ fibers and the slower polymodal C fibers working in concert causes a painful stimulus to deliver a "double" sensation of pain—initially a fast, sharp pain sensation that is available to initiate an immediate reaction; then a slower, lasting, burning pain sensation. This slow, burning pain tends to become more intense over time, and if the stimulation is not relieved, it may evolve into chronic pain. Unlike other sensory receptors in the body, nociceptors have a limited ability to adapt. As a painful stimulus continues, the excitation of pain receptors becomes greater, with increasing afferent signal transmission. Hyperalgesia is the result [6].

Spinal cord

The primary afferent nerve fibers from each of the peripheral nociceptors enter the dorsal spinal cord from the dorsal spinal root ganglion. Many afferent fibers synapse with the second-order neuron at that same spinal level in the dorsal horn; however, portions of these fibers can ascend or descend one to three spinal segments before terminating. These ascending/descending afferent fibers travel in the in the tract of Lissauer, located posterior to the dorsal horn of the cord gray matter. This distribution of the afferent signals over several spinal segments contributes to the difficulty in precisely localizing a painful sensation [3].

The dorsal horn of the spinal cord is divided anatomically into six distinct layers or laminae, with each receiving specific types of afferent nerve fibers. Lamina I is referred to as the lamina lamginalis, and laminae II and III are collectively called the substantia gelatinosa. It is within these laminae that the majority of the Aδ and C fibers synapse. Some Aδ fibers do extend into the deep dorsal horn and synapse in laminae V. Glutamate and the glutamate receptor—designated the alpha-amino-3-hydroxy-5-methylisoxazole-4-propionic-acid (AMPA) receptor—constitute the main neurotransmitter/receptor combination in acute pain neurons [7,8].

Projection neurons, inhibitory neurons, and excitatory neurons are found within the dorsal horn, and affect the propagation of an afferent pain signal. Inhibitory and excitatory neurons function specifically to modulate the flow of afferent traffic to higher centers, and projection neurons forward afferent sensations to higher centers. Three physiological subtypes of projection neurons are known. Nociceptor-specific neurons respond only to noxious stimuli and have small receptive fields. They are mostly located in lamina I, but can also found in small numbers in laminae II and V. Located in laminae III and IV, low threshold (LT) neuron responds to innocuous. Wide dynamic range (WDR) neurons are the most plentiful neurons in the dorsal horn, and predominate in laminae V. WDR neurons are also found in lesser concentrations in laminae I. This neuronal type responds to a large range of sensory stimuli, and require a combination of multiple signals to activate. WDR neurons receive converging inputs from many sensory modalities and posses large receptor fields [9].

Ascending pathways

There are several pathways for afferent pain signals to traverse through the ascending spinal cord to the cortex. The spinothalamic pathway is regarded as the most important pathway, and can be subdivided into the neospinothalamic (lateral spinothalamic) pathway and the paleospinothalamic (medial spinothalamic) pathway. The neospinothalamic is the primary pathway for sensations initiated by fast pain signals. The thinly mylenated Aδ fibers transmit the sensations of mechanical and thermal pain and enter the spinal cord, terminating in the lamina marginalis of the spinal cord's dorsal horn. The nociceptive signal can then continue through to the second-order neurons in the neospinothalamic tract. The neospinothalamic fibers cross immediately to the opposite side of the spinal cord through the anterior commisure, and pass upward toward the cortex in the anterolateral area of the spinal cord.

The neospinothalamic nerve fibers travel to the thalamus, with only a few fibers terminating in the reticular area of the brainstem. In the thalamus, a majority of the fibers terminate in the ventrobasal complex, with a few fibers ending in the posterior nuclear group. From these areas, the signals propagate to the somatic sensory cortex and other basal areas of the brain.

The neospinalthalamic tract is responsible for transmitting the discriminating aspects of pain, such as location, intensity, and duration. The localization of the Aδ fast/sharp pain sensation is much more accurate than with the polymodal C receptors, because of the simultaneous stimulation of both pain receptors and tactile receptors during injury. If only pain receptors are stimulated, sensations are poorly localized to an area of about 10 cm. With the added stimulation of tactile receptors, the location of origin can be exactly identified [9].

The paleospinothalmaic pathway is principally for the transmission of unmylinated, type C fibers that are conductive of slow or chronic pain sensations. The autonomic and unpleasant emotional perceptions travel this pathway as well [3]. These peripheral fibers enter the spinal cord and terminate in the substantia gelatinosa of the dorsal horn. These signals then pass through one or several other short neurons before landing in lamina V of the dorsal horn. From lamina V, the majority of neurons then join with the fibers from the fast pathway and cross at the anterior commisure, then ascend to the cortex in the same anterolateral columns as the neospinothalamic fibers. Some of the paleospinothalamic fibers do not cross, but ascend in the spinal cord ipsilaterally to the cortex in the anterolateral columns. This multisynaptic ascending route is another reason for the inability to specifically localize these pain sensations to a greater degree than the general body region of the sensation. Substance P is believed to be the main neurotransmitter of the paleospinothalamic pathway in the dorsal horn, and therefore the main neurotransmitter associated with slow pain sensations. This synaptic transmitter has the typical synaptic neuropeptide characteristics: slow buildup within the synapse, with a more delayed resolution. This is shown by the progressive intensity of slow type pain, as well as the persistence of this type of pain after the removal of the painful stimulus [10].

The polymodal C fibers have a large area terminal distribution, with only one tenth to one fourth of the fibers ending in the thalamus. This area is comprised mainly of the reticular nuclei of the medulla, pons, and mesencephalon: the tectal area of the mesencephalon, and the periaqueductal gray region surrounding the aqueduct of silvius [2]. From the reticular area of the brain stem, the signals continue to the thalamus, hypothalamus, and other areas of the basal brain.

The spinomesencephalic pathway modulates afferent information, and is not vital for the perception of pain. The spinomesencephalic pathway also plays a role in the activation of descending control systems and endogenous opiod systems. It begins with the nociceptors in laminae I and V, and terminates in the roof of the midbrain and the periaqueductal gray matter [9]. Ongoing research has identified additional pathways, including the spinopontoamygdaliod [11], as well as a pathway for visceral pain ascending to the posterior funiculus [12].

Cerebral interpretation

The lateral and medical thalamus initiate the interpretations of most noxious stimuli, then forward the stimuli to the cerebral cortex. The cortical structures involved in interpretation of pain sensations are the primary somatosensory cortex, secondary somatosensory cortex, pariental operculum, insula, anterior cingulated cortex, and prefrontal cortex [10]. Recent achievements have evolved defining central mechanisms of pain processing from the use of positron emission tomography (PET) and functional MRI scans [13]. These advanced imaging techniques have the ability to detect alterations in blood flow that can be then correlated to metabolic activity. These technological advancements support the idea that pain sensations arrive in the cortex only after thalamic processing has been abandoned. Some examples of direct cortical processing include: the coding of pain intensity in the periventricular white matter and posterior cingulated cortex; the encoding of pain and unpleasantness to the posterior sector of the anterior cingulated cortex; and the gating function reflected by the pain threshold in the anterior cingulate gyrus, the frontal cortex, and thalamus [3].

Modulation and antinociception response

Within the nervous system there is a pain-inhibitory or antinociceptive response system. The periaqueductal gray area, the raphe magnus nucleus, and the pain inhibitory complex in the anterior horn provide the body with the ability to overcome debilitating painful stimuli while simultaneously allowing the commencement of survival functions. This response consists of multiple component parts, including competitive inhibition, endogenous opiods, and other chemicals released within the nervous system, such as norepinephrine, relaxin, gamma-aminobutyric acid, oxytocin, and dynorphin.

Competative inhibition caused by sensory nerves has been identified and described with the gate control theory. This is an example of modulation occurring at the spinal cord level. The gate control theory states that the larger Aβ sensory fibers transmitting sensory information from the periphery inhibit the signals of the smaller Aδ and C fibers in the substancia gelatinosa, thereby decreasing the amplitude of the afferent pain signal. Additionally, it has been demonstrated that WDR neurons can be inhibited by noxious stimulation in other noncontiguous areas of the body [14]. This is the physiologic explanation for why use of transcutaneous electrical nerve stimulation, the simple rubbing of an injury site, or the use of a topically applied liniment can relieve pain.

Endorphins, enkephalins, and dynorphin are three subtypes of endogenous opioids that are responsible for another important part of the antinociceptive response. These opioids are released throughout the brain and spinal cord by supportive neuronal cells responding to a painful stimulation. Additionally, the receptors for these opioids are the site of action for exogenously administered opioids. The article on chronic pain previously cited offers a detailed discussion of each specific opioid, defining its mechanism and place of action.

Visceral pain

Visceral pain has several specific characteristics that differentiate it from pain felt by direct cutaneous stimulation. Direct trauma to skin and superficial structures typically produces pain; however, when direct trauma is applied to healthy visceral organs, no pain is appreciated. Nevertheless, with diffuse stimulation of visceral pain receptors, pain sensation can be extremely severe. This can be demonstrated by the pain caused from gut ischemia. Visceral pain is often difficult to localize and is diffuse, and as time increases it is often referred to more superficial structures. Radiation of the pain can travel over a considerable distance. Lastly, the site of the referred pain may develop hyperalgesia, as may the affected viscera [15].

The four specific causes to for true visceral pain are ischemia, chemical stimulation, spasm of a hollow viscus as well as overdistention of a hollow viscus. The liver parenchyma and the alveoli of the lungs are almost entirely insensitive to pain, but though their associated structures—the liver capsule and bile ducts and the bronchi and parietal pleura—identification of inflammation and injury can occur [3].

Summary

The method by which the body detects, interprets, and responds to painful stimulation is tantamount to an orchestral concert, with each individual instrument contributing a subtle yet important element composing the finished product. The polymodal peripheral receptors initiate unpleasant sensations that can be modulated in the dorsal horn and the anterior columns of the spinal cord before reaching the cerebral cortex. Despite similar neurological "wiring," pain sensations from the skin are not the same in character as those from visceral organs. A reaction of pain is based upon interpretation in specific cerebral centers and the resultant motor function. With the advent of functional MRI and PET scanners, the understanding of the cerebral interpretation of pain is expanding. Remember as well that emotional and psychological factors are crucial in pain perception, and are the starting points for any individual's perception of a painful circumstance.

References

[1] Byres MR, Bonica JB. Peripheral pain mechanisms and nocciceptor plasticity. In: Loser JD, Butler SH, Champion CR, et al, editors. Bonica's management of pain. 3rd edition. Philadelphia: Lippencott Williams and Wilkins; 2001. p. 32–3.

[2] Guyton AC. Somatic sensations. II. Pain, headache, and thermal sensations. In: Guyton AC, editor. Textbook of medical physiology. 8th edition. Philadelphia: WB Saunders Company; 1991. p. 520.

[3] Beaulieu P, Rice AS. Applied physiology of nociception. In: Rowbotham DJ, Macintyre PE, editors. Clinical Management of Acute Pain. New York: Arnold Publishers; 2003. p. 4–14.

[4] Schmidt RF. The articular polymodal receptor nociceptor in health and disease. In: Kumaza T, editor. The polymodal receptor—gateway to pathological pain. Progress in brain research, vol. 113. Amsterdam: Elsevier; 1996. p. 53–81.

[5] Fields HL. Pain. New York: McGraw-Hill; 1987.

[6] Myer RA, Campbell JN, Srinivasa NR. Peripheral neural mechanisms of nociception. In: Wall PD, Melzack R, editors. Textbook of pain. 3rd edition. New York: Churchill Livingstone; 1994. p. 14–9.

[7] Rexed B. The cytoarchitectonic organization of the spinal cord in the cat. J Comp Neurol 1952;96:415–95.

[8] Parent A. Carpenter's human neuroanatomy. Baltimore (MD): Williams & Wilkins; 1996.

[9] Terman GW, Bonica JJ. Spinal mechanisms and their modulation. In: Loser JD, Butler SH, Champion CR, et al, editors. Bonica's management of pain. 3rd edition. Philadelphia: Lippencott Williams and Wilkins; 2001. p. 84–122.

[10] Guilbaud G, Bernard JF, Besson JM. Brain areas involved in nociception and pain. In: Wall PD, Melzack R, editors. Textbook of Pain. 3rd edition. New York: Churchill Livingstone; 1994. p. 113–20.

[11] Hirshberg RM, Al-Chaer ED, Lawand NB, et al. Is there a pathway in the posterior funiculus that signals visceral pain? Pain 1996;67:291–305.

[12] Levine JD, Fields HL, Basbaum AI. Peptides and the primary afferent nociceptor. J Neurosci 1993;13:2273–86.

[13] Tolle TR, Kaufmann T, Seissmeier T, et al. Region-specific encoding of sensory and affective components in the human brain: a positron emission tomography correlation analysis. Ann Neurol 1999;45:40–7.
[14] Melzack R, Wall PD. Pain mechanisms: a new theory. Science 1965;150(699):971–9.
[15] McMahon SB. Mechanisms of cutaneous, deep and visceral pain. In: Wall PD, Melzack R, editors. Textbook of pain. 3rd edition. New York: Churchill Livingstone; 1994. p. 129–30.

ELSEVIER
SAUNDERS

Emerg Med Clin N Am 23 (2005) 285–295

EMERGENCY
MEDICINE
CLINICS OF
NORTH AMERICA

Pain Assessment Instruments for Use in the Emergency Department

Knox H. Todd, MD, MPH

Department of Emergency Medicine, Pain and Emergency Medicine Institute, Beth Israel Medical Center, First Avenue at 16th Street, New York, NY, 10003

The field of health measurement has a relatively brief history. Most developed countries have collected national statistical data, including health-related data, for little more than a century. It is important to understand that the decision to collect particular health-related data or health indicators is ultimately driven by social concerns. The effort is not an isolated intellectual exercise. The selection of particular health indicators reflects the perceived importance of a problem at a particular historical point in time, and the results of such measurements commonly become tools, or even ammunition, for those promoting social reforms. Thus this article has been published, and perhaps you are reading it, to focus attention on the problem of inadequately treated pain and improve our collective practice.

One definition of measurement is "the assignment of numbers to objects or events to represent quantities of attributes according to rules" [1]. The process of measuring health involves asking standardized questions about a particular condition, and assigning numbers to the responses. Many such questions may be aggregated into a cumulative score, intended to reflect some aspect of health. Although physicians record patients' histories routinely, the difference between history-taking and health measurement is the standardized nature of the questions and the assigning of numerical scores to such results.

Barriers to assessment

Pain is inherently subjective and inevitably complex. Our patients experience pain and suffering as individuals; we assess it only indirectly.

This work is supported, in part, though a generous grant from The Mayday Fund, New York, New York.

E-mail address: ktodd@bethisraelny.org

0733-8627/05/$ - see front matter
doi:10.1016/j.emc.2004.12.002

emed.theclinics.com

Our clinical and research task is to use a commonly understood vocabulary and classification system in assessing pain, so that our findings can be communicated consistently. Only by quantifying the pain experience in meaningful ways can we move beyond myth and idiosyncratic opinions toward a more scientific approach to questions regarding the pain experience.

This challenge of understanding another's internal experience is at the root of our difficulties in treating pain; thus issues surrounding pain assessment have primacy in our approach to understanding. Only when we use comparable methods in assessing pain can we begin to accumulate the scientific evidence that should drive our practice.

The most common response of physicians confronted by a patient's pain report is skepticism. The validity of patient self-report is often questioned, and attempts to objectify the pain experience are sought. This search is bound to disappoint the querulous clinician, because neither blood tests, tissue pathology, diagnostic imaging, physical assessments, nor patient behaviors reliably reflect the internal pain experience.

Before beginning a discussion of specific pain assessment instruments, we should consider who the users of such information might be, and how the perspectives of different user groups might differ (Fig. 1). At the level of the patient–clinician encounter, pain intensity and pain relief are of primary importance. Adverse effects may be viewed differently by patient and provider, particularly when the provider is concerned with the medicolegal ramifications of his or her therapeutic decisions. Functional impairment and satisfaction may have disparate meanings as well to the patient and provider.

Beyond the level of the clinical encounter, third-party payers and managed care organizations are likely to have very different opinions as to the importance of specific pain-related outcomes. Enrollees' health-care use patterns have important implications for the managed care or health

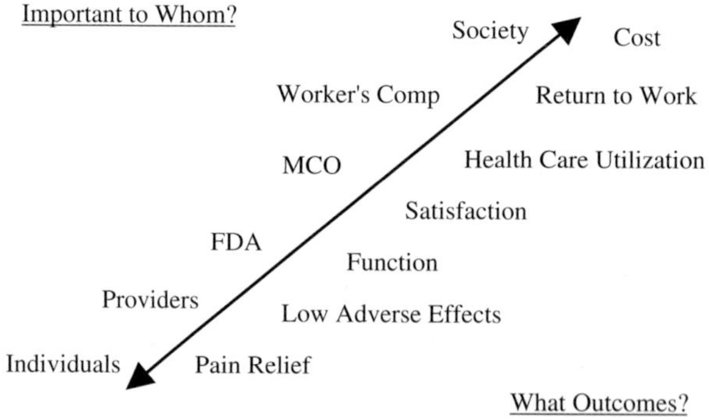

Fig. 1. Differing perspectives on pain.

maintenance organization's profitability, whereas workers' compensation entities may be much more concerned about level of function and return to work. Finally, society is concerned with global cost-effectiveness. How do we, as a society, ration our resources in the face of the seemingly continuous rise in health care costs? The measures required for communicating to each of these stakeholders differ, and we must select our instruments with knowledge of their disparate needs for information.

Reliability and validity

As the author discusses specific measurement instruments, he will refer often to validity and reliability. Validity asks the question: "Does this instrument measure what it is supposed to measure?" Common aspects of validity that can be assessed include content validity, criterion validity, or predictive validity. In judging content validity, we question how relevant specific questions are to the aims of the instrument. This is often done informally by asking experts their opinions of the instrument content's relevance to intended measurement goals, resulting in statements concerning face validity. Another concept of validity is criterion validity. Where an older gold standard exists, how well does the newer measure agree with the accepted instrument? The higher the correlation between the two, the greater the criterion validity of the new measure.

Finally, predictive validity refers to how well the instrument of interest predicts certain outcomes. An instrument possessing predictive validity should result in lower pain intensity scores after a patient in pain receives an analgesic of known efficacy, and higher scores when the patient has suffered disease progression from a disease that is known to be associated with pain, such as cancer. Distinct from validity, reliability concerns the replicability of an instrument's results. In assessing pain, our major concerns regarding reliability are whether an instrument's results remain stable over time when a patient's pain intensity has not changed. This feature is termed test-retest reliability.

Pain intensity

We will consider four single-item instruments used to rate pain intensity: the numerical rating scale (NRS), visual analog scale (VAS), graphical rating scale (GRS), and verbal rating scale (VRS). The integration of pain intensity as a "vital sign" within health care institutions has been promoted with some success by the Joint Commission on the Accreditation of Health Care Organizations (JCAHO), and in most US emergency departments today, a single-item rating of pain intensity (usually some form of NRS) is elicited and documented, often at the time of triage.

The numerical rating scale

A typical NRS consists of a range of numbers, from which one is selected by the patient as most representative of their level of pain intensity (Fig. 2). Although the range of numbers used is usually 0 to 10, other ranges may be used, such as 0 to 20, or 0 to 100. Patients are told that zero represents "no pain" and that the highest number represents some maximal measure of pain. The verbal descriptor for this extreme state may vary; however, phrases such as "pain as intense as you can imagine" or "worst pain possible" are commonly used. Patients may be asked to respond verbally to an NRS, or it may be administered as a written instrument. The former feature facilitates its use in a wide variety of clinical care settings.

Although the NRS has enjoyed less use as a research tool than the VAS (see discussion below), this practice may be changing. In fact, NRS scales are used increasingly in clinical trials. They have acceptable reliability and validity, and their psychometric properties are very similar to those of the VAS [2–11]. The NRS is sensitive to the short-term changes in pain intensity associated with emergent care [10,12].

The visual analog scale

The VAS typically consists of a 100-mm line, oriented horizontally and bounded at each end by verbal descriptors of pain intensity severity (Fig. 3). The descriptor "no pain" is situated to the left of the line, and a phrase describing an upper pain intensity limit, such as "worst pain possible" or "pain as bad as it could be," appears to the right of the line. Patients are asked to place a mark at the point on the line that best represents their pain intensity level. The distance from the left of the line to the mark is measured and pain intensity is reported in millimeters (range 0 to 100). Unlike the NRS, the VAS requires written materials. The VAS, like the NRS, has been shown to be a reliable and valid measure of pain intensity in the ED setting and elsewhere [5,6,8,10].

Visual analog scale versus numerical rating scale

Given the similar psychometric properties of the VAS and NRS, which instrument is preferred? As mentioned above, the VAS has been used more frequently in the past; however, patients appear to prefer the NRS, and

No Pain 0 1 2 3 4 5 6 7 8 9 10 *Worst Pain Possible*

Circle one number from 0 to 10

Fig. 2. The numerical rating scale.

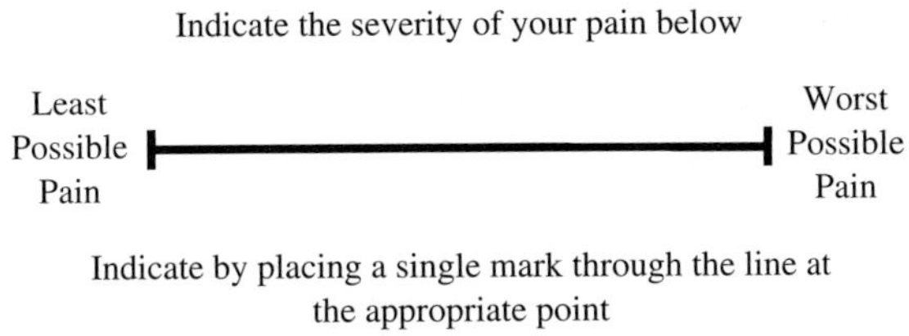

Fig. 3. The visual analog scale.

comprehension of the VAS is problematic in the elderly population and in those with cognitive impairments. Patients unable to complete the VAS were found to be older than those able to complete the measure (73 versus 54 years) [6]. Other investigators have found that patients prefer the NRS, and it is more often successfully completed than the VAS [10]. In one emergency department study [13], failure rates for the VAS were 15% versus 0% for the NRS. Thus, in both clinical and research settings, the NRS has much to commend it over the VAS.

Picture scales

These instruments include a series of facial images or illustrations of facial expressions meant to represent various pain states [14]. They are presented to the patient, who is asked to choose the facial expression that best matches his or her pain intensity. Each image is assigned a number, which becomes the patient's pain intensity score (Fig. 4).

Picture scales demonstrate both criterion and predictive validity, and may be particularly useful for populations with limited literacy, including children [15,16]. In one study of patients who have advanced cancer and pain [17], 81% were able to complete a picture scale, whereas only 75% could complete the VAS. In another study [18], the authors noted that male patients were uncomfortable with scales depicting severe pain using tears. Picture scales with such depictions might profitably be avoided, because they may be biased in the direction of less severe pain in male patients.

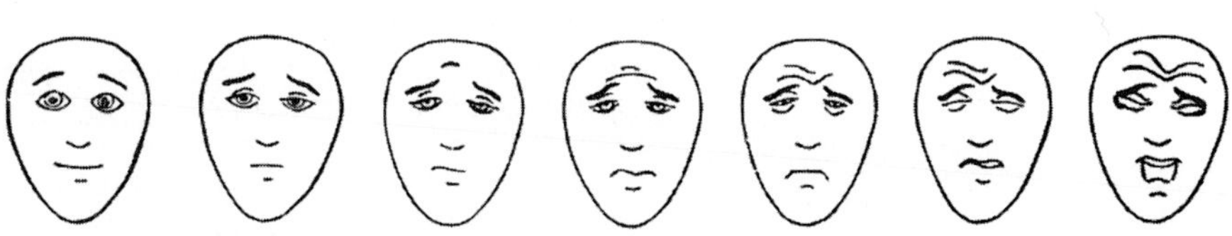

Fig. 4. The Faces Pain Scale. (*From* Bieri D, Reeve RA, Champion GD, et al. The Faces Pain Scale for the self-assessment of the severity of pain experienced by children: development, initial validation, and preliminary investigation for ratio scale properties. Pain 1990;41(2):144; with permission.)

Verbal rating scales

Verbal rating scales (VRS) consist of a number of adjectives or phrases describing increasing pain intensities (Fig. 5). Patients are told to choose the adjective or phrase that best describes their pain intensity. The pain intensity score is the number assigned to the descriptor chosen by the patient. The number of descriptors used has ranged from four (none, mild, moderate, severe) [7] to 15 [19]. The four-descriptor scale is widely used in clinical settings, is easy to administer, and has demonstrated validity and reliability [10]. For patients who have limited literacy or cognitive impairment, use of these scales may be difficult, and they do not provide the number of choices available with the VAS or NRS, thus potentially limiting precision [20].

Temporal characteristics

Pain in the emergent setting tends to be severe; thus measures of time to pain relief are of particular importance. These measures are relatively underused in pain research, and are a promising area of investigation for emergency medicine pain researchers. For emergency medical in general, and pain management in particular, minutes count.

One method of assessing this temporal quality of pain experience uses a "double stopwatch" technique [21–26]. Patients are given two stopwatches at the time of analgesic administration, and are asked to stop the first watch on noticing any analgesic effect and the second then they experience "meaningful" pain relief. Respectively, these times are labeled "time to analgesic onset" and "time to meaningful pain relief." Currently little used in emergency medicine pain research, these measures should be considered for any analgesic comparison trial planned in our practice setting.

Pain-related physical function—the Brief Pain Inventory

Pain is a multidimensional experience. The impact of pain on the patient's function and mood is particularly important to understand and has relevance to multiple stakeholders, including his or her family, social contacts, and employer, and workmen's' compensation entities. Although measures of physical function are commonly incorporated into studies of chronic pain, the author was unable to identify emergency medicine studies

None **Mild** **Moderate** **Severe**

Choose the word that best describes your pain.

Fig. 5. Verbal rating scale.

assessing the impact of pain on function. Given that emergency medicine pain research rarely extends beyond the emergency department episode itself, this is perhaps not surprising. As our research efforts evolve, emergency medicine investigators should become familiar with instruments assessing pain related function and mood states. One such instrument is the Brief Pain Inventory (Fig. 6) [27]. It is discussed in the following paragraphs.

The BPI is a self-administered, validated questionnaire available in many languages (including English, French, and Spanish) and requires less than 5 minutes to complete [28–33]. It was originally used to assess pain intensity

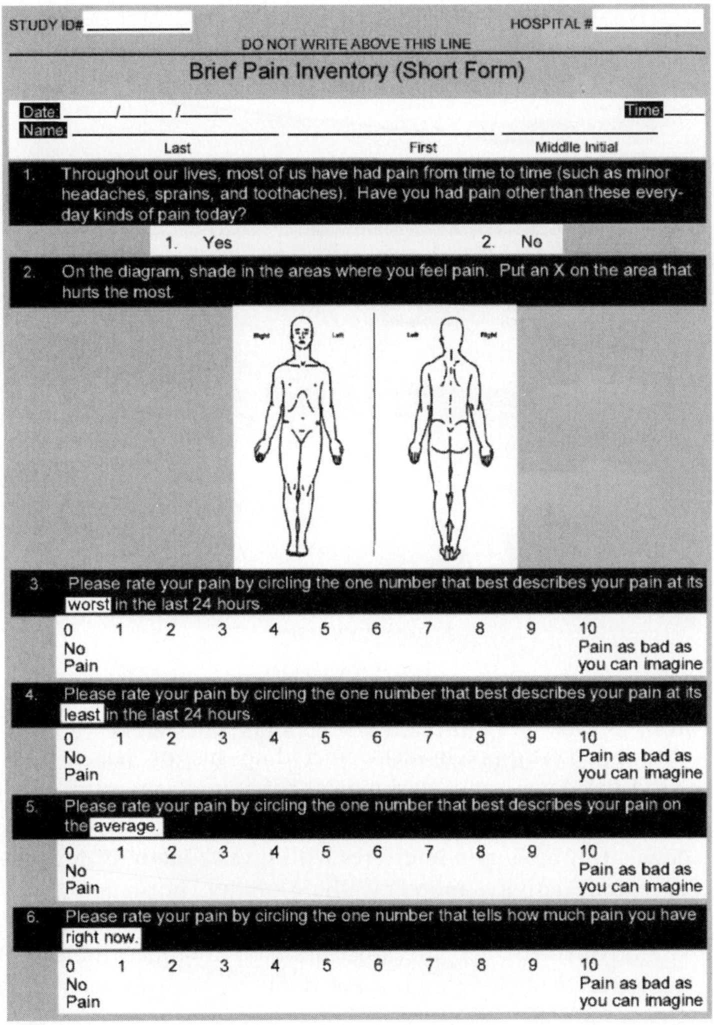

STUDY ID# ____________ HOSPITAL # ____________

DO NOT WRITE ABOVE THIS LINE

Brief Pain Inventory (Short Form)

Date: ____/____/____ Time: ____

Name: ____________ ____________ ____________
Last First Middle Initial

1. Throughout our lives, most of us have had pain from time to time (such as minor headaches, sprains, and toothaches). Have you had pain other than these every-day kinds of pain today?
   1. Yes 2. No

2. On the diagram, shade in the areas where you feel pain. Put an X on the area that hurts the most.

3. Please rate your pain by circling the one number that best describes your pain at its **worst** in the last 24 hours.
   0 1 2 3 4 5 6 7 8 9 10
   No Pain — Pain as bad as you can imagine

4. Please rate your pain by circling the one nuimber that best describes your pain at its **least** in the last 24 hours.
   0 1 2 3 4 5 6 7 8 9 10
   No Pain — Pain as bad as you can imagine

5. Please rate your pain by circling the one number that best describes your pain on the **average**.
   0 1 2 3 4 5 6 7 8 9 10
   No Pain — Pain as bad as you can imagine

6. Please rate your pain by circling the one number that tells how much pain you have **right now**.
   0 1 2 3 4 5 6 7 8 9 10
   No Pain — Pain as bad as you can imagine

Fig. 6. The Brief Pain Inventory. (*From* the M. D. Anderson Department of Symptom Research. Available at http://www.mdanderson.org/pdf/bpisf.pdf; with permission.)

7. What treatments or medications are you receiving for your pain?

8. In the last 24 hours, how much relief have pain treatments or medications provided? Please circle the one percentage that most shows how much **relief** you have received.

0% No Relief | 10% | 20% | 30% | 40% | 50% | 60% | 70% | 80% | 90% | 100% Complete Relief

9. Circle the one number that describes how, during the past 24 hours, pain has interfered with your:

A. General Activity

0 Does not Interfere | 1 | 2 | 3 | 4 | 5 | 6 | 7 | 8 | 9 | 10 Completely Interferes

B. Mood

0 Does not Interfere | 1 | 2 | 3 | 4 | 5 | 6 | 7 | 8 | 9 | 10 Completely Interferes

C. Walking Ability

0 Does not Interfere | 1 | 2 | 3 | 4 | 5 | 6 | 7 | 8 | 9 | 10 Completely Interferes

D. Normal Work (includes both work outside the home and housework)

0 Does not Interfere | 1 | 2 | 3 | 4 | 5 | 6 | 7 | 8 | 9 | 10 Completely Interferes

E. Relations with other people

0 Does not Interfere | 1 | 2 | 3 | 4 | 5 | 6 | 7 | 8 | 9 | 10 Completely Interferes

F. Sleep

0 Does not Interfere | 1 | 2 | 3 | 4 | 5 | 6 | 7 | 8 | 9 | 10 Completely Interferes

G. Enjoyment of life

0 Does not Interfere | 1 | 2 | 3 | 4 | 5 | 6 | 7 | 8 | 9 | 10 Completely Interferes

Fig. 6 (*continued*)

and location as well as pain-related functional interference among cancer patients. The functional interference section of the BPI assesses the impact of pain on various aspects of daily functioning. Using a 0 to 10 scale (0 = does not interfere, 10 = completely interferes), the patient is asked to rate the degree to which pain interferes with seven functions during the past 24 hours: general activity, mood, walking ability, normal work (includes both work outside the home and housework), relations with other people, sleep, and enjoyment of life. Investigators have modified the original BPI interference scale to include additional domains such as recreational and social activities as well as self-care [34,35].

The BPI interference scale has been shown to be internally consistent and reliable. In an analysis involving data from four countries, the scale displayed internal stability coefficients from 0.86 to 0.91 [36]. Test-retest reliability at 30 minutes was found to be excellent in one German study ($r = 0.97$) [31]. The BPI interference scale is sensitive to treatment effects. One study conducted within the Veterans Administration system documented significant and sustained reductions in pain interference scores after implementation of cancer pain guidelines [37].

In addition to an extensive literature involving cancer patients, the interference scale of the BPI was found to be sensitive to treatment effects in five randomized studies of noncancer pain, including HIV-related and non-HIV related neuropathy, osteoarthritis, temporomandibular joint syndrome, and Fabry disease [38–42]. Although use of the BPI has not been reported in the emergency medicine literature, the author and colleagues are currently using the interference scale in a multicenter epidemiologic study involving emergency departments in the United States and Canada.

Summary

Each patient's pain experience is uniquely his or her own. Standardized pain assessment methodologies and procedures provide a window to this experience and constitute a necessary first step to our understanding of pain, in both clinical and research settings. All too often, emergency department pain assessment is cursory—performed more to satisfy regulatory requirements than to guide our therapies or evaluate our practices. This article provides information on a number of assessment techniques that are appropriate for clinical and research use. Their use should inform our practice and lead to continuous improvements in our management of pain.

References

[1] Chapman CR. Measurement of pain: problems and issues. In: Bonica JJ, Albe-Fessard D, editors. Advances in pain research and therapy, Vol. 1. New York: Raven Press, 1976;345–53.

[2] Berthier F, Potel G, Leconte P, et al. Comparative study of methods of measuring acute pain intensity in an ED. Am J Emerg Med 1998;16(2):132–6.

[3] Bijur PE, Latimer CT, Gallagher EJ. Validation of a verbally administered numerical rating scale of acute pain for use in the emergency department. Acad Emerg Med 2003;10(4):390–2.

[4] Jensen MP, Karoly P, O'Riordan EF, et al. The subjective experience of acute pain. An assessment of the utility of 10 indices. Clin J Pain 1989;5(2):153–9.

[5] Singer AJ, Kowalska A, Thode HC Jr. Ability of patients to accurately recall the severity of acute painful events [comment]. Acad Emerg Med 2001;8(3):292–5.

[6] Kremer EF, Atkinson JH Jr, Ignelzi RJ. Measurement of pain: patient preference does not confound measurement. Pain 1981;10:241–8.

[7] Seymour RA. The use of pain scales in assessing the efficacy of analgesics in post-operative dental pain. Eur J Clin Pharmacol 1982;23:441–4.

[8] Ekblom A, Hansson P. Pain intensity measurements in patients with acute pain receiving afferent stimulation. J Neurol Neurosurg Psychiatr 1988;51:481–6.

[9] Wilkie D, Lovejoy N, Dodd M, et al. Cancer pain intensity measurement: concurrent validity of three tools—finger dynamometer, painintensity number scale, visual analogue scale. Hosp J 1990;6:1–13.
[10] Paice J, Cohen F. Validity of a verbally administered numeric rating scale to measure cancer pain intensity. Cancer Nurs 1997;20:88–93.
[11] Sze FK, Chung TK, Wong E, Lam KK, Lo R, Woo J. Pain in Chinese cancer patients under palliative care. Palliat Med 1998;12:271–7.
[12] Farrar JT, Cleary J, Rauck R, et al. Oral transmucosal fentanyl citrate: randomized, double-blinded, placebo-controlled trial for treatment of breakthrough pain in cancer patients. J Nat Cancer Inst 1998;90:611–6.
[13] Stahmer SA, Shofer FS, Marino A, et al. Do quantitative changes in pain intensity correlate with pain relief and satisfaction. Acad Emerg Med 1998;5:851–7.
[14] Bieri D, Reeve RA, Champion GD, et al. The Faces Pain Scale for the self-assessment of the severity of pain experienced by children: development, initial validation, and preliminary investigation for ratio scale properties. Pain 1990;41(2):139–50.
[15] Breyer JE, Knott CB. Construct validity estimation for the African-American and Hispanic versions of the Oucher Scale. J Pediatr Nurs 1998;13:20–31.
[16] Bellamy N, Campbell J, Syrotuik J. Comparative study of self-rating pain scale in osteoarthritis patients. Curr Med Res Opin 1999;15:113–9.
[17] Shannon MM, Ryan MA, D'Agostino N, et al. Assessment of pain in advanced cancer patients. J Pain Sympt Manage 1995;10:274–8.
[18] Ramer L, Richardson JL, Zichi Cohen M, et al. Multimeasure pain assessment in an ethnically diverse group of patients with cancer. J Trans Nurs 1999;10:94–101.
[19] Gracely RH, McGrath P, Dubner R. Ratio scales of sensory and affective verbal pain descriptors. Pain 1978;5:5–18.
[20] Ferraz MD, Quaresma MR, Aquino LRL, et al. Raliability of pain scales in the assessment of literate and illiterate patients with rheumatoid arthritis. J Rheumatol 1990;17:1022–4.
[21] Chang DJ, Desjardins PJ, Chen E, et al. Comparison of the analgesic efficacy of rofecoxib and enteric-coated diclofenac sodium in the treatment of postoperative dental pain: a randomized, placebo-controlled clinical trial. Clin Ther 2002;24(4):490–503.
[22] Desjardins P, Black P, Papageorge M, et al. Ibuprofen arginate provides effective relief from postoperative dental pain with a more rapid onset of action than ibuprofen. Eur J Clin Pharmacol 2002;58(6):387–94.
[23] Doyle G, Jayawardena S, Ashraf E, et al. Efficacy and tolerability of nonprescription ibuprofen versus celecoxib for dental pain. J Clin Pharmacol 2002;42(8):912–9.
[24] Medve RA, Wang J, Karim R. Tramadol and acetaminophen tablets for dental pain. Anesth Progress 2001;48(3):79–81.
[25] Moller PL, Norholt SE, Ganry HE, et al. Time to onset of analgesia and analgesic efficacy of effervescent acetaminophen 1000 mg compared to tablet acetaminophen 1000 mg in postoperative dental pain: a single-dose, double-blind, randomized, placebo-controlled study. J Clin Pharmacol 2000;40(4):370–8.
[26] Olson NZ, Otero AM, Marrero I, et al. Onset of analgesia for liquigel ibuprofen 400 mg, acetaminophen 1000 mg, ketoprofen 25 mg, and placebo in the treatment of postoperative dental pain. J Clin Pharmacol 2001;41(11):1238–47.
[27] Cleeland CS, Ryan KM. Pain assessment: global use of the Brief Pain Inventory. Ann Acad Med 1994;23:129–38.
[28] Caraceni A, Mendoza TR, Mencaglia E, et al. A validation study of an Italian version of the Brief Pain Inventory (Breve Questionario per la Valutazione del Dolore). Pain 1996;65: 87–92.
[29] Ger LP, Ho ST, Sun WZ, et al. Validation of the Brief Pain Inventory in a Taiwanese population. J Pain Symptom Manage 1999;18:316–22.

[30] Klepstad P, Loge JH, Borchgrevink PC, et al. The Norwegian Brief Pain Inventory questionnaire: translation and validation in cancer pain patients. J Pain Symptom Manage 2002;24:517–25.
[31] Radbruch L, Loick G, Kiencke P, et al. Validation of the German version of the Brief Pain Inventory. J Pain Symptom Manage 1999;18:180–7.
[32] Saxena A, Mendoza T, Cleeland CS. The assessment of cancer pain in north India: the validation of the Hindi Brief Pain Inventory—BPI-H. J Pain Symptom Manage 1999;17: 27–41.
[33] Wang XS, Mendoza TR, Gao SZ, et al. The Chinese version of the Brief Pain Inventory (BPI-C): its development and use in a study of cancer pain. Pain 1996;67:407–16.
[34] Tyler EJ, Jensen MP, Engel JM, et al. The reliability and validity of pain interference measures in persons with cerebral palsy. Arch Phys Med Rehabil 2002;83:236–9.
[35] Jensen MP, Ehde DM, Hoffman AJ, et al. Cognitions, coping and social environment predict adjustment to phantom limb pain. Pain 2002;95:133–42.
[36] Serlin RC, Mendoza TR, Nakamura Y, et al. When is cancer pain mild, moderate or severe? Grading pain severity by its interference with function. Pain 1995;61:277–84.
[37] Chang VT, Hwang SS, Kasimis B. Longitudinal documentation of cancer pain management outcomes. A pilot study at a VA medical center. J Pain Symptom Manage 2002;24:494–505.
[38] Evans S, Fishman B, Spielman L, et al. Randomized trial of cognitive behavior therapy versus supportive psychotherapy for HIV-related peripheral neuropathic pain. Psychosomatics 2003;44:44–50.
[39] Semenchuk MR, Sherman S, Davis B. Double-blind, randomized trial of bupropion SR for the treatment of neuropathic pain. Neurology 2001;57:1583–8.
[40] Roth SH, Fleischmann RM, Burch FX, et al. Around-the-clock, controlled-release oxycodone therapy for osteoarthritis-related pain: placebo-controlled trial and long-term evaluation. Arch Intern Med 2000;160:853–60.
[41] Thie NM, Prasad NG, Major PW. Evaluation of glucosamine sulfate compared to ibuprofen for the treatment of temporomandibular joint osteoarthritis: a randomized double blind controlled 3 month clinical trial. J Rheumatol 2001;28:1347–55.
[42] Schiffmann R, Kopp JB, Austin HA III, et al. Enzyme replacement therapy in Fabry disease: a randomized controlled trial. JAMA 2001;285:2743–9.

ELSEVIER
SAUNDERS

Emerg Med Clin N Am 23 (2005) 297–306

EMERGENCY
MEDICINE
CLINICS OF
NORTH AMERICA

Changing Attitudes About Pain and Pain Control in Emergency Medicine

David E. Fosnocht, MD*, Eric R. Swanson, MD, MS, Erik D. Barton, MD

Division of Emergency Medicine, University of Utah School of Medicine, 1150 Moran Building, 175 North Medical Drive, East Salt Lake City, Utah 84132, USA

Emergency department (ED) lore has countless humorous and often self-deprecating stories about the treatments of pain and the seekers of pain relief encountered on a daily basis. A culture of suspicion, limited research, diverse and often difficult patient populations, and challenging clinical environments have plagued our specialty in its approach to analgesia. Additionally, the limited use of advances in analgesia by other medical specialties has afforded emergency medicine the opportunity to lead the efforts for effective patient pain management.

As emergency physicians, our focus is often on the underlying diagnosis of painful complaints; however, the single-minded attention on the diagnosis of the underlying cause of pain has resulted in ignoring the pain that prompted the patient to seek care in the first place. Analgesia is often an afterthought to diagnosis and disposition. To improve our treatment of pain in the ED, a fundamental change in the way we practice is required. Treatment of pain should parallel the search for diagnosis of a patient's underlying condition, and has now become the standard of care. Pain is now considered the "fifth vital sign," and should be addressed in the same manner as other time-sensitive events we manage every day. For example, response to pain can be likened to the approach and treatment of myocardial ischemia. Today's well-trained ED physician would not ignore or fail to appropriately treat a 55-year-old male who has substernal chest pain suffering from an acute MI with nitrates, aspirin, beta-blockers, and angioplasty or thrombolytics. Why does other pain not warrant a similar emergent response, such as the hip pain of a 67-year-old female after a fall, the neck pain of a 22-year-old male after

* Corresponding author.
E-mail address: davefosnocht@comcast.net (D.E. Fosnocht).

doi:10.1016/j.emc.2004.12.003 ***emed.theclinics.com***

a rear-end motor vehicle accident, or the back pain of a 35-year-old male after lifting a couch? Is it difficult to change the focus from the diagnosis of the hip fracture, the cervical strain, or the acute muscle spasm to the treatment of the pain that brought the patient to the ED? Emergency medical personnel should consider changing focus from the immediate diagnosis of the pain to the immediate relief of the pain. The first step in changing provider attitudes in pain management is the acknowledgment and accurate measurement of the initial pain experienced by the patient. Subsequent measures of patients' responses to analgesics are needed to assess treatment adequacy and to guide further therapy. With these changes in attitudes, providers can enhance not only overall care and satisfaction for the patients, but also job satisfaction for the providers.

"Oligoanalgesia" in the emergency department

Pain is the most common chief complaint of patients presenting to the ED [1]. This is not surprising to anyone working in an ED. What is surprising is the fact that emergency physicians have not established themselves as champions in the treatment of acute pain. In 1989, Wilson and Pendleton coined the term "oligoanalgesia in the ED" to describe the poor treatment by emergency physicians for patients presenting with pain [2]. In this landmark paper, 44% of patients in the ED with pain received analgesic medication. In addition, underdosing of narcotic analgesics was common. Since 1989, awareness of inadequate analgesia within the setting of emergency medicine has increased. The findings of the proceedings from the first international symposium on pain research in emergency medicine were published in the Annals of Emergency Medicine in 1996 [3], and report this increase in awareness of pain and use of adequate analgesia in the ED. Despite this increase in awareness and attention, there is little evidence that oligoanalgesia in the ED has changed significantly over the last 15 years. Four articles from various practice settings since 1989 report that only 30% to 63% of patients presenting with pain received analgesic medications within the ED [4–7].

Recent federal guidelines require the assessment of pain for all patients, including those presenting to the ED. This regulatory incentive should be expected to increase the assessment of pain; however, Singer and colleagues [8] found that undertreatment of pain in the ED is common, even when providers recognize the severity of pain.

Research and pain management in the emergency department

A lack of research and practice guidelines for the emergency physician has been reported as one reason for poor treatment of pain in the ED [9]. In 1996, Afilalo and coauthors [10] reported finding 60 articles on pain and emergency medicine in a literature search, representing 1.7% of the research in emergency medicine at that time. Performing a similar search in 2003 with PubMed using the same search terms (pain and emergency medicine, emergency medical services, or emergency department) revealed 318 articles, an increase of over 400%. The few pain treatment initiatives published have shown modest results. In the United Kingdom, Goodacre and Roden [11] described the use of a pain protocol to improve analgesia for ED patients who have fractures. Those receiving analgesia increased from 9% to 31%. A pediatric pain protocol showed an improvement from 34% to 55% of patients receiving pain medication within 30 minutes of arrival [12]. Another triage pain protocol showed an improvement in the time to analgesia for patients who have acute musculoskeletal pain, but no differences in the mean pain intensity at discharge [13]. Similarly, an educational intervention showed no change in the percentage (56% preintervention and 54% postintervention) of patients receiving analgesia in a large-volume ED [14]. Based on these conflicting study results, it is unclear if the recent increased research efforts have truly made significant progress in the clinical treatment of pain within the ED.

Patient attitudes: expectations and satisfaction with pain treatment in the emergency department

If an increase in research does not result in improved pain management, we should consider factors related to the patients themselves. It is recognized that in the postoperative setting, patients have low expectations for pain relief. This results in overall high levels of patient satisfaction with pain management, despite high levels of postoperative pain [15]; however, ED patients do not appear to share these low expectations for pain relief. ED patients expect mean pain relief of 72%, and 18% of ED patients expect complete (100%) relief of their pain [16]. ED patients also expect analgesia soon after ED arrival. The mean expectation for time to analgesic administration for ED patients is 23 minutes, compared with actual mean time to analgesic administration of 78 minutes [4].

Patient satisfaction correlates poorly with initial pain intensity, discharge pain intensity, and change in pain intensity between presentation and discharge [17–20]; however, patients who report that their needs for pain relief have been met in the ED have higher mean satisfaction (83/100), than those in whom needs for pain relief are not met (51/100) [4]. Overall, these findings suggest that pain intensity and pain relief in the ED indirectly impact patient satisfaction. Meeting patient expectations for pain relief likely plays a larger role than absolute pain intensity or change in pain intensity. In addition, an attitude or expression of caring about the patients' pain may be as meaningful as providing the pain medication itself [21–24]. This may explain in part the seemingly contradictory findings that whereas only 45% of ED patients in pain receive analgesic medication, 70% report that their needs for pain relief were met at discharge [4].

Barriers to treatment of pain in the emergency department: ethnic, cultural, and gender bias

Physician and nursing attitudes may have a disproportionate impact upon the treatment of pain for various subgroups within the ED. Todd reported that both Hispanic and Black patients who have fractures are less likely to receive analgesia in the ED that nonHispanic whites [25,26]; however, several recent reports have demonstrated no differences in analgesic treatment among minority groups [27,28]. Raftery and coworkers [29] reported that female patients describe more pain and receive more analgesic medication than male patients in the ED; however, female patients do not appear to have different expectations for pain relief when compared with male patients [16]. Cultural bias in the expression of pain and cultural differences between patients and practitioners may also influence attitudes toward the treatment of pain in the ED setting. This has not been extensively studied. Todd et al [30] reported no differences in physician estimates of pain between Hispanic and nonHispanic white patients who have long bone fractures, concluding that other explanations for the differences in treatment between these two groups must be found. At a minimum, this requires understanding that differences in cultural norms for the expression, reporting, and expectations for the treatment of pain exist and must be considered when treating pain in patients from other cultures.

Barriers to treatment of pain in the emergency department: the emergency department environment

Another potential barrier to treatment of pain in the ED is the environment of the ED itself. Chisholm and coauthors [31] eloquently reported on the number of interruptions and the nature of the multitasking that are seen in the ED. Over a 180-minute period, emergency physicians experience a mean of 30 interruptions and 20 events requiring them to switch tasks. The number of interruptions and breaks in task correlated with the number of patients simultaneously managed. This environment might be expected to contribute to poor pain management; however, an analysis of the number of physicians per patient, nursing staff per patient, physicians per acuity-weighted patients, and nursing staff per acuity-weighted patients found no differences in the percentage of patients who received pain medication while present in the ED [32]. This suggests that emergency physicians do a poor job of providing analgesia, regardless of whether the emergency department is busy or slow. The response that "it is too busy" remains a poor excuse for not providing pain relief in the ED.

The nursing and physician dichotomy of assessment and treatment of pain may also play a role in the poor treatment of pain in the ED. Beel and coworkers [33] found that ED patients who had fractures were willing to have nursing staff administer pain medication before physician evaluation; however, in most departments, the process of pain medication administration requires a large number of independent steps, and represents a formidable obstacle to timely analgesia. These steps may include patient presentation and registration, nursing assessment and triage, placement in a treatment room, primary nurse assessment and documentation, physician evaluation, physician ordering of pain medication, nursing obtaining pain medication, and finally, after these seven independent steps, nursing administration of pain medication. Overcoming this process requires that analgesia be given a high priority for triage and treatment at the earliest phase of a patient visit to the ED.

Barriers to treatment of pain in the emergency department: opioids

Opiophobia (prejudice against the use of opioid analgesics) is used to describe another barrier to the use and prescription of narcotic analgesics. Regulatory and licensing concerns, suspicion of "drug-seeking" behavior, concern for addiction or dependence, and lack of follow-up or continuity of care produce a culture in which adequate treatment of pain is difficult to achieve. Weinstein and colleagues [34] found that working physicians have significant opiophobia, display lack of knowledge about pain and its treatment, and have negative views about patients who have chronic pain. Emergency physician rating of suspicion for drug addiction correlates poorly with drug abuse screening testing [35]. Many ED physicians suspect drug-seeking behavior among patients in pain, particularly in high-risk urban environments. In addition, patients who do not respond to analgesia are viewed with an increased suspicion of drug-seeking behavior [36]. Clinically, this often results in a patient exhibiting pseudoaddictive behavior, with demands for analgesia and increased demonstrations of pain. The typical reaction of ED personnel to this scenario is often a refusal of analgesia rather than a chance to relieve the pain causing the behavior.

The typical "limited prescription" for opioid analgesia at ED discharge may also reflect an attitude of opiophobia. A prescription for one to two hydrocodone/acetaminophen tablets every 4 to 6 hours as required by pain, dispense #20, will last less than 2 days if the maximum dose is taken as directed. The common beliefs that the primary care physician should prescribe all opioids, or that limiting the number of pills dispensed will "ensure" follow-up are poor excuses for the undertreatment of pain after ED discharge. Reluctance to prescribe opioids also results in few prescriptions for long-acting opioids following ED discharge; however, the scheduled use of long-acting opioids with as-needed dosing of short-acting opioids for breakthrough pain is well-established, and results in better pain control when compared with as-needed dosing alone. The benefits of sustained release opioids in improving pain control have also been shown to be superior to as-needed dosing of short-acting opioids for pain relief in the 3 days following anterior cruciate ligament (ACL) repair [37]. As the treating physicians for a large number of severely painful diagnoses, emergency physicians have the opportunity to embrace the principles used in postoperative settings, and to provide analgesia with both a long-acting analgesic and an as-needed medication when making a discharge plan for pain management.

Barriers to treatment of pain in the emergency department: emergency department culture

There is a large arsenal of analgesic choices available to emergency physicians. Similarly, the range of painful afflictions seen by emergency physicians spans the scope of all medical specialties. One is left to wonder why everyone receives the same doses of morphine, and why discharge options are limited to short-acting combination narcotics and ibuprofen. The preprinted prescriptions found in many EDs for ibuprofen and hydrocodone/acetaminophen work for many, but not all. The prevailing attitude of one-size-fits-all is not an effective strategy for pain control. The convenience of preprinted prescriptions and the drive for efficient discharge of patients often leaves ED discharge lacking in pain management. The lack of follow-up may also contribute to a false sense of adequate treatment. The skepticism of the staff toward a patient who calls back to the ED after returning home with inadequately controlled pain presents yet another barrier to effective pain management. How is the patient who calls back to the ED needing "something more" for pain triaged at your ED? Is he turned down by the clerk, chastised by the registered nurse, or told that he will have to return to the ED and wait to see the doctor? The prevailing mindset is "patients abuse the ED system" rather than "the ED pain management system is broken and needs repair." As an example, meperidine continues to be used more commonly than all other abortive therapy for treatment of migraine headache in the ED. This occurs despite strong recommendations against the use of this agent [38]. Does this behavior result from the attitude that this is really what the patient wants, or is this just the fastest and easiest way to get the patient out of the ED? We must consider changing our mindset to embrace educational opportunities for providing appropriate and medically sound analgesia.

Barriers to treatment of pain in the emergency department: provider education

Pain management is infrequently taught within the medical school framework, and the treatment of acute pain, which is typically encountered in the ED, is almost never given a format for formal teaching. This lack of education was demonstrated in a survey of medical students as freshmen and then repeated as seniors. Weinstein et al [39] found that prejudice toward the use of opioid analgesics had increased during the 4 years of medical school training. Emergency medicine residency training focuses upon the diagnosis and treatment of the underlying medical or surgical causes of pain; the treatment of pain is often secondary to establishing a diagnosis. When pain relief is addressed, it is often inadequate, with little regard to pathophysiology and the pharmacology of analgesics available. On a positive note, an educational intervention performed within an emergency medicine residency program framework resulted in significant improvement in pain relief for ED patients [40].

Changing the practice patterns of established physicians remains extremely difficult. Nationwide distribution and publication of practice guidelines for the treatment of chest pain and back pain have shown poor results in changing behavior among working physicians [41,42].

These findings suggest that opportunities to affect change in behavior and improve treatment of pain in the ED should focus on medical students and residency training programs. Unfortunately, effective training tools to change attitudes about pain and pain control among practicing physicians have yet to be described.

Consequences of inadequate pain management in the emergency department

The ED is both the first and last resort medical point of access for many traumatic and nontraumatic painful conditions. This is true for patients who have acute and chronic pain. It is easy to fall into the belief that "pain never killed anyone" and attend to other pressing issues in the ED; however, relief of pain is one of the primary physician responsibilities, and one of the greatest services that a physician can provide to a patient. This is an opportunity that is often ignored or overlooked by emergency physicians. Many of us have heard and now ignore the wisdom of Albert Schweitzer:

> "We must all die. But that I can save a person from days of torture, that is what I feel is my great and ever-new privilege. Pain is a more terrible lord of mankind than even death itself."

Beyond the relief of suffering, however, inadequate treatment of acute pain has also been shown to contribute significantly to the development of chronic pain [43,44]. Opportunities to save lives within the ED are rare, but opportunities to relieve pain are nearly infinite within the practice of emergency medicine. A change in attitude regarding pain may allow emergency physicians to take advantage of these opportunities.

Treatment of pain in the ED and the prescription of opioid analgesics is often a source of mistrust and dissatisfaction for both the patient and the emergency physician. A paradigm shift that challenges the prevailing culture and focuses on the relief of pain will result in improved care for the patient, and improvement in satisfaction for both the patient and the physician.

Summary

Oligoanalgesia continues to be a large problem in the ED. An attitude of suspicion, a culture of ignoring the problem, and an environment that is not conducive to change in practice combine to present formidable obstacles for effective pain management in the emergency setting. Overcoming these obstacles for effective analgesia in the ED is not beyond the capabilities of the individual ED, the emergency physician, or the specialty of emergency medicine. Changing the attitudes of emergency medical providers about pain assessment and management will require attention in several areas of research, education and training.

Oligoanalgesia remains a global problem within emergency medicine; however, this awareness is often not felt to be present "in my ED." Individual ownership of the problem may contribute to improvements in pain control. The last 15 years have seen a substantial increase in ED research focused on pain and pain management. Continued research efforts and focused clinical application of these efforts are still required. A better understanding of patient needs and expectations for pain relief, as well as continued efforts at patient education regarding pain, will also improve our treatment of pain in the ED. Recognition by providers of the ethnic, cultural, and gender differences in the expression, reporting, and expectations for treatment of pain should also continue to be a priority in changing attitudes toward pain and pain control. These goals must be realistic within the chaotic and unpredictable environment that defines emergency medicine. Practical and time-sensitive approaches to pain and pain management will continue to be a challenge to enact and enforce in our EDs.

The stigma of opioids, in combination with the transient nature of the emergency physician/patient relationship, may be the largest hurdles to overcome for effective pain management not only in the ED, but also following ED discharge. Improvement in provider education of the realities, myths, and misunderstandings of opioid management may provide insight into this problem.

The consequences of oligoanalgesia in the ED are not insignificant. To improve our treatment of pain in the ED, a fundamental change in attitude toward pain and the control of pain is required. This is unlikely to occur until pain is adequately addressed and treated appropriately as a true emergency.

References

[1] Burt CW, McCaig LF. Trends in hospital emergency department utilization: United States, 1992–99. Vital Health Stat 2001;13(150):1–34.

[2] Wilson JE, Pendleton JM. Oligoanalgesia in the emergency department. Am J Emerg Med 1989;7(6):620–3.
[3] Ducharme J. Proceedings from the first international symposium on pain research in emergency medicine: foreword. Ann Emerg Med 1996;27(4):399–403.
[4] Fosnocht DE, Swanson ER, Bossart P. Patient expectations for pain medication delivery. Am J Emerg Med 2001;19(5):399–402.
[5] Lewis LM, Lasater LC, Brooks CB. Are emergency physicians too stingy with analgesics? South Med J 1994;87(1):7–9.
[6] Petrack EM, Christopher NC, Kriwinsky J. Pain management in the emergency department: patterns of analgesic utilization. Pediatrics 1997;99(5):711–4.
[7] Selbst SM, Clark M. Analgesic use in the emergency department. Ann Emerg Med 1990; 19(9):1010–3.
[8] Singer AJ, Richman PB, Kowalska A, et al. Comparison of patient and practitioner assessments of pain from commonly performed emergency department procedures. Ann Emerg Med 1999;33(6):652–8.
[9] Bonica J. Foreword. In: Paris PM, Stewart RD, editors. Pain management in emergency medicine. West Hartford (CT): Appleton-Lange; 1987. p. xi–ii.
[10] Afilalo M, Cantees K, Ducharme J. Current pain-control practices and research. Ann Emerg Med 1996;27(4):404–7.
[11] Goodacre SW, Roden RK. A protocol to improve analgesia use in the accident and emergency department. J Accid Emerg Med 1996;13(3):177–9.
[12] Somers LJ, Beckett MW, Sedgwick PM, et al. Improving the delivery of analgesia to children in pain. Emerg Med J 2001;18(3):159–61.
[13] Fosnocht DE, Swanson ER, Bossart PJ. Triage pain protocol: effects on patient satisfaction and change in pain intensity. Ann Emerg Med 2001;38(4):s90.
[14] Singer AJ, Chisum E, Stark MJ. An educational intervention to reduce oligoanalgesia in the emergency department. Ann Emerg Med 2003;42(4):s41.
[15] Kuhn S, Cooke K, Collins M, et al. Perceptions of pain relief after surgery. BMJ 1990; 300(6741):1687–90.
[16] Heaps ND, Fosnocht DE, Swanson ER. The effect of age, gender, and pain magnitude on patient expectations for pain relief in the ED. Ann Emerg Med 2001;38(4):s88.
[17] Blank FS, Mader TJ, Wolfe J, et al. Adequacy of pain assessment and pain relief and correlation of patient satisfaction in 68 ED fast-track patients. J Emerg Nurs 2001;27(4): 327–34.
[18] Stahmer SA, Shofer FS, Marino A, et al. Do quantitative changes in pain intensity correlate with pain relief and satisfaction? Acad Emerg Med 1998;5(9):851–7.
[19] Thompson DA, Yarnold PR. Relating patient satisfaction to waiting time perceptions and expectations: the disconfirmation paradigm. Acad Emerg Med 1995;2(12):1057–62.
[20] Ward SE, Gordon DB. Patient satisfaction and pain severity as outcomes in pain management: a longitudinal view of one setting's experience. J Pain Symptom Manage 1996; 11(4):242–51.
[21] Bursch B, Beezy J, Shaw R. Emergency department satisfaction: what matters most? Ann Emerg Med 1993;22(3):586–91.
[22] Hall MF, Press I. Keys to patient satisfaction in the emergency department: results of a multiple facility study. Hosp Health Serv Adm 1996;41(4):515–32.
[23] Yarnold PR, Michelson EA, Thompson DA, et al. Predicting patient satisfaction: a study of two emergency departments. J Behav Med 1998;21(6):545–63.
[24] Trout A, Magnusson AR, Hedges JR. Patient satisfaction investigations and the emergency department: what does the literature say? Acad Emerg Med 2000;7(6):695–709.
[25] Todd KH, Deaton C, D'Adamo AP, et al. Ethnicity and analgesic practice [comments]. Ann Emerg Med 2000;35(1):11–6.
[26] Todd KH, Samaroo N, Hoffman JR. Ethnicity as a risk factor for inadequate emergency department analgesia [comments]. JAMA 1993;269(12):1537–9.

[27] Fuentes EF, Kohn MA, Neighbor ML. Lack of association between patient ethnicity or race and fracture analgesia. Acad Emerg Med 2002;9(9):910–5.
[28] Yen K, Kim M, Stremski ES, et al. Effect of ethnicity and race on the use of pain medications in children with long bone fractures in the emergency department. Ann Emerg Med 2003; 42(1):41–7.
[29] Raftery KA, Smith-Coggins R, Chen AH. Gender-associated differences in emergency department pain management. Ann Emerg Med 1995;26(4):414–21.
[30] Todd KH, Lee T, Hoffman JR. The effect of ethnicity on physician estimates of pain severity in patients with isolated extremity trauma [comments]. JAMA 1994;271(12):925–8.
[31] Chisholm CD, Collison EK, Nelson DR, et al. Emergency department workplace interruptions: are emergency physicians "interrupt-driven" and "multitasking"? Acad Emerg Med 2000;7(11):1239–43.
[32] Hollifield MB, Fosnocht DE, Swanson ER. Effect of patient volume and acuity on pain management in the ED. Acad Emerg Med 2003;10:483–4.
[33] Beel TL, Mitchiner JC, Frederiksen SM, et al. Patient preferences regarding pain medication in the ED. Am J Emerg Med 2000;18(4):376–80.
[34] Weinstein SM, Laux LF, Thornby JI, et al. Physicians' attitudes toward pain and the use of opioid analgesics: results of a survey from the Texas Cancer Pain Initiative. South Med J 2000;93(5):479–87.
[35] Kelly AM, Dang CT, Phan V, et al. Analgesia and addiction in ED patients with acute exacerbations of chronic pain. Ann Emerg Med 2003;42(4):s67.
[36] Miner JR, Kruse S, Biros MH. Physician perception of drug seeking behavior and ethnicity. Ann Emerg Med 2003;42(4):S67.
[37] Reuben SS, Connelly NR, Maciolek H. Postoperative analgesia with controlled-release oxycodone for outpatient anterior cruciate ligament surgery. Anesth Analg 1999;88(6): 1286–91.
[38] Vinson DR. Treatment patterns of isolated benign headache in US emergency departments. Ann Emerg Med 2002;39(3):215–22.
[39] Weinstein SM, Laux LF, Thornby JI, et al. Medical students' attitudes toward pain and the use of opioid analgesics: implications for changing medical school curriculum. South Med J 2000;93(5):472–8.
[40] Jones JB. Assessment of pain management skills in emergency medicine residents: the role of a pain education program. J Emerg Med 1999;17(2):349–54.
[41] Lewis LM, Lasater LC, Ruoff BE. Failure of a chest pain clinical policy to modify physician evaluation and management. Ann Emerg Med 1995;25(1):9–14.
[42] Di Iorio D, Henley E, Doughty A. A survey of primary care physician practice patterns and adherence to acute low back problem guidelines. Arch Fam Med 2000;9(10):1015–21.
[43] Perkins FM, Kehlet H. Chronic pain as an outcome of surgery. A review of predictive factors. Anesthesiology 2000;93(4):1123–33.
[44] Strassels SA, Chen C, Carr DB. Postoperative analgesia: economics, resource use, and patient satisfaction in an urban teaching hospital [table of contents]. Anesth Analg 2002; 94(1):130–7.

ELSEVIER
SAUNDERS

Emerg Med Clin N Am 23 (2005) 307–338

EMERGENCY MEDICINE CLINICS OF NORTH AMERICA

Management of Chronic Pain in the Acute Care Setting

George R. Hansen, MD

Department of Emergency Medicine, Sierra Vista Regional Medical Center, 1010 Murray Avenue, San Luis Obispo, CA 93405, USA

The management of chronic nonmalignant pain is challenging in any setting. Chronic pain is commonly associated with a complex interaction of physical, psychological, and social components. Consequently, the evaluation and management of chronic pain requires a long-term relationship and an investment of time beyond what is normally available to acute care physicians. Opioid medications are commonly used in the treatment of chronic pain, but they can further complicate the management of chronic pain, possibly worsening pain through N-methyl-D-aspartate (NMDA)-receptor mediated tolerance and descending pain facilitation. Moreover, opioids are intrinsically self-reinforcing, which can cause them to be taken compulsively even as they contribute to the worsening of the patient's condition.

The purpose of this article is to describe the unique pathophysiology of chronic pain, the function and limitations of opioids, alternative treatments, and strategies through which acute care physicians can participate in the care of chronic nonmalignant pain patients in ways that contribute positively to their long-term management.

Definition of chronic pain

The American Chronic Pain Association defines chronic pain as that which "continues beyond the usual recovery period for an injury or an illness. It may be continuous or come and go" [1]. Other definitions include "persistent or episodic pain of a duration or intensity that adversely affects the function or well being of the patient, attributable to any nonmalignant etiology" [2], and "pain and disability far out of proportion to the

E-mail address: cingemanor@aol.com

0733-8627/05/$ - see front matter
doi:10.1016/j.emc.2004.12.004 ***emed.theclinics.com***

peripheral stimulus," with significant psychological factors [3]. Severe pain from acute injuries, including fractures, rarely persists longer than 2 weeks. When patients present with complaints of severe pain beyond this time period, then one should consider the possibility of a developing chronic pain syndrome [4].

Prevalence

At the emergency department of an urban teaching hospital, approximately 11% of the patients presented for treatment of chronic pain [5]. A Gallup survey found that 89% of Americans age 18 and older have pain at least once a month; 15% of them have severe pain monthly. Among people aged 65 and older, 55% have pain daily [6]. "Chronic pain," by these criteria, is a ubiquitous condition that will affect the majority of the population at some time. The implication of this is that any missteps in the treatment of chronic pain are likely to affect many millions of people, with profound consequences.

Special biological considerations in chronic pain

The function of normal pain is to influence us to protect ourselves from injury. Congenital or acquired insensitivity to pain results in destructive processes such as the Charcot joint [7].

The majority of people have similar pain thresholds; however, it has been shown that the threshold of pain can be increased 50% in most people through acupuncture, relaxation, hypnosis, or imagery [8]. Pain tolerance also varies, and appears to have a genetic component [9]. Some patients are simply less willing or able to cope with moderate levels of pain [10]. A numerical level quantifies how much pain patients tell us they feel, but does not quantify the intensity of noxious physiologic stimulus.

The perception of pain can be divided into three components: sensory, affective (how it affects you emotionally), and evaluative (what you think about the pain and what it means to you) [11]. The pathophysiology of acute pain is covered in the article by Fink elsewhere in this issue.

Chronic pain pathways

There are different kinds of chronic nonmalignant pain with different etiologies. Pain may be felt from stimuli that are not normally painful, referred to as "allodynia." Alternatively, a patient may feel a level of pain that is out of proportion to the level of noxious stimulus, referred to as "hyperalgesia." Both of these are present in many chronic pain syndromes [12].

Pain secondary to nerve injury, sometimes referred to as "causalgia" [12], occurs when damaged nerves can fire spontaneously, producing neuropathic pain. When large-diameter sensory fibers are damaged, the patient may experience numbness, whereas small-diameter C-fiber nociceptors can still transmit pain [13]. This accounts for the paradoxical complaint of feeling both numbness and pain at the same site.

Deafferentation, or the loss of sensory input from afferent nerves, can produce pain. Normal afferent fibers inhibit pain transmission by inhibiting second- and third-order neurons in the spinal cord. Injury to these sensory afferent fibers and the loss of sensory input can result in increased irritability and firing of second- and third-order neurons up the chain [12–14]. After an amputation, deafferentation causes remapping to occur in the subcortical areas of the brain, resulting in "phantom limb pain" [15].

Complex regional pain syndrome (CRPS) is an uncommon type of chronic pain. In Type I CRPS, there is no known nerve injury. Type II CRPS is associated with a known nerve injury. Subsets of each type have been referred to as "sympathetically maintained," because of apparent improvement with a sympathetic block [16], although some studies have shown the efficacy of sympathetic blocks to be no better than placebo [17]. A review of 145 cases [18] found no correlation between pain and autonomic dysfunction, and 41% of the cases had a history of chronic pain before they developed CRPS.

It has been shown that inactivity produces concurrent myofascial pain [12], and that prolonged immobilization is a predisposing factor for Type I CRPS [16]. Some patients, in response to injury or discomfort, are unwilling to move the extremity or tolerate any stimulation of it. One may speculate that they are effectively self-deafferenting, and that they are contributing to the development of a chronic pain syndrome. This may in part explain the effectiveness of physical therapy in some chronic pain syndromes, or the effectiveness of vigorous sensory stimulation of the affected part in complex regional pain syndrome in children [19].

Central sensitization and N-methyl-D-aspartate receptor activation

Central sensitization, or "wind up," has been implicated in the development of chronic pain syndromes. Central sensitization itself is a normal physiologic response to repetitive noxious stimulation. Following the persistent or large-scale activation of alpha-amino-3-hydroxy-5-methylisexazole-4-propionic-acid (AMPA) receptors, a second glutamate receptor, designated as the NMDA receptor, depolarizes the cell, opens the NMDA-associated Na+ and Ca++ channels, and raises the intracellular Ca++ level [20–22]. This process is mediated by protein kinase C [23].

NMDA receptor activation also induces the synthesis of nitric oxide (NO) which diffuses back to nociceptors. There, NO causes the release of the peptide neurotransmitter substance P, which binds neurokinin-1 (NK-1) receptors in the spinal cord, and amplifies the pain signal [21].

Presumably, central sensitization exists to force us to pay attention to whatever is causing the repetitive noxious stimuli, and to alter our behavior.

At this stage it is not pathological, and is not chronic pain; however, persistent activation of NMDA-receptors results in persistent substance P release, which stimulates nerve growth and regeneration within the spinal cord. The remodeling and the formation of new connections with other nerves produces "allodynia." Persistent NMDA-receptor activation may also cause apoptosis (loss) of neurons, resulting in further remodeling [21].

It is important to note that the new neural connections that are formed lack mu-receptors, making them resistant to opioid pain relievers; however, drugs that antagonize NMDA-receptors, such as ketamine, phencyclidine, dextromethorphan, and methadone, can effectively relieve chronic pain [21]. Some anticonvulsant drugs, even though they lack anesthetic properties, are often effective in treating many kinds of chronic pain, particularly neuropathic pain [24]. Because of the different pathophysiology, opioids frequently produce little or no analgesia in chronic pain.

Antinociceptive response

Our endogenous pain-inhibitory antinociceptive response system is a normal part of how our bodies process a pain signal, modulating the transmission of the signal and its effect on the brain. It exists to override the pain stimulus on order to allow vital survival functions such as fighting, escaping, or even hiding ("fight, flight, or hide") in the presence of injury. It is an important and often overlooked aspect of the perception and treatment of pain, particularly in chronic pain, in which psychological and physiological factors may interfere with antinociceptive function. Chronic opioid use also may compromise the antinociceptive response.

The system consists of several parts. Wide dynamic range (WDR) neurons in the dorsal horn can be inhibited by noxious stimuli in noncontiguous areas of the body, contributing to the "gate" response [20]. This may contribute to the mechanism by which rubbing an area after injury or pinching the skin at a distant site reduces the pain from that injury. Vagus and sympathetic nerve stimulation also decreases pain [21].

The endogenous opioids are a very important part of the antinociceptive response, and are particularly relevant as they function at the site of action of opioid medications. Endogenous opioids bind receptors coupled to G proteins on their target cells. Receptor activation decreases the influx of calcium and inhibits adenylate cyclase, resulting in decreased activity of protein kinase A. Receptor activation also alters gene expression and the phosphorylation or other proteins [25].

There are three different types of endogenous opioids: endorphins, enkephalins, and dynorphin.

Endorphins are released in the periaqueductal gray matter of the brain. Beta-endorphin is the most potent endogenous opioid [26]. Endorphins bind mu-opioid receptors on presynaptic terminals of nociceptors and post-synaptic surfaces of dorsal horn neurons, and inhibit the propagation of pain signals [21]. Mu-receptors are in the highest concentration in the brain. Although mu-receptors are present in the spinal cord, activation of mu-receptors is mostly involved with analgesia above the level of the spinal cord [26]. Mu-receptor activation produces both analgesia and euphoria [27].

Enkephalins are involved in spinal analgesia [26]. They are released in the nucleus raphe magnus of the brain stem. They bind delta-opioid receptors on inhibitory interneurons in the substantia gelatinosa of the dorsal horn, causing the release of gamma-aminobutyric acid (GABA) and other substances, dampening pain signals in the spinal cord. Delta-receptors are stored in the same presynaptic vesicles with the neurotransmitters, so that when the neurotransmitters for pain are released, delta-receptors are simultaneously incorporated into the presynaptic cell membrane. This produces increased sensitivity to the antinociceptive effects of enkephalins at the same time the cells are transmitting a pain signal [21], demonstrating the tight linkage between pain signal propagation and modulation.

Following the release of enkephalins, other pain signal inhibitory molecules, including norepinephrine, oxytocin, and relaxin, are released from spinal cord cells [21].

Dynorphin, released from spinal interneurons, also produces spinal analgesia. It activates Kappa-receptors, leading to the closure of N-type calcium channels in the spinal cord cells that normally relay pain signals to the brain [21]. Kappa-receptor activation reduces pain with less respiratory depression than mu-receptor activation, and less dependence [28], but may also be pronociceptive [29]. Kappa-receptors are the site of action of opioid agonist-antagonists [26].

Within the medulla, there are "on-cells" that augment the transmission of pain, and "off-cells" that block it. On-cells are activated by the anticipation of pain even before it is painful. Morphine inhibits on-cells and produces continuous firing of off-cells, inhibiting the transmission of the pain stimulus signal. Giving naloxone or withdrawing morphine produces activation of on-cells to a level higher than before morphine was given, causing rebound pain [11].

Physiologic and painful stressors induce an increased tolerance of pain. Congenital differences in this stress-induced analgesia system and the endogenous opioid system appear to account for part of the genetic variation in pain tolerance [9].

While in a state of central sensitization, endorphins and exogenous opioids are less effective [21]. There are also systems within the brain that modulate the antinociceptive response and appear to contribute to the tolerance that develops to opioid medications. This counter-antinociception exists to keep pronociceptive and antinociceptive processes in balance [29]. Presumably, this functions to protect us from further injury.

It is important to note that the endogenous opioid system is only part of the neuromodulary system. Although some pain does not respond well to opioids, it may respond to other measures [28].

Psychological and social considerations

Psychological and social aspects of pain are described in detail in the chapter by Hansen et al elsewhere in this issue. Chronic pain patients commonly have problems with these psychosocial aspects [30]. Pre-existing psychological factors have been shown to be very important in many types of chronic pain [18,31–35]. There is a vicious cycle in which pain causes disability and stress, which in turn worsens pain perception [36]. An unhealthy lifestyle, lack of social support, depressive illness, and substance abuse are predisposing factors [37].

Acute care physicians should understand the role that attention and distraction have in the perception of pain, and encourage patients to distract themselves from the pain rather than focus their attention on it. Physicians can improve their patients' outcomes by raising their expectations of improvement, encouraging them to act as usual and not let themselves become debilitated or deconditioned [38].

Other psychosocial issues, such as patients' beliefs about their pain [39], tendency to "catastrophize" [40], involvement in the "sick role" [41], and "pain behavior" [42], should be appreciated. Physicians should be careful to avoid reinforcing dysfunctional beliefs and behavior.

Overall, some psychiatric morbidity is present in up to 67% of chronic pain patients [43]. Physicians should be aware of the high prevalence of personality and mood disorders in chronic pain patients, and insure that they are referred to a program in which these issues will be evaluated and addressed appropriately.

The role of opioids in chronic pain

Although opioids are now widely accepted for the treatment of acute pain and cancer, the long-term use of opioids for chronic nonmalignant pain remains controversial. Many studies show that some patients' pain and function improve with long-term opioid therapy [44–48]; however, the use of opioids in the treatment of chronic pain is more complicated than is commonly appreciated. Their efficacy for chronic pain is also controversial, as is reviewed below. Prescribing opioids for chronic pain, particularly in the acute care setting, has been discouraged in the past [49,50]. It has been stated that for the most common type of chronic pain patient, opioids do more harm than good [3], and that the use of opioids for chronic pain is associated with poor treatment outcomes [51]. This can become a problem when chronic pain patients demand opioids on a regular basis, particularly when better modalities are available [52].

Function of opioids

To appreciate the actions and limitations of opioids, it is important to understand their mechanism of action. In general, opioid medications work at the sites of endogenous opioids in the central nervous system's pain control and reward centers. In the spinal cord, they bind opioid receptors, and inhibit the propagation of the pain signal [21]. The analgesic effect occurs mainly at the dorsal horn of the spinal cord, and is not dependent on supraspinal centers or on descending inhibition [53]. The spinal and supraspinal effects of opioids are said to be synergistic [54].

Within the brain, opioids function by both producing analgesia and by altering the emotional components of pain [55]. Opioids have been found to be less effective in relieving experimental pain induced in controlled laboratory conditions. This is because anxiety and context, which are very important parts of the experience of pain, are greatly diminished in a controlled experimental setting [56].

Efficacy

There are genetic differences in the metabolism of opioids, in their effectiveness as analgesics, and in their psychological effects [57]. Codeine is normally metabolized to morphine, which is the form by which it produces what little effect it has. Approximately 10% of Caucasians are deficient in the enzyme for this transformation [9]. Morphine is converted to a more potent form, morphine-6-glucuronide, in the liver and kidney [28]. There are genetic differences in the rate of this conversion as well [57].

Codeine has been shown to be a poor analgesic. Combining 60 mg codeine with acetaminophen adds at most 5% more pain relief to acetaminophen alone, which is lost after the first week [58]. Even 120 mg codeine has been shown to be no better than placebo [52]. Even where codeine was found to have poor efficacy and substantial side effects, many patients requested it as long-term therapy [59]. This demonstrates codeine's self-reinforcing properties despite its poor efficacy.

Propoxyphene is another frequently prescribed opioid analgesic, but is also very weak, with little advantage over non-opioids, and few indications for use [60]. 100 mg of propoxyphene napsylate has been shown to be no more effective than 32 mg codeine, and alone it is no more effective than aspirin or acetaminophen [61]. Not only is propoxyphene no better than aspirin or acetaminophen, it has addictive potential and a risk of renal toxicity [62]. A propoxyphene metabolite produces central nervous system (CNS) excitation and seizures [27].

The opioid agonist tramadol has been found to have no more analgesic properties than codeine or propoxyphene [61].

Some studies of codeine [63], propoxyphene [47], and tramadol [64] have reported relief of chronic pain with these medications. In view of the fact that they have poor analgesic efficacy that is likely to become worse with time, it is probable that the perceived benefits are primarily from the psychological side effects. Even these psychological effects will be lost with the development of tolerance, after which patients will be taking the medications solely as treatment for withdrawal symptoms.

A review of studies of various opioids yielded highly variable results, with an average pain relief of around 32% [65]. Some studies have found adequate pain relief in some patients, but little or no improvement in employment or social function [46], and worsening among those whose pain did not improve [66].

Opioids have been found to be poorly effective, and were not recommended for chronic pain associated with multiple sclerosis [67], or for "sympathetically maintained pain" [12]. At 2 years follow-up of the long-term intrathecal morphine treatment for low back pain, one half of the patients had less then 25% pain relief [68].

A study was done in which idiopathic pain patients, who believed that opioids were effective for their pain, were blinded and given either an opioid or placebo. When they learned that they did not get significant pain relief from opioids compared with placebo, they became motivated for detoxification and rehabilitation, and decreased their dependence on opioids [69].

Other studies have shown good responses to opioids, but still a substantial percentage of patients received little or no improvement in their pain [47,48,70,71]. Of those patients who appear to improve, it is difficult to distinguish between psychological effects and true analgesic benefit. Again, many patients may have actually been self-treating withdrawal caused by physiologic dependence to medications that initially provided little analgesia.

Neuropathic pain

Neuropathic pain is particularly unresponsive to opioids [54,69,71,72]. This may be in part due to the presence of neurological remodeling, in which the new neural connections generally lack mu-receptors, making them resistant to opioids [21]. In postherpeutic neuralgia, controlled-release oxycodone produced a mean pain relief of only 19 out of 100 points on the visual analog scale; 76% reported side effects [73].

Because of the generally poor response of neuropathic pain to opioids, some authors state that the condition usually should not be treated with these agents [14,71], or that patients who already are on opioids should be detoxified [12].

Side effects

Some degree of sedation and impaired performance commonly occurs when opioid analgesic drugs are initiated, until tolerance to them develops [74]. Respiratory depression may occur if opioids are started at a high dose. Constipation occurs frequently and is potentially serious [47]. The physician should consider prescribing a stool softener along with the opioid.

Tolerance

Tolerance has been defined as a physiologic adaptation to the effect of a drug, with diminished effectiveness at constant dosage, or requiring an increased dosage to maintain the same intensity and duration [75]. This does not necessarily imply addiction, because tolerance is a normal physiologic process [44].

Tolerance to the analgesic effect of opioids occurs commonly [55,61,76,77]. In one study of chronic pain patients [71], 69% of the patients developed some degree of tolerance, and required a steadily increasing dose; 47% of the patients had mild tolerance, but in 22% it was marked and limited treatment. In a formal treatment program, 4% of the patients developed rapid, progressive tolerance with poor improvement in pain, and required discontinuation of their opioid medication [70].

Tolerance occurs through multiple mechanisms. Chronic opioid administration activates pronociceptive descending pathways via upregulation of cholecystokinin (CCK) in the rostral ventromedial medulla. This process, in addition to causing resistance to the analgesic effects of opioids, increases the patient's pain [29]. Opioid tolerance has also been shown to involve a functional uncoupling of opioid receptors to internal mechanisms within neurons [78], along with up-regulation of adenylate cyclase activity [79]. It is detectable after just 1 hour of continuous infusion of alfentanil in rats [80]. Ominously, this process involves the activation of protein kinase C (PKC) and results in increased NMDA-receptor activation—the same process that has been implicated in the development of chronic pain [23].

In rats given morphine injections once daily for 8 days, tolerance has been shown to activate not only these pain-facilitating processes, but also the nuclear repair enzyme Poly (ADP ribose) synthetase (PARS). Activation of PARS leads ultimately to cell death and neuronal remodeling, with irreversible changes similar to those seen in chronic pain syndromes [81].

The clinical consequences of tolerance are significant. Tolerance-induced hyperalgesia in rats is similar to that produced by a thermal burn [22], with a substantially decreased ability to tolerate mechanical painful stimuli [54].

In humans, paradoxical opioid-induced pain has been observed after a single infusion [29]. The ability to tolerate pain has been found to be two times worse in actively-using opioid addicts compared with those who are abstinent. Poor pain tolerance persists even in addicts maintained on methadone, and worsens with increased dose [82]. A low pain threshold and poor pain tolerance persist even in former addicts [83,84]. In this way, the chronic use of opioids can increase the patient's sensitivity to pain, leading to a vicious cycle of increased pain and increased medication requirements [85].

Tolerance also develops if opioid receptors are blocked without coactivation of substance P receptors, and is reversed by stimulating the substance P receptors, suggesting that there must be a balance between opioid receptor activation and painful stimuli [86]. This implies that giving opioids for mild or psychological pain may induce neuroplastic changes in the patient, resulting in increased pain.

Paradoxically, tolerance to opioids is worse with short-acting opioids than with long-acting opioids. This may be due to the dual effect of opioid receptor occupation plus NMDA-receptor activation by glutamate when the opioid has worn off [87].

In addition to developing tolerance to the analgesic and physiological effects of opioids, tolerance develops to the psychological effects as well, namely sedation and possibly euphoria. This generally occurs more rapidly than the tolerance to analgesic effects [88]. Tolerance to the psychological effects actually complicates the use of opioids further, because the psychological effects are in many cases the only reason many patients prefer them to other types of pain control. Some may interpret the loss of these effects as worsening pain, and this may cause them to seek higher doses.

Ultimately, there is an upper limit to which you can increase the dose of opioids to try to stay ahead of this tolerance [88]. Some authors maintain that if tolerance is mild, then opioids can be continued. If there is a rapid escalation of dose, then opioids should be tapered and discontinued [71].

There is some evidence that cross-tolerance between opioids is incomplete. It is recommended that if the patient is to try a different class of opioid, then it should be started at one half of the equivalent dose [26].

Studies suggest that giving an NMDA-receptor antagonist along with an opioid can prevent tolerance. If tolerance is already present, then giving multiple NMDA-receptor antagonist treatments over several days may reverse the tolerance [22].

Physiologic dependence

Physiologic dependence is closely related to tolerance. It is defined as a physiologic state of adaptation, usually characterized by development of withdrawal symptoms when the drug is discontinued [75]. It develops in the majority of patients who take opioids chronically [89]. In one study [47], it was found to be present in all of 52 patients treated with long-term opioids. Clinical dependence can be detected after just a few days of continuous use [55,90,91]. Subclinical physiologic dependence can be detected after a single dose of morphine in the analgesic range, 10 to 30 mg [92].

Physiologic dependence has a high degree of genetic heritability [93]. In addition to cellular changes seen in opioid tolerance, the mechanism of dependence involves activation of the pain-transmitting on-cells of the medulla. Withdrawal results in a level of activity in these cells higher than before opioids were started, producing rebound pain [11]. A rebound increase in acetylcholine levels in the nucleus accumbens has also been demonstrated, and was shown to persist beyond the period of withdrawal symptoms. This represents long-lasting adverse neuroadaptive effects after even a relatively short period of opioid administration [94].

Withdrawal symptoms include deep bone pain, muscle aches, and back pain [92], and may result in an increase in a chronic pain patient's usual pain [88,95]. It also produces marked increases in depression, hypochondriasis, anxiety, irritability, and feelings of weakness and sickness [96].

Withdrawal symptoms start 8 to 12 hours after the last dose of a short-acting opioid, peak at 48 hours, and subside over 5 to 7 days. Withdrawal to long-acting opioids such as methadone starts after 36 to 48 hours, peaks at 4 to 6 days, and may persist over 14 days. Drug craving may persist even after protracted abstinence [92].

The frequent use of short-acting opioids on a regular basis produces withdrawal symptoms between doses [88], and thereby worsens the patient's condition. This may involve the rebound stimulation of NMDA-receptors by glutamate that is worse with short-acting opioids, similar to the problem of short-acting opioids and tolerance [87].

Dependence may compel patients to seek opioids for withdrawal even if pain has resolved [97]. It has been noted that patients on opioids rarely reduce their doses when the pain improves [50], and that the quantity of opioids taken is dependent on supply rather than on levels of pain [76].

Because of the phenomena of tolerance, dependence, and withdrawal, we should use caution in interpreting the results of studies using long-term opioids to treat chronic pain. For example, a study which claimed excellent relief of chronic pain with codeine [98] also found that patients taking it for longer than 3 months had better relief than those taking it for less time. In view of the known poor efficacy of codeine and the loss of efficacy that occurs with time, it is likely that such patients ultimately find themselves treating withdrawal symptoms rather than their primary pain disorder.

Problems with psychological dependence, abuse, addiction, and pseudoaddiction are reviewed in the chapter by Hansen elsewhere in this issue. They are important issues, but they are controversial, and do not necessarily affect the decision whether or not to use opioids for chronic pain. It is more important to understand the limitations of the true analgesia provided by opioids in chronic pain, and the potential harm done to patients through physiologic dependence, descending pain facilitation, and tolerance-induced, NMDA-receptor mediated worsening of their pain.

The "pain-opioid downhill spiral"

It has been the experience of many pain treatment clinics that the long-term use of opioids makes some patients' conditions worse. This starts with a painful injury, for which opioids prescribed. The pain, however, does not resolve as expected. More opioids are then given, and tolerance develops, with subtle withdrawal and psychosocial changes. Full-blown addiction occurs in predisposed individuals. As psychosocial dysfunction gets worse, the perceived pain worsens. This, therefore, is iatrogenically worsened pain. The problem becomes opioid maintenance rather than pain management [3].

Many chronic pain patients actually have improvement in their pain when they are weaned off opioids, or when their dose is decreased [3,76,88,95,99–101]. In one series [102], pain decreased 18% to 89%, with an average decrease of 57%. Some patients' pain resolves completely with stopping opioids [95,103]. This is especially likely to occur when patients have been taking short-acting opioids [97,104].

Poor improvements in psychological and functional status have been observed, despite good improvement in pain, presumably due to learned behavior [43]. The global functioning of some patients has also been shown to be worse with the long-term use of opioids, and to improve after withdrawal [3,104].

Long-term opioid therapy for chronic nonmalignant pain appears to be effective for some patients, but clearly some patients are made worse. Consequently, acute care physicians should exercise caution in initiating opioid therapy in chronic pain patients, because many of them may ultimately require detoxification. Detoxification can be very difficult, particularly if the patients have developed psychological or physiological dependence. Moreover, some of the neuroplastic changes may be irreversible.

Are physicians required to provide opioids?

There is a common misconception that the 2001 Joint Commission on the Accreditation of Health care Organizations (JCAHO) pain standards [105] require that all patients' complaints of pain must be completely eliminated, and that physicians are thus compelled to use opioids if the patient demands them. Although the standards state that "patients have the right to appropriate assessment and management of pain" [105], there are no specific references to opioids, nor is any degree of relief specified. Rather, the intent of these standards is that a patient's pain should be evaluated and treated in the best way possible, which does not necessarily include opioids [106]. Treating pain "aggressively and effectively" may include the use of opioids for acute or postsurgical pain, but may exclude opioids for many chronic pain patients.

The term "oligoanalgesia" has been used to describe the undertreatment of pain, which has been reported to occur in emergency departments [107]. Opioids are very effective for treating pain during the relatively brief acute and recovery phases of injury or illness. Chronic pain is far more complicated, however. Rarely should rapid-onset, short-acting opioids be used. Many patients should not be given opioids at all, particularly in the acute care setting. The goal in the treatment of chronic pain is improved function and long-term pain management. Attempts to eliminate pain in the short term can interfere with these goals. Consequently, the term "oligoanalgesia" should not be applied to the treatment of chronic pain in the acute care clinic.

Conditions for long-term opioid use

Carefully selected chronic pain patients can benefit from long-term opioid therapy when it is managed appropriately; however, multiple studies have shown that non-opioid therapy works for the majority of pain patients. It has been recommended that other therapies be used first before considering long-term opioid therapy [48,70,108]. Ideally, chronic pain patients should not be started on opioid medications without an opioid trial to test for analgesic efficacy, and only after a thorough evaluation, to include a drug history and consideration of behavioral strategies [71,109]. This approach has been tested in a blinded study [69] to determine in advance if opioids would be efficacious for particular chronic pain patients.

Multidisciplinary therapy

When opioids are used for chronic nonmalignant pain, it is usually recommended that they be used in combination with other modalities, including physical and psychological therapies [3,65,66,110–112]. It is important that opioids not be offered as an alternative to multidisciplinary therapy. If the use of opioids is made contingent on the failure of nonopioid therapy, then some patients will not be motivated to pursue it [51].

To maintain control and optimize the patient's drug usage, opioids should be prescribed by only one physician or one chronic pain treatment team whenever possible [90]. Because patients commonly express a preference for medications or treatments that are less effective for long-term pain control, the treating physician or group must have a good understanding of the multiple aspects of chronic pain treatment, and a there must be a good physician–patient relationship, in order to direct the patient toward the most effective pain control strategies.

Complete assessment

It has been stated that opioids should not be started or maintained in chronic pain patients without a complete assessment [90,113]. The JCAHO Pain Standards for 2001 [105] state that the assessment should include physical, cognitive, behavioral, communicative, and emotional and social status, and include substance use and emotional and behavioral disorders. This is similar to the requirements stated by the American Academy of Pain Medicine [109] and the American Society of Anesthesiologists Task Force on Pain Management [2]. This obligates acute care physicians to either complete this assessment themselves, or to ensure that it either has already been done or will be done at follow-up, before opioids are continued.

Patient selection

Appropriate patient selection is vital in the decision to use chronic long-term opioids.

There are studies showing that such a carefully selected subgroup of patients can have reasonably good relief with opioids, with a low frequency of problematic use. Patients who have a well-defined physical etiology are good candidates [60], particularly those near the end of life [74]. Other patients require greater scrutiny. Psychogenic pain should be ruled out or treated appropriately [66]. Patients should have a stable work and family situation, and there should be no history of substance abuse [50]. The risk of addiction approaches 50% in patients who are actively abusing illicit drugs, are not in a recovery program, or have poor social support [114]. All patients should be willing to participate in other treatment modalities and to adhere to the conditions of a contract [110].

Opioids should not be used unless psychosocial issues are also addressed. Even in those chronic pain patients for whom opioids provide pain relief, it is frequently found that psychological and functional status is not improved [46,115]. Cognitive/behavioral and physical therapy should be maintained during opioid maintenance therapy to improve function [46,70,109].

It has been stated that opioids can be used in patients with a history of addiction, but only if the addictive disorder has been treated [88]. In these and other patients who are unable to control or regulate their opioid use, it may be necessary for a pain management clinic to dole their medications out to them on a daily basis.

Set goals

It is also important to establish realistic goals of opioid therapy. For many patients, opioids will not provide the degree of relief that they are seeking [74]. Patients should be informed that the goal of therapy is to improve function, with the intention of tapering the medication to the minimally effective dose. If function is not shown to improve, then opioids are not considered worth their associated risks [114].

Dose and duration

When opioids are used in chronic pain patients, they should be used at the lowest dose that provides reasonable pain relief [99] and improved function [116]. This may also minimize tolerance and opioid-induced NMDA-receptor activation. If moderate or moderately high doses of opioids do not effectively improve pain, then it would be better to gradually withdrawn them, rather than increase to a very high dose [117]. Patients should be made to understand that even though high-dose opioids may give them some psychological relief, it will quickly be lost to opioid tolerance, whereupon they will have developed physiological dependence and possibly worse pain.

The opioid chosen should be long-acting. Short-acting drugs should be used only for acute pain, or for the titration phase of long-term opioid treatment for chronic pain [118]. Many patients' pain improves just by switching to a long-acting medication [108]. Methadone has been used successfully in younger patients, who are at lower risk for drug accumulation [50]. Controlled-release morphine sulfate has been studied in cancer patients [119] and chronic nonmalignant pain patients [120], and has been shown to improve pain and quality of life.

For chronic pain, opioids should be given around the clock rather than as needed for pain [99,121]. It should be noted that even in patients whose pain was decreased and whose mood was stabilized when their opioids were given on a fixed interval, the majority stated a preference for the on-demand schedule [122]. One can anticipate that patients will seek on-demand medications even though they are less effective for pain relief and functional improvement.

The medication should also be slow-onset, to minimize the reinforcing effect of pairing the narcotic effect with the perception or expression of pain. Rapid-onset medication should be avoided in the treatment of chronic pain, particularly when a long-acting medication is given around the clock [28]. Parenteral opioids are the ultimate rapid-onset, short-acting form, even when given intramuscularly. This not only causes a problem with reinforcing pain behavior, but it also provides a short-lived flood of psychological relief or euphoria. When one considers that many patients will get at most 30% relief of their pain even with opioids, then it will be difficult for many of them to resist seeking the psychological effects of an injection. This will only complicate the long-term management of these patients. The use of parenteral opioids for chronic pain should be minimized, if not avoided entirely.

If the dose of medication is increased, it should be done in a gradual manner, by no more than 30% to 50% [27]. If the patient is rapidly developing tolerance with a rapid escalation of dose, then opioids should be tapered and discontinued [71].

"Rescue" medications provided for breakthrough pain should be limited to six to eight extra doses per month for unexpected exacerbations. If the patient consistently requests additional doses, then there needs to be a reassessment of the dose and schedule, and a consideration of psychosocial issues [60]. To avoid reinforcement issues, rescue medications should not be dispensed on an urgent basis, but prophylactically, by the patient's physician or clinic [97].

To maintain control and optimize the patient's drug usage, opioids should be prescribed by only one physician or one chronic pain treatment team whenever possible [90]. Because patients commonly express a preference for medications or treatments that are less effective for long-term pain control, the treating physician or group must have a good understanding of the multiple aspects of chronic pain treatment, and a there must be a strong physician–patient relationship, in order to direct the patient toward the most effective pain control strategies.

Pain contracts

A pain contract should also be made when opioids are used frequently for chronic pain, to include documentation of the patient's understanding of the limitations of opioid therapy, treatment objectives, risk of dependence, and need for other treatment modalities [70,110]. Such contracts usually limit the patient to obtaining prescriptions only through the pain clinic, and limit replacements for "lost or stolen" prescriptions [123]. Some contracts specifically prohibit the patient from seeking opioid medication from the emergency room [113].

Preventing chronic pain

Greater attention needs to be paid to the prevention of chronic pain. In surgical patients, there is some evidence that preemptive analgesia with opioids may prevent postoperative pain and the development of chronic pain [124,125]. Preoperative lumbar epidural blockade has been shown to be highly effective in preventing postamputation phantom limb pain [126].

Early recognition of pain and aggressive treatment can help prevent unnecessary functional impairment, secondary physical and psychosocial disability, and chronic pain [37]. Because the self-reinforcing effect of opioids may contribute to the development of chronic pain after acute injury, opioids should be prescribed for a predetermined amount of time [121]. Severe pain from acute injuries, including fractures, rarely persists longer than 2 weeks [4]. If patients seem to need opioids beyond the normal healing period for an acute injury or illness, then they should be considered to be at risk for chronic pain or opioid dependence. Opioids should be discontinued or restricted to a low dose. These patients should be referred to a multidisciplinary pain clinic [127].

Liability

There is potential liability for physicians who prescribe opioids for chronic or poorly defined pain outside of a multidisciplinary pain clinic. Physicians are being sued for causing addiction [77]. A physician was found liable for refilling an opioid despite the fact that the patient had a contract that prohibited it. The patient had a known history of noncompliance, and overdosed on the medication [123].

Follow up

Physicians should always keep in mind that long-term opioid therapy can make some patients' pain worse. Patients should be monitored to ensure that they are not having accelerated tolerance, and that physical and psychological therapies are maintained.

Nonopioid therapy

There are many alternative treatments to opioid medications that can be very effective in chronic pain patients. It has been established that the majority of people have similar pain thresholds, but this threshold can be raised by 50% using such techniques as acupuncture, relaxation, hypnosis, and imagery. [8] Women in active labor show a sharp decline in pain and negative mood if they have attended a Lamaze childbirth preparation class, relative to controls [128]. Nearly 90% of women can go through labor without medication using relaxation techniques [129]. These methods should be applicable to chronic pain patients, and they should be encouraged to use them and minimize their reliance on medications.

Psychological treatments

Cognitive-behavioral techniques have been applied in the treatment of chronic pain. Re-educating patients about how they should think about their pain and how they should respond to it has been shown to be very helpful in improving patients' pain and function [38]. Operant conditioning [130], relaxation training [131], and the medication technique "mindfulness" [132] have also been used successfully; however, it has been noted that cognitive therapy approaches generally do not work well in isolation from other aspects of multidisciplinary treatment [133].

Physical treatments

Physical therapy reinforces adaptive efforts and extinguishes maladaptive pain behaviors [134], produces improvements in activity and well-being, and tends to reduce the use of opioids [135]. It is also thought to retrain the nervous system to re-establish normal neural connections. Pain levels generally do not improve until patients have begun reconditioning, and have increased their activity levels [136].

Many studies have shown that nonspecific or placebo treatments can produce improvement equivalent to physical therapy [137], suggesting that there is therapeutic value in merely getting patients to engage in any form of physical activity, rather than allowing them to be sedentary and avoid movement and stimulation.

Other physical treatments such as manual therapies, acupuncture, and exercise have been also found to be effective. The application of cold raises the threshold of pain for up to 12 hours. Many of these therapies may be effective based on the activation of descending pain inhibitory systems [138]. Acupuncture appears to work through the stimulation of endogenous opioids [25]. This raises the concern that acupuncture and other physical treatment modalities could be made less effective by tolerance to concurrently administered opioids.

Multidisciplinary pain clinics

Psychological and physical approaches are much more effective in combination. The management of chronic pain frequently requires a combined multidisciplinary approach, including education, psychological counseling, behavior modification, and physical medicine [139,140]. There must also be a "positive physician–patient relationship" [141]. Patients should be referred to a pain clinic within weeks to a few months of the development of chronic or persistent pain, to prevent progressive pain, associated morbidity, and increased costs [127].

Even simple chronic pain requires multiple modalities of treatment, including a psychological evaluation and possible treatment. "Complex" chronic pain, with complex interactions of legal, psychological, medication, and family, requires more intensive psychological and social interventions [142]. Geriatric patients also benefit from multidisciplinary care [74].

A review of multiple studies [130] has shown that combined treatment produces moderately to markedly improved pain, with decreased medication use and increased functioning in the majority of chronic pain patients. Most of the improvements were maintained at follow-up years later. The condition of patients not in multidisciplinary care tends to worsen [143].

Despite the effectiveness of multidisciplinary pain clinics, some patients choose not to participate in them, and prefer instead to seek care at emergency rooms and urgent care facilities; however, it has been noted that those patients who are dissatisfied or who do not complete multidisciplinary pain treatment programs tend to be those who have the greatest drug dependence and psychological pathology [49,144–146]. These patients have the greatest need for multidisciplinary care, and are the worst candidates for chronic opioid therapy outside of the clinic.

Drugs for chronic pain

Acetaminophen and cyclooxygenase inhibitors

Acetaminophen is a safe, effective analgesic for mild to moderate pain. It has a maximal "ceiling" of pain relief, at which increased dosage will not provide more analgesia. Its efficacy is often downplayed because it is commonly available; however, when one considers that nearly all of the pain relief provided by acetaminophen/codeine combinations is derived from the acetominophen, then its efficacy can be better appreciated. Patients should be encouraged to use acetaminophen, but not to exceed the recommended dose, nor to use it in addition to other medications that include it.

Nonsteroidal anti-inflammatory drugs (NSAIDS) have not been shown to be significantly better for musculoskeletal pain than acetaminophen. In osteoarthritis or "tendonitis," there is little or no chronic inflammatory component. NSAIDS are commonly used nonetheless. If there is a risk of gastrointestinal bleeding, a cyclooxygenase-2 (COX-2) inhibitor should be considered [147].

Nonanalgesic drugs

There are many drugs for use in chronic pain that were not originally used as analgesics. These include baclophen (a $GABA_B$-agonist), and clonidine (an alpha-2 adrenergic agonist) [21]. Tapered doses of steroids have been advocated for neurogenic back pain and complex regional pain syndromes [4].

Antidepressants and anticonvulsants may be started in the acute care clinic, preferably in consultation with a pain specialist or personal physician [4]. Carbamazepine has been used successfully in the treatment of neuropathic pain. In a study of carbamazepine used to treat chronic pain patients who were also depressed [148], the patients' pain improved from 8.2 to 4.0 (51%), but the depression improved only 26%. The starting dose of carbamazepine is 100 to 200 mg twice a day [4].

Gabapentin (an N-type calcium channel inhibitor) has also been used successfully for neuropathic pain [4]. In postherpeutic neuralgia, the dose can be slowly increased by up to 300 mg/day, to a target dose of 1800 to 2400 mg/day, up to 3600 mg/day, divided three times daily. Side effects include somnolence and dizziness in approximately 20% and 35%, respectively [149].

Some of the most promising drugs for chronic pain are the NMDA-receptor antagonists. These include ketamine, dextromethorphan, amantadine, and methadone [150]. Morphine sulfate (MS) combined with dextromethorphan (1:1) reduces the amount of morphine required for relief of cancer and other chronic pain by as much as one half [151]. Unfortunately, NMDA receptors are found in high density in the cerebral cortex and hippocampus, and drugs that block these receptors can cause psychological side effects [24].

In summary, there are many effective ways to treat chronic pain that do not involve opioid medications, and do not expose the patient to the risk of tolerance-induced increased pain or physical and psychological dependence. Because long-term opioid therapy often interferes with the management and rehabilitation of chronic pain patients [3], emergency and urgent care physicians should encourage patients to seek nonopioid treatment for their chronic pain. Informing patients about the problems with opioids and their generally poor effectiveness in chronic pain, may help motivate them to seek nonopioid treatments [69].

The role of the acute care physician

Emergency and urgent care physicians have an important role in the care of chronic pain patients. Not only are they immediately available to treat acute exacerbations and are available after hours and on weekends, but they are often the first provider that the patient sees. Moreover, they provide an alternative to the patient's personal physician or pain clinic when the patients are dissatisfied with their care, for better or worse. Acute care physicians should be careful that their practices contribute to the solution and not to the problems associated with chronic pain.

The message

Physicians should emphasize that improved function is vitally important in the treatment of chronic pain [152]. They should inform chronic pain patients that, although there is no quick fix for their condition, they will improve if they take an active role in their therapy [1,101,153]. Chronic pain patients should not be given the false expectation that any single mode of therapy will "cure" their condition [74,106], because this leads them to seek short-term relief at the expense of long-term improvement.

Telling patients to "let pain be your guide" commonly leads chronic pain patients to become deconditioned [121], which in turn can produce concurrent myofascial pain [12]. Instead, physicians should encourage chronic pain patients to increase their levels of activity.

Physicians should be sympathetic and supportive toward their patients, but they should be careful not to overstate the severity or consequences of their condition. It has been shown in a randomized trial that when "idiopathic pain" patients are told that there is no evidence of illness and that they do not require treatment, they are substantially better at follow-up than those who are given a symptomatic diagnosis and a prescription [154]. Patients who have minor whiplash injuries have been shown to have a better outcome if they are told that the actual physical damage is minimal, and that the injury itself does not cause long lasting pain. They should be encouraged to return to normal activity and go back to work as early as possible [38].

Physicians should be careful not to overemphasize medications and testing, because it tends to reinforce patients' perception that their pain is purely physical [121]. This is particularly problematic in patients who have somatization [155].

Consultation and disposition

It is very important that emergency and acute care physicians work closely with the local pain management clinic, or with the patient's personal physician. Physicians should understand that many treatments for chronic pain require a considerable amount of time and commitment on the part of the patient. Trying to make these treatments work without the coordinated efforts of a pain clinic may result in failure, and a loss of confidence by the patient.

The pain clinic or personal physician should be consulted whenever possible before opioids are given. Ideally, a strategy should be worked out in advance for new patients. This should include a plan for analgesia to help the patient through the period of time until he can be seen in the clinic, but should not establish a pattern of opioid use that may generate the expectation that opioids will be continued indefinitely. Such patterns, once established, are difficult to change, and may result in irreversible adverse changes in the patient's endogenous pain control system.

Close follow up should be arranged after discharge. Hospital admission is rarely indicated for chronic pain control [4].

Documentation

Physicians should document pain levels according to the JCAHO guidelines; however, this should not make physicians feel compelled to use opioids in patients in whom they are not appropriate. In one study [156], the documentation of pain assessment after treatment was associated with a trend for improved patient satisfaction, but it did not achieve statistical significance.

Patients who over-rely on the acute care clinic

The distinction between therapeutic opioid users and recreational drug-seekers is discussed in detail in the chapter by Hansen elsewhere in this issue; however, labeling patients with either designation has not been shown to help them [4]. It is far more important that the acute care physician remember that the frequent use of opioids can be harmful to either class of patients. Unfortunately, emergency and urgent care physicians have been shown to be very poor at restricting opioids in patients in whom they are inappropriate. In a study in which 30 drug-seeking patients were identified [157], 17 were told that they would receive no further narcotics from the facility, but 71% of those patients were given opioids anyway within 2 years.

Habitual patient files

A "habitual patient file" can help identify those patients who are at risk for addiction or tolerance-induce worsening of their chronic pain. Such files can be used in a way that is consistent with state laws, the Health Insurance Portability and Accountability Act of 1996 (HIPPA), and the JCAHO [158].

These are reviewed in greater detail in the chapter by Hansen elsewhere in this issue on drug-seeking patients.

Proactive arrangements

There are many ways in which an acute care facility can improve the care of frequent narcotic users and chronic pain patients who have legitimate needs and well-controlled opioid use. These include patient tracking systems, "narcotic contracts," and pain management letters that inform frequent users that they will be denied narcotics unless they have a detailed letter from their personal physician. One emergency department (ED) reports a system in which frequent narcotic users are referred to the emergency department's care manager. The manager then reviews the patient's history, checks with the patient's doctor, and creates a care plan for the patient. This may include helping the patient with follow-up, arranging referrals to multidisciplinary pain or drug treatment clinics, and educating the patient about alternative treatments, as well as specifying what drugs may be given to the patient when he presents. This system provides much better and more consistent care for both legitimate chronic pain patients and for drug seekers, decreases the number of visits to the ED by both types of patient, and improves the morale of the ED staff. The time invested by the care manager is more than made up by improved care [159].

A system has been proposed to identify pain patients who over-rely on the ED, and direct them toward appropriate outpatient care. Patients presenting to the ED for opioid treatment of a chronic pain problem 10 times in 1 year were reviewed for entry to a chronic pain registry. To be accepted into the registry, they had to have a primary care physician who could be contacted (or have back-up call) 24 hours a day, go to just one ED for treatment of the chronic pain problem, and be willing to undergo evaluation by a physician with expertise in chronic pain and drug dependence issues. Those patients who did not qualify or refuse to enter the registry would be denied opioids at the ED [160].

Whatever system is employed, it is important that the long-term benefit to the patient be kept in mind, and that it be consistent with the practices of the local pain management clinic or with the patient's personal physician (assuming that physician has reasonable expertise in the care of chronic pain).

Specific chronic pain syndromes

Complex regional pain syndrome

Physical therapy, including gentle desensitization and other measures, is one of the few interventions that have been shown to be effective in controlled studies of CRPS [161]. It produced a nearly 50% decrease in pain with effort at 3 months [162].

Physical therapy has been shown to very effective in the treatment of CRPS in children [19]. The majority of the children in the study were using crutches or wheelchairs, and had chronic changes secondary to maintaining the extremity immobile in a dependent position. The patients were treated solely with intensive physical therapy and vigorous toweling to provide sensory stimulation. The contralateral side was immobilized to force use of the affected side. By the end of therapy, 12 out of 20 had complete resolution of their symptoms. Two others had occasional discomfort and intermittent swelling. All had normal function, and none required a wheel chair or crutches. They were followed for average of 2.4 years, and there was only one recurrence.

Myofascial pain syndrome

Myofascial pain syndrome improves with multidisciplinary therapy [163]. Treatment should include specific musculoskeletal treatments, including physical therapy and trigger point injections. If not treated appropriately, myofascial pain syndrome may progress to a complex chronic pain syndrome, with sleep disturbances, fatigue, and psychosocial difficulties [164]. Trigger-point injections can be done in the acute care setting by physicians who are familiar with the technique.

Fibromyalgia

Aerobic exercise and cardiovascular fitness training produce long-term improvement. Although fitness training may make the patient feel worse initially, it is vital to prevent further deconditioning. Patients tend to be skeptical initially, and proven benefits are lost in the long run if patients are noncompliant [165,166]. Antidepressants [165] and acupuncture can be very effective in fibromyalgia, and may be synergistic [167]. Reducing fibromayalgia patients' "catastrophic" thoughts, and convincing them that they have the capacity to be more functional can have a substantial impact on their pain and function [34].

Low back pain

Early, aggressive rehabilitation programs can prevent disability in low back pain [90,168,169]. Nonspecific exercise has been found to be as effective as conventional physiotherapy [170]. Low back pain patients have been found to have poor aerobic capacity. Improving their fitness can improve their pain and disability to the point where they rate it as minimal [171]. Spinal cord stimulation [68] and percutaneous electrical nerve stimulation (PENS) [172] have been shown to produce approximately a 50% decrease in pain, with improved activity. Therapeutic massage was shown to improve discomfort 32% at 4 weeks; 74% of the subjects rated it "very helpful" [173].

A review of the efficacy of multidisciplinary pain clinics in relieving low back pain found that pain decreased 37%, compared with only 4% in control subjects. Prescription medication use, overall pain behaviors, and activity levels improved 65% [174]. Some programs report a success rate of over 80% back-to-work, compared with approximately 40% in controls [175,176].

The most important variable in the successful treatment of chronic low back pain appears to be the reduction of the patient's subjective feelings of disability [177]. It is therefore better if physicians and patients focus on function rather than pain. This encourages patients to be more active, and decreases avoidance behavior and maladaptive attempts to gain sympathetic attention [153].

Osteoarthritis

In a study of the treatment of hip and knee osteoarthritis [178], quadriceps-strengthening exercises produced a 30% improvement in pain. Aerobic exercise and strengthening produced a 24% increase in activity, with substantially decreased pain and use of medication. No flare-ups were observed.

Rheumatoid arthritis

Patients who present for acute exacerbations of rheumatoid arthritis may benefit from a short course of steroids; however, once steroids are started, it is often difficult to discontinue them. Long-term use may produce undesirable side effects without preventing the destructive process of the disease [179]. Consequently, it is important to consult a rheumatologist before initiating this treatment.

Chronic headaches

Chronic daily headaches are commonly caused by overuse of analgesic and other medications [180]. Acute care physicians should be careful not to contribute to this problem. The common practice of administering a short-acting opioid is frequently unsuccessful. In a follow-up study of headaches treated in the ED [181], as few as 13% of the patients treated had sustained headache relief, and almost half of the patients were unable to return to work the next day. Physicians should emphasize abortive or long-term treatment.

In another study [182], placebo plus lying in a quiet darkened room for 60 minutes produced good pain relief, equivalent to or better than meperidine or ketorolac plus an antiemetic. This should serve to remind us that in some diseases, improvement will occur without aggressive analgesia.

Summary

Chronic nonmalignant pain requires evaluation and treatment different from acute pain. The pathophysiology is different, and there is commonly some degree of psychosocial dysfunction. Opioids tend to be much less effective as analgesics for chronic pain, and may increase the sensitivity to pain when given long-term. Because they are self-reinforcing, opioids may be sought and be reported to improve chronic pain, even when they may make the condition worse over time. There are many effective alternatives to opioids for the treatment of chronic pain, but their use is complicated and may require considerable time and effort to determine which ones work. Patients, particularly those who have already been prescribed opioids, may resist these alternatives. An extensive physical and psychosocial evaluation is required in the management of chronic pain, which is difficult if not impossible to achieve in the emergency or urgent care settings. Consequently, emergency and urgent care physicians should work closely with the patient's pain management specialist or personal physician. Systems should be set up in advance to identify those patients whose frequent use of acute care services for obtaining opioids may be compromising their long-term management, putting themselves at risk for psychological and tolerance-induced adverse effects of frequent opioid use. Opioids may be used in carefully selected patients in consultation with their pain management specialist or personal physician, but care must be exercised not to initiate or exacerbate psychological or tolerance-related complications of chronic pain.

References

[1] American Chronic Pain Association. Available at: http://theacpa.org. Accessed Aug 6, 2001.

[2] The American Society of Anesthesiologists. Practice guidelines for chronic pain management. A report by the American Society of Anesthesiologists Task Force on Pain Management, Chronic Pain Section. Anesthesiology 1997;84(4):995–2004.

[3] Schofferman J. Long-term use of opioid analgesics for the treatment of chronic pain of nonmalignant origin. J Pain Symptom Manage 1993;8(5):279–88.

[4] Cline DM. Management of patients with chronic pain. In: Tintinalli JE, Kelen GD, Stapczynski JS, editors. Emergency medicine, a comprehensive study guide. 5th edition. New York: McGraw-Hill; 1999. p. 274–80.

[5] Cordell WH, Keene KK, et al. The high prevalence of pain in emergency medical care. Am J Emerg Med 2002;20(3):165–9.

[6] Gallup, Inc. Pain in America: highlights from a Gallup survey. June 9, 1999. Also available at Arthritis Foundation website: http://www.arthritis.org/conditions/speakingofpain/factsheet.asp. Accessed Aug 6, 2001.

[7] Mannik M, Gilliland BC. Miscellaneous arthridities and extraarticular rheumatism. In: Petersdorf RG, et al, editors. Harrison's principles of internal medicine. 10th edition. New York: McGraw Hill; 1983. p. 2006–10.

[8] Rogers C, Thompson TL. Pain problems in primary care medical practice. In: Tollison CD, Satterthwaite JR, Tollison JW, editors. Handbook of pain management. 2nd edition. Baltimore (MD): Williams and Wilkins; 1994.

[9] Mogil JS, Sternberg WF, et al. The genetics of pain and pain inhibition. Proc Natl Acad Sci USA 1996;93:3048–55.
[10] Hadler NM. MRI for regional back pain. Need for less imaging, better understanding. JAMA 2003;289(21):2863–5.
[11] Fields H. Depression and pain: a neurobiological model. Neuropsychiatry Neuropsychol Behav Neurol 1991;4(1):83–92.
[12] Lipman AG. Analgesic drugs for neuropathic and sympathetically maintained pain. Clin Geriatr Med 1996;12(3):501–15.
[13] Belgrade MJ. Following the clues to neuropathic pain. Postgrad Med 1999;106(6):127–40.
[14] Sindrup SH. Opioids. A way to control central pain? Neurology 2002;58(4):517.
[15] Davis KD, et al. Phantom sensations generated by thalamic microstimulation. Nature 1998;391:385–7.
[16] Lederhaas G. Complex regional pain syndrome: new definintions, new emphasis. Emerg Med 2000;18–22.
[17] Ochoa J. Reflex sympathetic dystrophy: fact and fiction. Am Fam Physician 1997;56(9): 2182–5.
[18] Birklein F. Neurological findings in complex regional pain syndromes—analysis of 145 cases. Acta Neurol Scand 2000;101(4):262–9.
[19] Bernstein BH, et al. Reflex neurovascular dystrophy in childhood. J Pediatr 1978;93(2): 211–5.
[20] Sosnowski M. Pain management: physiopathology, future research and endpoints. Support Care Cancer 1993;1:79–88.
[21] Brookoff D. Chronic pain: 1. A new disease? Hosp Pract 2000;45–59.
[22] Mao J, et al. Mechanisms of hyperalgesia and morphine tolerance: a current view of their possible interactions. Pain 1995;62(3):259–74.
[23] Chen L, Huang LYM. Protein Kinase reduces Mg + block of NMDA-receptor channels as a mechanism of modulation. Nature 1992;356:521–3.
[24] Bennett GJ. Neuropathic pain: new insights, new interventions. Hosp Pract 1998;33(10): 95–114.
[25] Simon EJ. Opiates: neurobiology. In: Lowinson J, Ruiz P, Millman R, editors. Substance abuse: a comprehensive text. Baltimore (MD): Williams and Wilkens; 1997. p. 148–58.
[26] Ferrante FM. Principles of opioid pharmacotherapy: practical implications of basic mechanisms. J Pain Symptom Manage 1996;11(5):265–73.
[27] Cherny NI. Opioid analgesics: comparative features and prescribing guidelines. Drugs 1996;51(5):713–37.
[28] Bushnell TG, Justins DM. Choosing the right analgesic. A guide to selecion. Drugs 1993; 46(3):394–408.
[29] Ossipov MH, Lai J, Vanderah TW, et al. Induction of pain facilitation by sustained opioid exposure: relationship to opioid antinociceptive tolerance. Life Sci 2003;73(6):783–800.
[30] Clark MR, Cox TS. Refractory chronic pain. Psychiatr Clin North Am 2002;25(1):71–88.
[31] Perkins FM, Kehlet H. Chronic pain as an outcome of surgery. A review of predictive factors. Anesthesiology 2000;93(4):1123–33.
[32] Epker J, Block AR. Presurgical psychological screening in back pain patients: a review. Clin J Pain 2001;17(3):200–5.
[33] Sherry DD. Psychological aspects of childhood reflex neuorvascular dystrophy. Pediatrics 1988;81(4):572–8.
[34] Bennett RM. Controversies in fibromyalgia and related conditions. Multidisciplinary group programs to treat fibromyalgia patients. Rheum Dis Clin North Am 1966;22(2): 351–67.
[35] Harper RC, Steger JC. Psychological correlates of frontalis EMG and pain in tension headache. Headache 1978;18:215–8.
[36] Barkin RL, et al. Management of chronic pain. Part II. Dis Mon 1996;42(8):457–507.

[37] Gallagher RM, et al. Chronic pain. Sources of late-life pain and risk factors for disability. Geriatrics 2000;55(9):40–4, 7.
[38] Ferrari R. Prevention of chronic pain after whiplash. Emerg Med J 2002;19(6):526–30.
[39] Jensen MP, et al. Relationship of pain-specific beliefs to chronic pain adjustment. Pain 1994;57(3):301–9.
[40] Rosenstiel AK, Keefe FJ. The use of coping strategies in chronic low back pain patients: relationship to patient characteristics and current adjustment. Pain 1983;17:33–44.
[41] Gamsa A. The role of psychological factors in chronic pain. II. A critical appraisal. Pain 1994;57:5–30.
[42] Romano JM, et al. Overt pain behaviors: relationship to patient functioning and treatment outcome. Behav Ther 1988;19:191–201.
[43] Compton P, Darakjian MA, Miotto K. Screening for addiction in patients with chronic pain and "problematic" substance use: evaluation of a pilot assessment tool. J Pain Symptom Manage 1998;16(6):355–63.
[44] Melzack R. The tragedy of needless pain. Sci Am 1990;262(2):19–25.
[45] McCarberg B. Managing the acute pain patient: alleviating the pain. Family Practice Recertification 2000;22(9):4–7.
[46] Portenoy RK, Foley KM. Chronic use of opioid analgesics in non-malignant pain: report of 38 cases. Pain 1986;25(2):171–86.
[47] Tennant F Jr, et al. Chronic opioid treatment of intractable non-malignant pain. NIDA Res Monogr 1988;81:174–80.
[48] Schofferman J. Long-term opioid analgesic therapy for severe refractory lumbar spine pain. Clin J Pain 1999;15(2):136–40.
[49] Boisaubin EV. The assessment and treatment of pain in the emergency room. Clin J Pain 1989;5(Suppl 2):S19–25.
[50] Murphy TM. Chronic opioids for chronic low back pain—solution or problem? J Am Board Fam Pract 1996;9(3):225–7.
[51] Halpern LM, Robinson J. Prescribing practices for pain in drug dependence: a lesson in ignorance. Adv Alcohol Subst Abuse 1985;1:135–62.
[52] Ducharme J. Emergency pain management: a Canadian Association of Emergency Physicians (CAEP) consensus document. J Emerg Med 1994;12(6):855–66.
[53] Duggan AW, North RA. Electrophysiology of opioids. Pharmacol Rev 1984;35(4):5–38.
[54] Chritensen D, Kayser V. The development of pain-related behaviour and opioid tolerance after neuropathy-inducing surgery and sham surgery. Pain 2000;88(3):231–8.
[55] Jaffe J, Martin W. Opioid analgesics and antagonists. In: Gilman A, et al, editors. The pharmacologic basis of therapeutics. New York: Macillan; 1980. p. 491–531.
[56] Sternbach RA. Pain. A psychophysiological analysis. New York: Academic Press; 1968.
[57] Belknap JK, O'Toole LA. Studies of genetic differences in response to opioid drugs. In: Crabbe JC, Harris RA, editors. The genetic basis of alcohol and drug actions. New York: Plenum Press; 1991. p. 225–52.
[58] De Craen AJM, Di Giulio G, et al. Analgesic efficacy and safety of paracetamol-codeine combinations versus paracetamol alone: a systematic review. BMJ 1996;313:321–5.
[59] Arkinstall W, et al. Efficacy of controlled-release codeine in chronic non-malignant pain: a randomized, placebo-controlled clinical trial. Pain 1995;62(2):169–78.
[60] Chernin T. The use of opioids for chronic nonmalignant pain. Pharm Times 1999;18–25.
[61] Drugs for pain. The Medical Letter on Drugs and Therapeutics 2000;42(1085):73–8.
[62] Ferrell BA. Pain management in elderly people. J Am Geriatr Soc 1991;39:64–73.
[63] Peloso PM, Bellamy N, et al. Double blind randomized placebo control trial of controlled release codeine in the treatment of osteoarthritis of the hip or knee. J Rheumatol 2000;27(3): 764–71.
[64] Mullican WS. Tramadol/acetaminophen combination tablets and codeine/acetaminophen combination capsules for the management of chronic pain: a comparative trial. Clin Ther 2001;23(9):1429–45.

[65] Turk DC. Combining somatic and psychosocial treatment for chronic pain patients: perhaps 1 + 1 does = 3. Clin J Pain 2001;17(4):281–3.
[66] Zens M, et al. Long-term oral opioid therapy in patients with chronic nonmalignant pain. J Pain Symptom Manage 1992;7(2):69–77.
[67] Kalman S, Osterberg A, et al. Morphine responsiveness in a group of well-defined multiple sclerosis patients: a study with i.v. morphine. Eur J Pain 2002;6(1):69–80.
[68] Anderson VC, Israel Z. Failed back surgery syndrome. Curr Rev Pain 2000;4(2):105–11.
[69] Arner S, Meyerson BA. Lack of analgesic effect of opioids on neuropathic and idiopathic forms of pain. Pain 1988;3(1):11–23.
[70] Burchman SL, Pagel PS. Implementation of a formal treatment agreement for outpatient management of chronic nonmalignant pain with opioid analgesics. J Pain Symptom Manage 1995;10(7):556–63.
[71] Bouckoms AJ, et al. Chronic nonmalignant pain treated with long-term oral narcotic analgesics. Ann Clin Psychiatry 1992;4:185–92.
[72] McQuay HJ, et al. Opioid sensitivity of chronic pain: a patient-controlled analgesia method. Anaesthesia 1992;47(9):757–67.
[73] Watson CP, Babul N. Efficacy of oxycodone in neuropathic pain: a randomized trial in postherpetic neuralgia. Neurology 1998;50:1837–41.
[74] American Geriatric Society Panel on Chronic Pain in Older Persons. AGS clinical practice guidelines: the management of chronic pain in older persons. J Am Geriatr Soc 1998;46:635–51.
[75] Rinaldi RC, et al. Clarification and standardization of substance abuse terminology. JAMA 1988;259(4):555–7.
[76] Streltzer J. Chronic pain and addiction. In: Leigh H, editor. Consultation-liaison psychiatry: 1990 and beyond. New York: Plenum Press; 1994. p. 43–51.
[77] Robinson RC, Gatchel RJ, et al. Screening for problematic prescription opioid use. Clin J Pain 2001;17(3):220–8.
[78] Collin E, Cesselin F. Neurobiological mechanisms of opioid tolerance and dependence. Clin Neuropharmacol 1991;14(6):465–88.
[79] Liu JG, Anand KJS. Protein kinases modulate the cellular adaptations associated with opioid tolerance and dependence. Brain Res Brain Res Rev 2001;38(1–2):1–19.
[80] Kissin I, Bright CA, et al. Acute tolerance to continuously infused alfentanil: the role of cholecystokinin and N-methyl-D-aspartate-nitric oxide synthase systems. Anesth Analg 2000;91(1):110–6.
[81] Mayer DJ, Mao J, et al. Cellular mechanisms of neuropathic pain, morphine tolerance, and their interactions. Proc Natl Acad Sci USA 1999;96:7731–6.
[82] Compton MA. Cold pressor pain tolerance in opiate and cocaine abusers: correlates of drug type and use status. J Pain Symptom Manage 1994;9(7):462–73.
[83] Martin JE, Inglis J. Pain tolerance and narcotic addiction. Br J Soc Clin Psychol 1965;4(3):224–9.
[84] Ho A, Dole VP. Pain perception in drug-free and in methadone-maintained human ex-addicts. Proc Soc Exp Biol Med 1979;162(3):392–5.
[85] Mao J, et al. Thermal hyperalgesia in association with the development of morphine tolerance in rats: roles of excitatory amino acid receptors and protein kinase C. J Neurosci 1994;14(4):2301–12.
[86] Foran SE. A substance P opioid chimeric peptide as a unique nontolerance-forming analgesic. Proc Natl Acad Sci USA 2000;97(13):7621–6.
[87] Ibuki T, et al. Effect of transient naloxone antagonism on tolerance development in rats receiving continuous spinal morphine infusion. Pain 1997;70(2–3):125–32.
[88] Savage SR. Long-term opioid therapy: assessment of consequences and risks. J Pain Symptom Manage 1996;11(5):274–86.
[89] American Academy of Pain Medicine, American Pain Society, American Sociey of Addiction Medicine. Consensus statement. Definitions related to the use of opioids for the

treatment of pain. February 2001. Available at: http://www.painmed.org/productpub/statements/index.html. Accessed December 22, 2001.
[90] Sees KL, Clark HW. Opioid use in the treatment of chronic pain: assessment of addiction. J Pain Symptom Manage 1993;8(5):257–64.
[91] Abramowicz M. Drugs for pain. The Medical Letter on Drugs and Therapeutics 1993; 35(887):1–6.
[92] Jaffe J. Opiates: clinical aspects. In: Lowinson J, Ruiz P, Millman R, editors. Substance abuse: a comprehensive text. Baltimore (MD): Williams and Wilkens; 1997. p. 158–66.
[93] McLellan AT, et al. Drug dependence, a chronic medical illness: implications for treatment, insurance, and outcomes evaluation. JAMA 2000;284(13):1689–95.
[94] Fiserova M, Consolo S, Krsiak M. Chronic morphine induces long-lasting changes in acetylcholine release in rat nucleus accumbens core and shell: an in vivo microdialysis study. Psychopharmacology (Berl) 1999;142(1):85–94.
[95] Brodner RA. Chronic pain exacerbated by long-term narcotic use in patients with nonmalignant disease: clinical syndrome and treatment. Mt Sinai J Med 1978;45(2):233–7.
[96] Haertzen CA, Hooks NT Jr. Changes in personality and subjective experience associated with the chronic administration and withdrawal of opiates. J Nerv Ment Dis 1969;148(6): 606–14.
[97] Savage SR. Opioid use in the management of chronic pain. Med Clin North Am 1999;83(3): 761–86.
[98] Ytterberg SR, et al. Codeine and oxycodeine use in patients with chronic rheumatic disease pain. Arthritis Rheum 1998;41:1603–12.
[99] Sternbach RA. Mastering pain. A twelve-step program for coping with chronic pain. New York: G.P. Putnam's Sons; 1987.
[100] Kudrow L. Paradoxical effects of frequent analgesic use. Adv Neurol 1982;33:335–41.
[101] Black RG. The chronic pain syndrome. Surg Clin North Am 1975;55:999–1012.
[102] Taylor CB, et al. The effects of detoxification, relaxation, and brief supportive therapy on chronic pain. Pain 1980;8:319–29.
[103] Finlayson RD, et al. Substance dependence and chronic pain: profile of 50 patients treated in an alcohol and drug dependence unit. Pain 1986;26:167–74.
[104] Streltzer J. Treatment of iatrogenic drug dependence in the general hospital. Gen Hosp Psychiatry 1980;2:262–6.
[105] Joint Commission on Accreditation of Healthcare Organizations. Pain Standards for 2001. Available at: http://www.jcaho.org/news + room/health + care + issues/pain + mono_npc.pdf, p. 77. Accessed December 21, 2001.
[106] Portenoy RK, quoted in: Hospitals face new standards on treating pain. The Press-Enterprise. December 26, 2000:A3.
[107] Blackburn P, Vissers R. Pharmacology of emergency department pain management and conscious sedation. Emerg Med Clin North Am 2000;18(4):803–27.
[108] Tennant F Jr, et al. Chronic opioid treatment of intractable non-malignant pain. Pain Management 1988;18–36.
[109] American Academy of Pain Medicine and American Pain Society. The use of opioids for the treatment of chronic pain. 1997. Available at: http://www.painmed.org/productpub/statements/opioids.pdf. Accessed February 20, 2005.
[110] Brown RL, et al. Chronic opioid analgesic therapy for chronic low back pain. J Am Board Fam Pract 1996;9(3):192–204.
[111] Goucke CR. Australian management strategies for oral opioid use in non-malignant pain. Eur J Pain 2001;5(Suppl A):99–101.
[112] American Pain Society. President's message. APS must advocate for policy improvements. Available at: http://ampainsoc.org/pub/bulletin/mar01/pres1.htm. Accessed August 6, 2001.
[113] Parrott T. Using opioid analgesicics to manage chronic noncancer pain in primary care. J Am Board Fam Pract 1999;12(4):293–306.

[114] Passik SD, Weinreb HJ. Managing chronic nonmalignant pain: overcoming obstacles to the use of opioids. Adv Ther 2000;17(2):70–83.
[115] Moulin DE, et al. Randomized trial of oral morphine for chronic non-cancer pain. Lancet 1996;347(8995):143–7.
[116] Helme RD. Chronic pain management in older people. Eur J Pain 2001;5(Suppl A):31–6.
[117] Ballantyne JC, Mao J. Opioid therapy for chronic pain. N Engl J Med 2003;349: 1943–53.
[118] McCarberg BH, Barkin RL. Long-acting opioids for chronic pain: pharmacotherapeutic opportunities to enhance compliance, quality of life, and analgesia. Am J Ther 2001;8(3): 181–6.
[119] Ferrell B, et al. Effects of controlled-released morphine on quality of life for cancer pain. Oncol Nurs Forum 1989;16(4):521–6.
[120] Cowan DT, et al. A pilot study into the problematic use of opioid analgesics in chronic non-cancer pain patients. Int J Nurs Stud 2002;39(1):59–69.
[121] Fordyce WE. Behavioral factors in pain. Neurosurg Clin N Am 1991;2(4):749–59.
[122] Berntsen D, Gotestam KG. Effects of on-demand versus fixed-interval schedules in the treatment of chronic pain with analgesic compounds. J Consult Clin Psychol 1987;55: 213–7.
[123] Fishman SM, et al. The opioid contract in the management of chronic pain. J Pain Symptom Manage 1999;18(1):27–37.
[124] McQuay HJ. Pre-emptive analgesia: a systematic review of clinical studies. Ann Med 1995; 27(2):249–56.
[125] Richmond CE, et al. Preoperative morphine pre-empts postoperative pain. Lancet 1993; 342(8863):73–5.
[126] Bach S, Noreng MF, Tjellden NU. Phantom limb pain in amputees during the first 12 months following limb amputation, after preoperative lumbar epidural blockade. Pain 1988;33:297–301.
[127] American Academy of Pain Medicine. Consensus statement. The necessity for early evaluation of the chronic pain patient. 2001. Available at: www.painmed.org/productpub/ statements/index.html. Accessed December 22, 2001.
[128] Leventhal EA, Leventhal H, et al. Active coping reduces reports of pain from childbirth. J Consult Clin Psychol 1989;57(3):365–71.
[129] Lieberman AB. Easing labor pain. The complete guide to achieving a more comfortable and rewarding birth. Garden City (NY): Doubleday & Company; 1987. p. 46.
[130] Turner JA, Chapman CR. Psychological interventions for chronic pain: a critical review. II. Operant conditioning, hypnosis, and cognitive-behavioral therapy. Pain 1982;12(1):1–21.
[131] Turner JA, Chapman CR. Psychological interventions for chronic pain: a critical review. Pain 1982;12(1):1–21.
[132] Kabat-Zinn J, et al. The clinical use of mindfulness meditation for the self-regulation of chronic pain. J Behav Med 1985;8(2):163–90.
[133] Gamsa A. The role of psychological factors in chronic pain. I. A half century of study. Pain 1994;57:5–16; 17–30.
[134] Follick MJ, Ahern DK, Aberger EW. Behavioral treatment of chronic pain. In: Blumethal JA, and McKee D, editors. Applications in Behavioral Medicine and Health Psychology: A Clinician's Source Book. Professional Resource Press; 1987, Sarasota, FL. p. 237–70.
[135] Large RG, Schug SA. Opioids for chronic pain of non-malignant origin—caring or crippling. Health Care Anal 1995;3(1):5–11.
[136] Marcus DA. Treatment of nonmalignant chronic pain. Am Fam Physician 2000;61:1331–8; 1345–6.
[137] Feine JS, Lund JP. An assessment of the efficacy of physical therapy and physical modalities for the control of chronic musculoskeletal pain. Pain 1997;71(1):5–23.
[138] Wright A, Sluka KA. Nonpharmacological treatments for musculoskeletal pain. Clin J Pain 2001;17(1):33–46.

[139] Katz WA. Approach to the management of nonmalignant pain. Am J Med 1996;101(1A): 54S–63S.
[140] Dersh J, Gatchel RJ, et al. Prevalence of psychiatric disorders in patients with chronic work-related musculoskeletal pain disability. J Occup Environ Med 2002;44(5): 459.
[141] Katz WA. The needs of a patient in pain. Am J Med 1998;105(1B):2S–7S.
[142] Weisberg MB, Clavel AL Jr. Why is chronic pain so difficult to treat? Postgrad Med 1999; 106(6):141–64.
[143] Allegrante JP. The role of adjunctive therapy in the management of chronic nonmalignant pain. Am J Med 1996;101(1A):33S–9S.
[144] Swanson DW, et al. Results of behavior modification in the treatment of chronic pain. Psychosom Med 1979;41:55–61.
[145] Finlayson RD, et al. Substance dependence and chronic pain: experience with treatment and follow-up results. Pain 1986;26:175–80.
[146] Swanson DW, et al. The dissatisfied patient with chronic pain. Pain 1977;4:367–78.
[147] Tissue-specific sports injuries. Analgesia in sports medicine [special report]. Phys Sportsmed 2003; Aug:13–27.
[148] Kudoh A, et al. Effect of carbamazepine on pain scores of unipolar depressed patients with pain: a trial of off-on-off-on design. Clin J Pain 1988;14(1):61–5.
[149] Rice ASC, Matan S, for the Postherpetic Neurology Study Group. Gabapentin in postherpetic neuralgia: a randomised, double blind, placebo controlled study. Pain 2001;94: 215–24.
[150] Hewitt DJ. The use of NMDA-receptor antagonists in the treatment of chronic pain. Clin J Pain 2000;16(Suppl 2):S73–9.
[151] Katz NP. MorphiDex (MS:DM) double-blind, multiple-dose studies in chronic pain patients. J Pain Symptom Manage 2000;19(Suppl 1):S37–41.
[152] Fe-Bornsteine M. Chronic pain in the elderly: an overview. Clin Geriatr Med 2002;10(1): 17–9.
[153] Mayer TG. Lower back pain. Rehabilitation. What do we do with the chronic patient? Neurol Clin 1999;17(1):131–47.
[154] Thomas KB. The consultation and the therapeutic illusion. BMJ 1978;20:1327–8.
[155] Ford CV. Dimensions of somatization and hypochondriasis. Neurol Clin 1995;13(2): 241–53.
[156] Eder SC, Sloan EP, Todd K. Documentation of ED patient pain by nurses and physicians. Am J Emerg Med 2003;21(4):253–7.
[157] Zednich AD, Hedges JR. Community-wide emergency department visits by patients suspected of drug-seeking behavior. Acad Emerg Med 1996;3(4):312–7.
[158] Geiderman JM. Keeping lists and naming names: habitual patient files for suspected nontherapeutic drug-seeking patients. Ann Emerg Med 2003;41(6):873–81.
[159] Do you give poor care to patients in pain? ED Manag 2003;65–7.
[160] MacLeod DB, Swanson R. A new approach to chronic pain in the ED. Am J Emerg Med 1996;14(3):323–6.
[161] Rho RH, Brewer RP, et al. Complex regional pain syndrome. Mayo Clin Proc 2002;77(2): 174–80.
[162] Oerlemans HM, et al. Pain and reduced mobility in complex regional pain syndrome I: outcome of a prospective randomised controlled clinical trial of adjuvant physical therapy versus occupational therapy. Pain 1999;83:77–83.
[163] Han SC, Harrison P. Myofascial pain syndrome and trigger-point management. Reg Anesth 1997;22(1):89–101.
[164] Kim BY, Brown S. Myofascial pain syndrome: don't let it sideline your patients. Your Patient and Fitness 1997;11(6):21–6.
[165] Simms RW. Controlled trials of therapy in fibromyalgia syndrome. Baillieres Clin Rheumatol 1994;8(4):917–34.

[166] Wigers SH, et al. Effects of aerobic exercise versus stress management treatment in fibromyalgia. A 4.5 year prospective study. Scand J Rheumatol 1996;25(2):77–86.
[167] Berman BM, et al. Is acupuncture effective in the treatment of fibromyalgia? J Fam Pract 1999;48(3):213–8.
[168] Frymoyer JW. Predicting disability from low back pain. Clin Orthop 1992;279:101–9.
[169] Justins DM. Management strategies for chronic pain. Ann Rheum Dis 1996;55(9):588–96.
[170] Carter IR. How effective are exercise and physical therapy for chronic low back pain? J Fam Pract 2002;51(3):209.
[171] Van der Velde G, Mierau D. The effect of exercise on percentile rank aerobic capacity, pain, and self-rated disability in patients with chronic low-back pain: a retrospective chart review. Arch Phys Med Rehabil 2000;81:1457–63.
[172] Ghoname EA, et al. Percutaneous electrical nerve stimulation for low back pain. A randomized crossover study. JAMA 1999;281(9):818–23.
[173] Cherkin DC, et al. Randomized trial comparing traditional Chinese medical acupuncture, therapeutic massage, and self-care education for chronic low back pain. Arch Intern Med 2001;161:1081–8.
[174] Flor H, et al. Efficacy of multidisciplinary pain treatment centers: a meta-analytic review. Pain 1992;49:221–30.
[175] Mayer TG, et al. A prospective two-year study of functional restoration in industrial low back injury. An objective assessment procedure. JAMA 1987;258(13):1763–7.
[176] Frymoyer JW. Back pain and sciatica. N Engl J Med 1988;318(5):291–300.
[177] Hildebrandt J, et al. Prediction of success from a multidisciplinary treatment program for chronic low back pain. Spine 1997;22(9):990–1001.
[178] Puett DW, Griffin MR. Published trials of nonmedicinal and noninvasive therapies for hip and knee osteoarthritis. Ann Intern Med 1994;121(2):133–40.
[179] Ruddy S. The management of rheumatoid arthritis. In: Kelley WN, Harris ED, Ruddy S, et al, editors. Textbook of rheumatology, vol. 1. 2nd edition. Philadelphia: W.B. Saunders; 1985. p. 979–92.
[180] Radat F, Irachabal S, Swendsen J, et al. Analgesic abuse and psychiatric comorbidity in headache patients. Encephale 2002;28(5 Pt 1):466–71.
[181] Sivilotti ML, et al. Studying emergency patients outside the emergency department. Ann Emerg Med 1996;27(4):442–7.
[182] Harden RN, et al. The placebo effect in acute headache management: ketorolac, meperidine, and saline in the emergency department. Headache 1996;36(6):352–6.

EMERGENCY MEDICINE CLINICS OF NORTH AMERICA

ELSEVIER SAUNDERS

Emerg Med Clin N Am 23 (2005) 339–348

The Psychology of Pain

George R. Hansen, MD[a,*], Jon Streltzer, MD[b]

[a]*Department of Emergency Medicine, Sierra Vista Regional Medical Center, 1010 Murray Avenue, San Luis Obispo, CA 93405, USA*

[b]*Department of Psychiatry, John A. Burns School of Medicine, University of Hawaii, 1356 Lusitana Street, Honolulu, HI 96813, USA*

The perception of pain involves far more than mere sensation. The affective and evaluative components of pain are often as important as the production and transmission of the pain signal. These emotional aspects are most prominent in chronic pain patients, but knowledge of the psychology of pain can greatly improve the treatment of acute pain as well.

Pain and its perception

The limbic system, where emotions are processed, modulates the amount of pain experienced for a given noxious stimulus. It has been shown in cancer patients [1] that the affective component of pain can be completely blocked by frontal lobectomy. Lobectomized patients still register severe pain, but it doesn't "bother" them. Pain can thus be viewed as merely a "signal" that something is wrong somewhere in the body, until it reaches the emotional brain, where this signal becomes what we feel as pain.

The emotional response to pain involves the anterior cingulate gyrus and the right ventral prefrontal cortex. These centers are also activated by social rejection. Serotonin and norepinephrine circuits are also involved in the modulation of sensory stimuli, which probably influence how depression and antidepressant medications affect the perception of pain [2].

Context

The perception of even acute pain is highly dependent on the context in which it occurs [3]. It has been found that the pain perceived in battle

* Corresponding author.

E-mail address: cingemanor@aol.com (G.R. Hansen).

doi:10.1016/j.emc.2004.12.005

wounds bears little relationship to the extent of the wounds [4]. There are reports of soldiers in battle who suffer a compound fracture, and report only twinges of pain [5]. In laboratory studies of experimental pain in which context, fear, and anxiety are controlled, the placebo effect and opioids are much less effective. This occurs because the reduction of both the fear and anxiety is a large part of the placebo effect and of the function of opioids [6].

Attention

Focusing one's attention on pain makes the pain worse [1]. Patients who have somatic preoccupation or hypochondriasis are overvigilant about bodily sensations. It has been found that by attending to these sensations, they amplify them to the point of feeling painful [7].

Conversely, distracting patients is highly effective in reducing their pain. Burn patients undergoing treatments or physical therapy experience excruciating pain, even after they have been given opioids. It has been shown that these patients report only a fraction of this pain if they are distracted with a virtual-reality type of video game during the procedure [8].

Anxiety

Anxiety, fear, and a sense of loss of control contribute to patient suffering. Treating anxiety and providing psychological support has been shown to improve pain and reduce analgesic use. Improving patients' sense of control and allowing them to participate in their care is also helpful [9]. Physicians should try to create an environment that is nonthreatening. For procedures, prepare needles and other equipment out of sight from the patient. In addition to assuring that procedures are performed in the least painful way possible, use nonthreatening terms such as "mild discomfort" instead of "pain." It is also helpful to distract patients with conversation about subjects that interest them, such as their hobbies or family [10].

Memory

Patients who have low levels of pain remember it as being worse than they originally reported, which tends to worsen with time. Almost all patients report relief with treatment, even when true measured changes in pain scale are not significant, and sometimes when measured pain is worse [11].

Learned pain

Pain can be a learned response, rather than a purely physical problem. Just as cancer patients can develop nausea as a learned response to treatment and experience it even before chemotherapy is administered, patients can learn to have pain even in the absence of a physical stimulus [12]. In some cases, pain can be entirely "in the mind," as in the case of a butcher who slipped and caught his arm on a meat hook, and was reported to be suffering in great agony. When he learned that the hook had merely caught on his sleeve and his arm was uninjured, his pain resolved [13].

Patients can learn to feel different amounts of pain just by viewing other people. When laboratory subjects were shown models demonstrating high pain tolerance, they required 3.48 times greater stimulus before they rated it as painful, compared with those subjects who observed models who showed poor tolerance. Nonaversive shock, usually described as "tingling," was rated as painful by only 3% of those who had viewed a tolerant model, compared with 77% of the subjects who viewed models who showed poor tolerance [14].

Expectations

Patients' expectations of how much pain they should have also influence how much pain they feel, their response to treatment [15], and whether or not the condition becomes chronic and disabling. The results of minor whiplash injuries have been shown to be highly variable in different regions. This has been attributed to the local cultures and expectations. Any messages that communicate to patients that they have a serious or debilitating injury may contribute to deconditioning and maladaptive postures that worsen their pain. Prescribing medications can contribute to the problem. Patients who are not given sick leave and are told to "act as usual" have much better outcomes [7].

The placebo effect is also influenced by patients' and physicians' expectations [15]. It can be assumed that the "nocebo" effect (ie, the perception of harm resulting from a patient's beliefs) can also result from messages that inadvertently increase the patient's anxiety and expectations of pain.

Beliefs and coping

Other psychosocial issues, such as what patients believe about their pain [16,17], their coping skills [18–21], their tendency to "catastrophize" [17,18,20], self-efficacy [17], locus or control [22], and their involvement in the "sick role" [13], all have an impact on how much pain patients feel, and how it affects them.

In successfully getting low back pain patients back to work, the most important factor identified has been a reduction in subjective feelings of disability [23]. Patients diagnosed with fibromyalgia have to stop catastrophizing to improve, and they must be persuaded that they have the capacity to be more functional [24]. Consequently, physicians should focus on improved function and long-term management. Patients should be led to understand that they themselves have an important role in distracting themselves, and that they can minimize the interference that pain has in their lives.

Chronic pain

Chronic pain patients commonly have problems with the psychological and emotional aspects of pain [25]. Preexisting psychological factors have been shown to be very important in the development of chronic pain after surgery [26,27] and in complex regional pain syndrome (CRPS) [28,29], tension-type headaches [30], and fibromyalgia [24]. The National Institutes of Health Technology Assessment Conference Statement [31] identified six factors that correlated with treatment failures of low back pain—all were psychosocial. Even chronic, episodic, low back pain may have a vital component of socioeconomic and psychological influences [32].

There is a vicious cycle in which pain causes disability and stress, which in turn worsens the perception of pain [21]. An unhealthy lifestyle, lack of social support, depressive illness, and substance abuse are predisposing factors to chronic pain [33]. Chronic pain has been referred to as "complex" when there are interactions of legal, psychological, medication, and family issues [34].

Behavior

Immobility may be a factor in adult "reflex sympathetic dystrophy," which some feel is overdiagnosed [35]. A study of reflex neurovascular dystrophy in children revealed that prominent swelling, skin changes, and decreased skin temperature were caused by maintaining the extremity in an immobile, dependent position. The prolonged immobility also caused chronic fibrosis of subcutaneous tissues and contractures of tendons and ligaments. This was effectively relieved with physical treatments, which included vigorous sensory stimulation and use of the affected extremity [36].

Inactivity is a serious impediment to improvement in chronic pain, and can produce concurrent myofascial pain [37]. Many fibromyalgia patients have been found to have a vicious cycle of maladaptive pain behavior, resulting in further deconditioning, social dysfunction, and subsequent worsening pain [24].

Obesity is also a problem in chronic pain. A review of patients at a rehabilitation clinic found that among those who could not be returned to gainful employment or function, 78% were grossly overweight [38]. Many low back pain patients have been found to be in the lowest quartile for aerobic capacity [39].

Pain behavior, such as guarding, bracing, rubbing, grimacing, and sighing, has been shown to be strongly influenced by psychological factors [40]. Some chronic pain patients demonstrate pain behavior only around staff [41], or decrease this behavior when they think no one is watching [42]. Reinforcing this behavior can cause some patients to perceive that they have more pain. Eliminating the behavior leads to improved pain [40]. It has been noted that if neuropathic pain patients are allowed to develop guarding and behavioral dysfunction, then drugs are not effective, and the patients require multidisciplinary pain treatment [37].

Pain can be a conditioned response similar to conditioned nausea associated with chemotherapy. The behavior begins purely in response to the presence of injury. It is then reinforced and becomes a conditioned response, an iatrogenic complication of treatment [12], particularly when rewards are made contingent on the expression of pain behavior [21]. The effect of reinforcement is illustrated by the case of a 10-year-old girl who had chronic daily abdominal pain for which no medical condition could be found. During episodes, her mother allowed her to rest in bed with her toys and watch television, and brought her food and drinks. After an hour or so, she would go back to play. After the mother stopped reinforcing the patient's pain behavior, the episodes rapidly diminished, as well as her use of belladonna and phenobarbital elixir [43].

Pain can result from conditioned fear reactions that persist even after the resolution of pain [42], phobic reactions to pain and to nonpainful activities [44], and posttraumatic stress disorder [45]. Some patients have had good improvement of their pain or function with desensitization therapy [46].

Psychiatric disease

Overall, some psychiatric morbidity is present in up to 67% of chronic pain patients [47]. Personality disorders have been found in 31% to 59% of chronic pain patients [48]. Among low back pain patients admitted to an inpatient multidisciplinary pain center, 70% were found to have a hysterical conversion disorder, and 8% had a sociopathic personality disorder [49].

Somatoform pain disorders

Somatoform disorders are conditions in which the presence of physical symptoms suggests a general medical condition, but cannot be explained by any such condition. Among the somatoform disorders, "pain disorder associated with psychological factors" is specified in the Diagnostic and Statistical Manual of Mental disorders, fourth edition (DSMIV) [50] as a clinical condition in which pain is the focus and in which psychological factors have the major role in the onset, severity, maintenance, or exacerbation The epidemiology of this condition is not known, but unexplained chronic pain that causes disability is common in general practice and is frequently seen in emergency rooms. Pain disorder associated with psychological factors was found in 88% of referrals to a pain clinic serving an indigent population [51]. Most somatoform patients had pain that spread to new areas from the site of injury, whereas this did not occur in the patients who had objective signs of injury. Compared with patients who had serious injuries involving long-term pain, mildly injured somatoform pain patients are more than five times as likely to use daily opioids [52]. Moreover, one program found a 30% incidence of abuse of opioids among those patients who had somatoform pain disorder, many times higher than that of the other patients [53].

Hypochondriasis, another kind of somatoform disorder that involves fear of having a disease when there is none, has also been identified in chronic pain patients [54]. It has been found to be worsened by the chronic medical use of morphine [55], and by its abuse [56].

Mood disorders

In a study of chronic pain patients on opioids, 61% were found to have major depression [57]. It appears that the pain causes depression at least as often as depression causes pain [58,59]. Nonetheless, depression is known to make the patient's pain feel worse [48]. In postsurgical pain after cholecystectomy, patients who had even subclinical depressive symptoms reported higher pain [60]. Treating depression can improve, and in some cases eliminate, chronic pain [6]. Whether depression is considered to be a cause or an effect of chronic pain, it should be considered at least a comorbid condition that requires concurrent treatment [61].

An anxiety disorder was found in 10.6% of chronic work-related musculoskeletal pain patients [62]. The lifetime risk of a major anxiety disorder in men who have chronic low back pain is 30.9%, compared with 14.3% in men who do not have low back pain [59]. It is likely that some "chronic pain" patients are actually using opioid medications to self-treat anxiety or depression, instead of relying on more effective anxiolytic or antidepressant agents [57]. These patients are not only using the wrong drug for their condition, but what little subjective benefit they initially feel is rapidly lost with tolerance, and replaced with dependence.

Evaluation

Because of the influence of psychological factors on chronic pain, at least brief screening should be done on initial evaluation. It is very useful to examine for Waddell signs or nonphysiological findings, which can be done quickly during the physical [63]. A particularly good test is the application of pressure on the top of the head when the patient is standing, to put stress on the spine. The low back pain patient who has a somatoform pain disorder will often complain of increased pain. If the pain were purely of spinal origin, this maneuver would not increase it.

Whenever psychiatric comorbidity is present or suspected, more comprehensive screening should include tests such as the Multidimensional Pain Inventory (MPI) and the Minnesota Multiphasic Personality Inventory 2 (MMPI-2) [21]. Such comprehensive testing is usually impractical in the emergency setting, and ideally should be done by a psychiatric consultant familiar with chronic pain [48]. Although acute care physicians are not likely to be doing this evaluation themselves, they should insure that it has already been completed, or that it will be done as soon as possible. Failing to address psychological issues in chronic pain patients may result in prolonged disability in a substantial number of patients [25].

The psychology of opioid dependence

The subject of opioid dependence in patients complaining of pain is controversial, and is discussed in further detail in the article by Hansen elsewhere in this issue on the drug-seeking patient. It should be noted that chronic opioid use, particularly in high doses, can produce a condition of enhanced pain sensitivity [64]. Patients dependent on daily doses feel worse when the medication wears off, and closer to baseline levels of pain temporarily when they take it, even though the overall pain condition fails to improve [65]. These patients may see opioids as necessary for survival. It may become difficult to control the use of opioids, and they visit the emergency room when they run out. They complain of increased pain from conditions that would not typically call for opioids. The patient who escalates demands for opioids when these are not forthcoming is typically opioid-dependent, and may have issues of problematic use.

The psychology of the physician also influences the use of opioids for chronic pain, and the interpretation of their effectiveness. Some patients are insistent that certain medications must be prescribed. They will exaggerate the benefits and deny adverse effects. Some physicians have difficulty setting limits. It is faster and easier to give in to the patient's demands than to institute an alternate course. The physician may realize that the prescription is in excess of normal practice, but rationalizes that for this particular patient, nothing else works. The emergency physician can anticipate these issues, and plan, with consultation if desired, how to deal with them.

Summary

Emotional and evaluative issues are very important in the evaluation and treatment of pain. Treating the physical pain alone can leave these issues unresolved, and possibly exacerbate them through reinforcement.

Understanding the impact of fear, expectations, and attention can help physicians deal more effectively with acute pain. Psychological issues are particularly prominent in chronic pain. Though acute care physicians my not be treating these psychological conditions, they can help by referring patients to the appropriate psychological or multidisciplinary setting.

References

[1] Fields H. Depression and pain: a neurobiological model. Neuropsychiatry Neuropsychol Behav Neurol 1991;4(1):83–92.
[2] Vastag B. Scientists find connections in the brain between physical and emotional pain. JAMA 2003;290(18):2389–90.
[3] Lambert WE, Libman E, Poser EG. The effect of increased salience of a membership group on pain tolerance. J Pers 1960;38:350–7.
[4] Beecher HK. Relationship of significance of wound to the pain experienced. JAMA 1956; 161:1609–13.
[5] Horstman J, Flax P. Controlling chronic pain. Hippocrates 1999; May:29–35.
[6] Sternbach RA. Pain. A psychophysiological analysis. New York: Academic Press; 1968.
[7] Ferrari R. Prevention of chronic pain after whiplash. Emerg Med J 2002;19(6):526–30.
[8] Hoffman HG, Patterson DR, et al. Effectiveness of virtual reality-based pain control with multiple treatments. Clin J Pain 2001;17(3):229–35.
[9] Ready LB. Acute perioperative pain. In: Miller RD, editor. Anesthesiology. 5th edition. Philadelphia: Churchill Livingstone; 2000. p. 2323–50.
[10] Paris PM, Stewart R. Analagesia and sedation. In: Emergency medicine: concepts and clinical practice. 3rd edition. St. Louis (MO): Mosby-Year Book, Inc.; 1992. p. 202–29.
[11] Feine JS, et al. Memories of chronic pain and perceptions of relief. Pain 1988;77(2):137–41.
[12] Fordyce WE. Behavioral factors in pain. Neurosurg Clin N Am 1991;2(4):749–59.
[13] Gamsa A. The role of psychological factors in chronic pain. II. A critical appraisal. Pain 1994;57:5–30.
[14] Craig KD. Social modeling influences on pain. In: Sternbach RA, editor. The psychology of pain. New York: Raven Press; 1978. p. 73–110.
[15] Turner JA, Deyo RA, Loeser JD, et al. The importance of placebo effects in pain treatment and research. JAMA 1994;271:1609–14.
[16] Jensen MP, et al. Relationship of pain-specific beliefs to chronic pain adjustment. Pain 1994; 57(3):301–9.
[17] Jensen MP, et al. Patient beliefs predict patient functioning: further support for a cognitive-behavioural model of chronic pain. Pain 1999;81(1–2):95–104.
[18] Turner JA, et al. Do beliefs, coping, and catastrophizing independently predict functioning in patients with chronic pain? Pain 2000;85(1–2):115–25.
[19] Gatchel RJ, Noe CE, et al. A preliminary study of multidimensional pain inventory profile differences in predicting treatment outcome in a heterogeneous cohort of patients with chronic pain. Clin J Pain 2002;18(3):139–43.
[20] Rosenstiel AK, Keefe FJ. The use of coping strategies in chronic low back pain patients: relationship to patient characteristics and current adjustment. Pain 1983;17:33–44.
[21] Barkin RL, et al. Management of chronic pain. Part II. Dis Mon 1996;42(8):457–507.
[22] Coughlin AM, et al. Multidisciplinary treatment of chronic pain patients: its efficacy in changing patient locus of control. Arch Phys Med Rehabil 2000;81(6):739–40.
[23] Hildebrandt J, et al. Prediction of success from a multidisciplinary treatment program for chronic low back pain. Spine 1997;22(9):990–1001.
[24] Bennett RM. Controversies in fibromyalgia and related conditions. Multidisciplinary group programs to treat fibromyalgia patients. Rhem Dis Clin North Am 1966;22(2):351–67.

[25] Clark MR, Cox TS. Refractory chronic pain. Psychiatr Clin North Am 2002;25(1):71–88.
[26] Perkins FM, Kehlet H. Chronic pain as an outcome of surgery. A review of predictive factors. Anesthesiology 2000;93(4):1123–33.
[27] Epker J, Block AR. Presurgical psychological screening in back pain patients: a review. Clin J Pain 2001;17(3):200–5.
[28] Birklein F. Neurological findings in complex regional pain syndromes—analysis of 145 cases. Acta Neurol Scand 2000;101(4):262–9.
[29] Sherry DD. Psychological aspects of childhood reflex neuorvascular dystrophy. Pediatrics 1988;81(4):572–8.
[30] Harper RC, Steger JC. Psychological correlates of frontalis EMG and pain in tension headache. Headache 1978;18:215–8.
[31] National Institute of Health. Integration of behavioral and relaxation approaches into the treatment of chronic pain and insomnia. NIH Technology Statement Online 1995, Oct 16–18, p. 1–34. Available at: http://odp.od.nih.gov/consensus/ta/017/017_statement.htm. Accessed August 6, 2001.
[32] Mayer TG. Lower back pain. Rehabilitation. What do we do with the chronic patient? Neurol Clin 1999;17(1):131–47.
[33] Gallagher RM, et al. Chronic pain. Sources of late-life pain and risk factors for disability. Geriatrics 2000;55(9):40–4, 7.
[34] Weisberg MB, Clavel AL Jr. Why is chronic pain so difficult to treat? Postgrad Med 1999; 106(6):141–64.
[35] Ochoa JL. Truth, errors, and lies around "reflex sympathetic dystrophy" and "complex regional pain syndrome." J Neurol 1999;246:875–9.
[36] Bernstein BH, et al. Reflex neurovascular dystrophy in childhood. J Pediatr 1978;93(2): 211–5.
[37] Lipman AG. Analgesic drugs for neuropathic and sympathetically maintained pain. Clin Geriatr Med 1996;12(3):501–15.
[38] Raskind R, Glover MB. Profile of a low back derelict. J Occup Med 1975;17:258–9.
[39] Van der Velde G, Mierau D. The effect of exercise on percentile rank aerobic capacity, pain, and self-rated disability in patients with chronic low-back pain: a retrospective chart review. Arch Phys Med Rehabil 2000;81:1457–63.
[40] Romano JM, et al. Overt pain behaviors: relationship to patient functioning and treatment outcome. Behav Ther 1988;19:191–201.
[41] Turner JA, Chapman CR. Psychological interventions for chronic pain: a critical review. II. Operant conditioning, hypnosis, and cognitive-behavioral therapy. Pain 1982; 12(1):1–21.
[42] Keefe FJ, et al. Observational methods for assessing pain: a practicle guide. In: Blumenthal JA, McKee DC, editors. Applications in behavioral medicine and health psychology: a clinician's source book. Sarasota (FL): Professional Resource Press; 1987. p. 67–94.
[43] Miller AJ, Kratchowill TR. Reduction of frequent stomach ache complaints by time-out. Behav Ther 1979;10:211–8.
[44] Follick MJ, Ahern DK, Aberger EW. Behavioral treatment of chronic pain. In: Blumenthal JA, McKee D, editors. Applications in Behavioral Medicine and Health Psychology. A Clinician's source book. Sarasota (FL): Professional Resource Press; 1987. p. 237–70.
[45] Sherman JJ, et al. Prevalence and impact of posttraumatic stress disorder-like symptoms on patients with fibromyalgia syndrome. Clin J Pain 2000;16(2):127–34.
[46] Muse M. Stress-related, posttraumatic chronic pain syndrome: behavioral treatment approach. Pain 1986;25(3):389–94.
[47] Compton P, Darakjian MA, Miotto K. Screening for addiction in patients with chronic pain and "problematic" substance use: evaluation of a pilot assessment tool. J Pain Symptom Manage 1998;16(6):355–63.
[48] Fishbain DA. Approaches to treatment decisions for psychiatric comorbidity in the management of the chronic pain patient. Med Clin North Am 1999;83(3):737–60.

[49] Seres JL, Newman RI. Results of treatment of chronic low-back pain at the Portland Pain Center. J Neurosurg 1976;45:32–6.
[50] American Psychiatric Association. Diagnostic and Statistical Manual of Mental disorders, fourth edition. Washington (DC): American Psychiatric Association; 1994.
[51] Anooshian J, Streltzer J, Goebert D. Effectiveness of a psychiatric pain clinic. Psychosomatics 1999;40:226–32.
[52] Streltzer J, Eliashof BA, Kline AE, et al. Chronic pain disorder following physical injury. Psychosomatics 2000;41:227–34.
[53] Wambach S, et al. Abuse of opioid therapy in somatoform pain disorder. A contribution from a psychosomatic/pain therapist point of view to the discussion of the indication of opioids in nonmalignant pain based on 8 cases. Schmerz 2001;15(4):254–64.
[54] Frymoyer JW. Back pain and sciatica. N Engl J Med 1988;318(5):291–300.
[55] Haertzen CA, Hooks NT Jr. Changes in personality and subjective experience associated with the chronic administration and withdrawal of opiates. J Nerv Ment Dis 1969;148(6): 606–14.
[56] Compton MA. Cold pressor pain tolerance in opiate and cocaine abusers: correlates of drug type and use status. J Pain Symptom Manage 1994;9(7):462–73.
[57] Bouckoms AJ, et al. Chronic nonmalignant pain treated with long-term oral narcotic analgesics. Ann Clin Psychiatry 1992;4:185–92.
[58] Merskey H. Psychological medicine, pain, and musculoskeletal disorders. Rheum Dis Clin North Am 1996;22(3):623–39.
[59] Atkinson JH, et al. Prevalence, onset, and risk of psychiatric disorders in men with chronic low back pain: a controlled study. Pain 1991;45:111–21.
[60] Taenzer P, et al. Influence of psychological factors on postoperative pain, mood and analgesic requirements. Pain 1986;24(3):331–42.
[61] Ducharme J. Acute pain and pain control: state of the art. Ann Emerg Med 2000;35(6): 592–603.
[62] Dersh J, Gatchel RJ, et al. Prevalence of psychiatric disorders in patients with chronic work-related musculoskeletal pain disability. J Occup Environ Med 2002;44(5):459.
[63] Waddell G. Volvo Award in Clinical Sciences: a new clinical model for the treatment of low back pain. Spine 1987;12:632–44.
[64] Ballantyne JC, Mao J. Opioid therapy for chronic pain. N Engl J Med 2003;349:1943–53.
[65] Streltzer J. Pain management in the opioid-dependent patient. Curr Psychiatry Rep 2001;3: 489–96.

ELSEVIER
SAUNDERS

EMERGENCY
MEDICINE
CLINICS OF
NORTH AMERICA

Emerg Med Clin N Am 23 (2005) 349–365

The Drug-Seeking Patient in the Emergency Room

George R. Hansen, MD

Department of Emergency Medicine, Sierra Vista Regional Medical Center, 1010 Murray Avenue, San Luis Obispo, CA 93405, USA

It has been estimated that an emergency department with 75,000 patients per year can expect up to 262 monthly visits from fabricating drug-seeking patients. Distinguishing drug seekers from patients who have a legitimate therapeutic need is not always possible in the acute care setting, yet physicians have the dual obligation to relieve pain and to protect susceptible patients from the consequences of abusing or becoming addicted to drugs [1]. Problems associated with frequent opioid use—for either recreational abuse or for pain control—make it imperative that physicians understand and appropriately manage patients who request psychoactive drugs.

In this article, the psychoactive properties of opioids, abuse, addiction, and pseudoaddiction are discussed, and various strategies for managing them are reviewed.

Psychoactive properties of opioids

The role of opioid medications in the treatment of pain, along with their physiologic and psychosocial limitations, is discussed in detail in other articles in this issue. Opioids, particularly mu-receptor agonists, produce psychological effects that cannot be separated from their analgesic properties. There are more mu-receptors in the brain than in the spinal cord, reflecting the role they play in the psychological aspects of pain and pain-control [2]. Euphoria and reward produced by mu-agonists and other addictive drugs are mediated through the stimulation of dopaminergic neurons in the ventral tegmental area in the midbrain. Experimental animals will rapidly learn to press a lever to inject morphine into this area [3], or electrically self-stimulate it to the point of ignoring their needs for food and water [4]. The reward and reinforcement properties of opioids persist even in the presence of analgesic tolerance, which is mediated through different parts of the central nervous system [5].

E-mail address: cingemanor@aol.com

doi:10.1016/j.emc.2004.12.006 **emed.theclinics.com**

When taken by normal patients at analgesic doses, opioids produce a change in mood and feeling typically described as decreased anxiety, drowsiness, and a sense of tranquility [6]. They "dull general discomfort" [7], or produce "a feeling of detachment from the responsibilities of the world" [8], even when they are not effective at relieving pain. Former addict volunteers usually report an elevation in mood and self-esteem. When taken intravenously (IV), some liken the opioid "rush" to sexual orgasm [6].

Prescription strength opioids are highly sought as drugs of abuse. The street value of prescription narcotics is greater than marijuana and heroin, and second only to cocaine [9]. The Drug Enforcement Administration (DEA) estimates that a third of illegal drug traffic is in the form of diverted prescriptions [10]. In drug treatment facilities, the principal drug abused is a prescription drug 9.4% of the time; the vast majority of these are obtained legally by prescription [11]. More than half of the patients who sought treatment or died of drug-related medical problems were abusing prescription drugs [12]. Short-acting, rapid-onset drugs produce a greater rush or "high," and therefore have a greater tendency to be abused [13,14]. Not all patients get high after taking moderate doses of opioids. A placebo-controlled study in which healthy volunteers were given moderate doses of various mu-receptor agonists revealed that equal numbers of subjects report disliking the effects as liking them [15]. Nonetheless, half the population does feel some degree of euphoria, and predisposed individuals will abuse opioids if given the opportunity.

Self-reinforcing properties of opioids

In addition to producing pleasant sensations or euphoria in many patients, opioids are intrinsically self-reinforcing. When the drug is paired with actions or other stimuli, it produces rapid and entrenched learning or conditioning. Repeated drug administration may produce permanent changes in the ventral tegmental area of the midbrain [4]. Furthermore, opioids reinforce behavior that leads to their administration [16], and can diminish other unrelated behaviors that have been learned or reinforced previously [17]. When opioids are given in response to the patient's complaint of pain, this self-reinforcing property may induce the patient to take the medication again, even if the patient's pain responds poorly to opioids, or even in the presence of adverse consequences [7].

Reinforcement is rarely a problem in patients who have acute pain or cancer [18], but may be more prominent among chronic nonmalignant pain patients [19]. When used for chronic pain, opioids can reinforce behavior that leads to their administration, while failing to reinforce behaviors that are supposed to decrease pain or improve function [20]. Moreover, when opioid use is made contingent on the experience of pain, opioids may reinforce the perception of pain at a level high enough to justify their use [21]. This has been observed in many patients whose pain is actually maintained by opioids [22], leading to a lifestyle that is "opioid centered" in addition to being pain centered [20]. Rapid-onset opioids, paired with the experience of pain, are greater reinforcers for pain and medication-taking than are slow-onset medications, and are more likely to increase the patient's perception of pain [21].

Abuse

The American Medical Association's Council of Scientific Affairs Panel on Alcoholism and Drug Abuse Task Force defines substance abuse as "use of a psychoactive substance in a manner detrimental to individual or society, but not meeting criteria for substance or drug dependence" [23]. This definition can be expanded to include use of an opioid for recreational purposes or for reasons other than pain control, whether or not the patient has a painful condition. Predisposing factors include chronic disease (possibly including chronic pain), an unhealthy lifestyle, lack of social support, and depression [24].

Drug abusers may insist on specific medications, claiming no other medications work [9], or may claim to be allergic to all pain medications except their drug of choice [25]. A preoccupation with opioids during the visit also tends to be associated with abuse [26]. Abusers may engage in various scams, such as faking kidney stones, to obtain narcotics [27]. Abusers tend to be younger. One study [28] reported that patients over age 65 were 10 times less likely to abuse drugs than those aged 18 to 44. In a study of drug-seeking patients that presented to an emergency room [11], the mean age was 34.3 years. These patients also averaged 12.6 visits per year, presenting to an average of 4.1 different hospitals, and used an average of 2.2 different aliases.

The prevalence of substance abuse among the general population in the United States is 6.1% in people aged 12 and older, and 9.9% among those 12 to 17 years old [29]; 9.3 million people used opioids nonmedically in 1999, including 1.6 million people who used them for the first time. This was increased from 500,000 in the 1980s [30]. Another study [31] found that 1.6% of the general population abuses pain medications.

The true prevalence of drug abuse among patients who complain of pain is difficult to determine, owing to problems distinguishing those who purely seek pain relief from those who seek the psychological effects [9]. In studies of chronic pain patients, the prevalence of abuse ranges from 2% [32] to 41% [33]. Much of the variation results from differences in the populations being studied, how abuse is defined, and at what point in time the researchers were looking for it. It has been shown that abusers tend to leave pain management programs early, and thus may not show up in reports of the prevalence of abuse in chronic pain patients [34].

The controversy over opioid abuse by chronic pain patients has been complicated further through inappropriate comparisons with acute pain and cancer patients [35], whose use is less likely to be problematic. Acute pain is more responsive to treatment with opioids than is chronic pain, and it generally lacks chronic pain's complex psychological and social issues, as noted in other articles in this issue. Cancer patients tend to be older, and older patients are less likely to abuse drugs [11,36,37]. Cancer patients also show little dose escalation (even when not explicitly prohibited) compared with patients who have nonmalignant pain [38]. Consequently, observations about low levels of narcotic abuse in acute pain or cancer patients cannot be applied to chronic nonmalignant pain patients.

Problematic use and dose escalation have been attributed to under-treated or increasing pain [18,39–43]; however, alcohol abuse has been found in up to 40.5% of chronic pain patients [44]. This, along with the known prevalence of drug abuse among non-pain patients, suggests that it is highly likely that a significant number of chronic pain patients abuse their medications, probably at a rate at least as high as the general population.

Screening for abuse

Screening for a history or predisposition for substance abuse is difficult even when the clinician has a large amount of time and resources to gather information [26]. Substance abusers present with complaints of pain, but there is no way to test for or confirm its presence or severity. Self-reporting of pain has been advocated as the only way to validate and determine a patient's pain level [45]; however, if you rely solely on self-report, you cannot distinguish those who have real pain from those who are lying or exaggerating to obtain opioids for psychological or recreational purposes. As noted previously with the operant conditioning of pain behavior and perception, giving opioids (particularly rapid-onset opioids) in response to patients' self-reports of pain can result in some patients exaggerating their complaints, and possibly worsen their perception of their pain [46].

Self-report of the amount of medication used has been found to be inaccurate. In an inpatient pain treatment program, chronic pain patients were found to be using 1.85 times more medication than their self-reported use. The discrepancy between self-reported and actual use was found to be substantially less for patients over 55 [36]. At a pain clinic in which patients were screened and selected for having no history of abuse (and were chosen as good candidates for long-term treatment by both the primary physician and a psychiatrist), 27% consistently took much more than prescribed [47]. Patients have been noted to have a greater tendency to overuse short-acting opioids [48].

A prior history of drug or alcohol abuse helps to identify patients at risk for the problematic use of opioids, but a lack of a history of abuse does not reliably exclude them [26,34]. Substance abusers tend not to be forthcoming about their histories. In a study of 244 consecutive chronic pain patients presenting to a pain clinic [49], 8.8% were proven to have lied about illicit drug use. In the emergency room, 90% of the patients who abuse opioids deny it [28].

Problems caused by drug abuse

There are many problems associated with the abuse of opioids, including those obtained by prescription. More than half of the patients who sought treatment for or died of drug-related medical problems in 1989 were abusing prescription drugs [12]. There are case reports of chronic pain patients biting and swallowing their transdermal fentanyl patches [50], including one patient who initially claimed to be medicating his pain, but later admitted to abusing the medication to get high. Despite being given a lower dose, he ultimately overdosed and died [51].

The cost of drug abuse on the American workplace was estimated at $100 billion in 1992, and is thought to be double that more recently [25]. Drug seekers account for a disproportionate share of emergency department services. One study found drug-seeking behavior (identified by the use of aliases, frequenting multiple hospitals for narcotics, and so on) in 2.3% of emergency room and urgent care patients. These patients accounted for 20% of the total visits, adding to the crowding and confusion already present in many emergency departments [11].

Recreational or psychologically motivated use of opioids, if allowed to occur with any degree of frequency, will result in physiologic dependence. There are few data that specifically address how often or frequently abuse must occur to substantially harm a patient; however, even short-term opioid infusions have been found to produce paradoxical opioid-induced pain, and longer exposures induce long-lasting adverse neuroplastic changes [52]. These are reviewed in greater detail in the article "The Psychology of Pain" by Hansen elsewhere in this issue.

Side effects, such as sedation, may interfere with the patient's quality of life. Some patients seek opioids to treat depression, anxiety, sleep disturbances, and other psychological problems, and misrepresent this to the prescribing physician [6,21]. Patients may then develop tolerance to the psychological effects they were seeking, increase the dose, and incur greater dependence.

For people who desire opioids for their psychological effects, pain is a socially acceptable stimulus that allows their use [8]. This may lead them to manipulate others in order to convince them that they are in pain, and they may adversely change their lifestyles for this purpose.

In those patients who have a real chronic pain condition and also abuse opioids for psychological or recreational purposes, it is important to note that opioid tolerance can increase chronic pain [52]. Most chronic pain problems will not improve significantly while the patient is actively abusing alcohol or illicit drugs [38,53]. Opioids have very little analgesic benefit for many chronic pain patients, and what little benefit they have gets lost due to tolerance, making the patients' condition worse. This also is reviewed in greater detail in the article "The Psychology of Pain" by Hansen.

There are liability issues regarding the unrestricted and poorly managed prescription of opioids. A physician in Massachusetts was found liable for being lenient and refilling an opioid prescription despite the patient having a contract that prohibited it. The patient had a known history of non-compliance, and overdosed [54].

It is important to consider that overt drug abuse for recreational purposes represents only one end of the spectrum. Although overt recreational abuse of opioids can lead to problems for the patient and should be discouraged, recreational drug abusers represent a relatively small percentage of the population. The greatest problem lies with those chronic pain patients who take opioids for their psychological effects. The intrinsically self-reinforcing aspect of opioids and the associated physiologic dependence contribute to their compulsive use, even when they provide little pain relief, and can result in worsening pain.

The meperidine problem

Meperidine, an opioid mu-receptor agonist, possesses the worst attributes of opioids. Parenteral meperidine has an onset within minutes of injection, but produces clinical analgesia for only 2 to 3 hours. This is not improved by giving it intramuscularly, but only made less predictable. It has a toxic metabolite, normeperidine, which causes central nervous system (CNS) excitation and seizures, and lasts 15 to 30 hours [55]. Like other rapid-onset opioid medications, when meperidine is paired with the complaint of pain, it reinforces pain and drug taking, and may consequently result in an increased perception of pain [21].

Meperidine has been shown to be the most "intoxicating" of the opioids, with the largest mean peak ratings of feeling "high," "floating," "confused," "drunk," "coasting," or "difficulty concentrating." It produced 67% more drug high than morphine at equivalent doses. Meperidine also produced more nausea [15]. Parenteral meperidine has been studied in hospitalized patients. One patient developed a mild degree of dependence after 21 doses of 75 mg over 16 days, and demonstrated craving on discontinuation. Another developed psychological dependence after just 4 doses of 100 mg [56].

Despite these limitations, meperidine is frequently given by physicians, and is very popular with many patients, presumably for its tendency to make them feel high; however, some nonopioid medications have been found to be as good or better for pain relief in migraine headaches [57,58], renal colic [59], and chronic pain [60].

There have been many studies comparing meperidine to morphine. Meperidine has not been found to be better for biliary or ureteral spasm—both drugs mildly increase biliary spasm, and there is no clinically significant difference between them [61]. Morphine has been shown to provide as good or better analgesia in a variety of other conditions [62–65]. In general, morphine is a better agent for most situations in emergency medicine that require a parenteral opioid analgesic [61]. In "idiopathic pain," however, there was only a minimal reduction in pain (compared with placebo) with either 20 mg morphine or 100 mg meperidine given intravenously [66].

Drug-seeking behavior and abuse can be reduced significantly if physicians limit the use of meperidine to special circumstances. Some facilities, such as Cedars-Sinai Medical Center in Los Angeles, prohibit the use of meperidine for any reason other than amphotericin-induced rigors or for documented intolerance to alternative narcotics [67]; however, despite the analgesic equivalence between meperidine and morphine, and the CNS side effects associated with meperidine, meperidine has been given to 60% of acute pain patients, and to 20% of chronic pain patients [57].

For those patients who cannot tolerate morphine but still require a parenteral mu-agonist opioid, methadone is an effective alternative [68].

Addiction

The tendency for opioids to cause addiction is well known. At the beginning of the 20th century, 1% of the population was addicted to opioids, leading opioids to be made controlled substances in 1914 [69]. Currently, addictive disorders affect 6% to 17% of the general population [70].

Opioid addiction has been defined as persistent dysfunctional opioid use with adverse consequences, or loss of control, or preoccupation, despite adequate analgesia [70]. The presence of physiologic dependence and tolerance, which are inherent in the long term use of opioids, do not necessarily mean that the patient is addicted [21,71]. They may be contributing factors, but are not required for a person to exhibit compulsive use or abuse of a drug. Physiologic dependence, tolerance, and withdrawal are discussed in detail in the chapter "Management of Chronic Pain in the Acute Care Setting" by Hansen elsewhere in this issue.

Psychological dependence, defined as an emotional craving for the positive effects of substance or to avoid negative effects, may be present without the presence of physiologic dependence [23]. It is associated with compulsive drug-seeking behavior leading to overwhelming involvement in drug use and to obtaining drugs [72]. Psychological dependence on kappa agonists has been observed, even though there are no physical withdrawal symptoms [73].

The signs of addiction overlap with those of abuse. They differ in that addiction involves persistent compulsive use, whereas abuse may be defined as the use of drugs for recreational or psychological purposes for which they were not intended. Addiction may arise from either abuse or from poorly managed medical use. In the latter instance, the prescribing physician is at least partially responsible.

Addiction in chronic pain patients

There is considerable controversy surrounding the issue of addiction in chronic pain patients. Behaviors associated with addiction include an inability to restrict medications or take them on an agreed-upon schedule, taking multiple medications together, doctor shopping, isolation from friends and family, the use of nonprescribed psychoactive drugs in addition to prescribed medications, inability to recognize psychosocial and psychological aspects of chronic pain, noncompliance with recommended non-opioid treatments or evaluations, a preoccupation with opioids, insistence on rapid-onset formulations and routes of administration, and reports of allergy or no relief whatsoever by any nonopioid treatments [13,21,74]. The frequent loss of prescriptions, concurrent abuse of other drugs, forgery, and selling, stealing, or getting drugs from the street are more strongly indicative of addiction [38].

Addiction is associated with loss of control or overwhelming involvement in obtaining opioids; however, mild psychological dependence may be present without evidence of overwhelming involvement. Because of the risk of psychological dependence, some authors recommend against the use of opioids for chronic pain, particularly parenteral opioids [75].

The presence of absence of tolerance does not reliably distinguish addicts from nonaddicted chronic opioid users. Patients may require moderate increases in dose as a normal result of tolerance. On the other hand, addiction can be present even when the dose has stabilized. Heroine addicts and experimental animals that self-administer narcotics ultimately reach a stable dose [19], similar to alcoholics who reach a stable intake level.

Rapid dose escalation, however, does imply addiction. Tolerance to the euphoric side effects of opioids develops faster than tolerance to the analgesic effects. Consequently, rapidly developing tolerance suggests that the patient is primarily seeking the drug's psychological effects [53].

Dose escalations have been attributed to worsening of the underlying condition or complications of the disease [42]; however, most of the patients in the study were taking codeine. Even at high doses, true analgesia from codeine is so poor that by itself it would not be an inducement for dose escalation [76]. Moreover, most forms of chronic pain have no objective evidence by which one can attribute worsening of the condition.

Because of confusion about the definition of opioid addiction in chronic pain patients, and the difficulty in distinguishing those who seek opioids for recreational or psychological purposes from those who are purely trying to relieve pain, it is difficult to determine the true prevalence of addiction among chronic pain patients. The prevalence of "psychological dependence and compulsive use" of substances by chronic pain patients has been found to be 3.2% to 16.5% [72]. The risk of addiction should be much lower for patients taking slow-onset, long-acting forms of opioids, but even among a group of patients taking sustained-release morphine, up to 120 mg/day,

4.3% reported craving [77]. The risk of addiction approaches 50% in chronic pain patients in patients who have contact with the "street culture," and who are actively abusing illicit drugs, are not in a recovery program, and have poor social support [78].

One report states that addiction is rare in patients treated with narcotics [79]; however, this was in fact only a brief follow-up report of a proposed surveillance system for adverse drug reactions [80], in which hospitalized patients received as little as a single dose, and no information was provided as to how they defined or identified addicts. Moreover, it is inconsistent with studies of true addicts, whose first exposure to opioids was medical use in 9% to 27% of cases [21]. It furthermore fails to address the chronic use of opioids for nonmalignant pain.

Because of the small but significant prevalence of true addiction among chronic pain patients, it is important to consider a dual diagnosis of chronic pain and addiction when patients demonstrate a preoccupation with opioid medications [20].

Screening for addiction

Screening for addiction is no easier than screening for abuse. One study found that the best predictor for "problematic use" is admission by the patient. Determining that the patient has an addictive disorder generally requires information from the personal physician and the family [70].

Problems with addiction

Addiction has serious consequences for both drug abusers and chronic pain patients. Even subtle addiction or psychological dependency may result in persistent sedation or intoxication due to overuse, functional impairment, irritability, apathy, anxiety, depression, and adverse legal, economic, and social consequences [74]. An example of this can be seen in the $5.2 billion class-action lawsuit filed against Perdue Pharma for pushing OxyContin, which caused addiction in some patients when used "exactly as their doctors prescribed it." One of the plaintiffs is a patient who abandoned her children "in the haze of her Oxy addiction" [81].

Other problems have been demonstrated in heroin addicts. They have been found to have a proneness to overreact, and be overly concerned about personal comfort, which improves with abstinence [82]. Their pain tolerance has been found to be lower than normal, as demonstrated by cold pressor tolerance [83]. Their pain threshold and tolerance remain abnormal even when they are maintained on methadone [84]. When addicts are in withdrawal, they suffer from hypochondriasis, depression, and lethargy [82].

It has been found that pain cannot be adequately managed, and may be made worse, when complicated by addictive disease [70]. On the other hand, treating opioid addiction in chronic pain patients has been shown to improve pain and well-being in the majority of patients, and they can return to work. Psychiatric illness cannot be treated until substance use is under control [85].

The problems with opioid addiction are worse with short-acting drugs, similar to the problem with abuse. These problems may resolve when the patient is switched to a long-acting drug [10].

There is a high relapse rate for patients that have been addicted [4,86]. It has been found that even a small quantity of drug similar to what they were abusing produces craving and relapse, even after 2 years of abstinence [86]. Consequently, caution should be used in prescribing small doses or weak opioids, or even agonist-antagonists, in patients who have been addicted to opioids in the past.

Patients and their families have blamed emergency physicians for their addiction, because they give them opioids every time they present [87]. There is concern that, since the Joint Commission on the Accreditation of Health care Organizations (JCAHO) has begun including checks on pain management for accreditation, physicians have become more liberal in their opioid prescription practices, resulting in an increase in the prevalence of addiction [25].

It is important to consider that overt addiction, like abuse, represents only a small part of the spectrum of problematic use. Many more patients have subtle psychological dependence that is not obvious to the physician or even to the patient. Although addiction and abuse are problems in themselves, the greatest threats to most patients are opioids' adverse effects on psychosocial function and pain control.

Pseudoaddiction

The term "pseudoaddiction" has been used to describe behavior similar to addiction that results from poorly managed pain. Pseudoaddicted patients may be overly focused on obtaining medications, "clock-watch," and appear to be drug-seeking. They may be deceptive and even use illicit drugs [74]. The natural progression of pseudoaddiction may include escalating analgesic demands associated with behavioral changes to convince others of the pain's severity [88].

It can be nearly impossible to distinguish pseudoaddiction from true addiction, particularly in the acute care setting. True addiction is probably present if the patient's function is deteriorating or if he is injecting oral formulations of narcotics [53]. Problematic use of poor analgesics such as codeine or propoxyphene probably represents addiction, because their psychological effects provide a far greater inducement for their use than their analgesic effects.

In pseudoaddicts, drug-seeking behaviors resolve when pain is effectively treated [74]. Pseudoaddicts demonstrate an improved level of function with appropriately managed opioids [21], particularly if they are switched to adequate doses of long-acting opioids [53].

The prevalence of pseudoaddiction among drug-seeking patients is not known. It is important to note that this concept was developed based on the behavior of a single cancer patient who was being under-treated with parenteral opioids [34]. For the acute care physician, it is important to understand that some patients who manifest drug-seeking behavior might actually be pseudoaddicts whose behavior may improve with better management of their pain; however, these patients need appropriate multidisciplinary care for their pain as much or more than any other pain patients. Prescribing higher doses of short-acting or injectable opioids may not only fail to help them, but may contribute to a true narcotic problem in addition to their poorly managed pain.

Managing drug-seeking patients in the acute care setting

Patients at risk for problems with opioids

Patients at risk for problems with opioids include anyone who frequently uses the emergency department or urgent care clinic to obtain opioids, whether it is for abuse or because his pain is not being appropriately managed as an outpatient. This is particularly important for patients who have psychosocial dysfunction. Some physicians believe it is better to give these patients the benefit of the doubt, and prefer to administer opioids to possible recreational drug abusers so as to avoid the risk of withholding them from patients who have legitimate pain [1]; however, physicians are also responsible for protecting patients from complications that arise from inappropriate or poorly managed opioid use [53,89].

Distinguishing patients as being either "legitimate" or "drug-seeking" is valuable only if the distinction is used to guide appropriate treatment. In designating patients as being legitimate, physicians should be careful not to imply that the emergency department is where they should be getting their treatment. Rather, they should reinforce that these patients are best served by having their pain managed comprehensively as outpatients [89].

True drug abusers and addicts should also be identified so that they might be given the help that they need. Studies have shown that although up to 27% of emergency room patients need drug or alcohol treatment, the problem is documented in only 1% [31]. The emergency department is in fact an excellent setting for the identification and referral of drug and alcohol abuse. The patient is already in a medical setting, and does not need to muster the additional motivation to seek help. The patient may also have had a drug-related accident, or be in some form of crisis involving use or supply, at which time he is most likely to consider change [90].

Habitual patient files

Some physicians will not prescribe an opioid until records from previous physicians are obtained and reviewed [53]. Such records are not always available, or they may be incomplete. An alternative is to keep a habitual patient file. Such files are allowed under the Health Insurance Portability and Accountability Act of 1996 (HIPPA), by the JCAHO, and by various state regulations, such as the Confidentiality of Medical Information Act in California. Patients should be selected in an appropriate and systematic manner. Information should be limited to what is necessary for the diagnosis or treatment of the patient, and should not contain any wording that is judgmental, demeaning or discriminating [1].

Management strategies

The treatment of drug addiction is beyond the scope of this article; however, various strategies are available to identify patients at risk for complications of frequent opioid use, and to improve their care. Some emergency departments use "narcotic contracts" or pain management letters that refuse narcotics to selected frequent users unless they have a detailed letter from their personal physician. One facility reports a tracking and management system for patients who request narcotics frequently. In this system, a "care manager" helps direct patients who have drug problems toward treatment programs, while assisting the department in providing optimal care for those who are therapeutic users. Systems such as these can help legitimate pain patients access optimal pain management, direct drug abusers and addicts to appropriate therapy, and improve emergency department use and staff morale [91].

A study was done [92] that identified frequent users of the emergency department, in an attempt to encourage them to use community services, where they can be managed more effectively. Denying a narcotic prescription in the emergency room, restricting prescriptions to one pharmacy, and supportive and addiction counseling for certain patients resulted in a 72% decrease in the use of the emergency department by the frequent users overall, from 26.5 visits to 6.5 visits per patient per year, with no increased use of other local hospitals.

Compassionate refusal

Some patients demand opioids when they are not appropriate. In such cases, the physician should express compassion for their condition while explaining that opioids, particularly those that are short-acting and rapid-onset, may do more harm than good for their long-term pain control. If they persist in their demands, the physician may "turn the tables." While expressing appropriate concern for their pain, the physician should review with them again that they are requesting a form of medication that may be harmful to them, and that there is a need to discuss issues of physiological and psychological dependence [9]. Many patients, particularly those who present with the expectation that they will be given an opioid, are highly resistant to any other recommendations. These expectations are not likely to change until multiple physicians have denied them narcotics.

If the physician decides to give an opioid for the patient's pain, methadone and long-acting morphine are considered good choices, and are less likely to reinforce drug-seeking behavior [93]. These drugs are particularly useful for patients who complain of pain and may be at risk for opioid withdrawal if they are not given an opioid. When prescribing methadone, documenting that it is being used for treating pain will avoid issues surrounding the treatment of addiction.

Summary

Drug-seeking patients include recreational drug abusers, addicts whose dependence occurred through abuse or the injudicious prescription of narcotics, and pseudoaddicts who have chronic pain that has not been appropriately managed. Opioids produce euphoria in some patients, providing the motivation for abuse, which can be detrimental even with occasional use. Even in the absence of overt euphoria, opioids are highly self-reinforcing and can be problematic in a large number of patients, requiring that acute care physicians exercise caution in whom they are administered. Habitual patient files, narcotic contracts, pain management letters, and patient tracking and management programs can be used for the benefit of both drug seeking-patients and chronic pain patients. For many patients, drug-seekers and chronic pain patients alike, withholding opioids may be an important part of their long-term management. For others, long-acting opioids such as long-acting morphine or methadone are a reasonable option.

References

[1] Geiderman JM. Keeping lists and naming names: habitual patient files for suspected nontherapeutic drug-seeking patients. Ann Emerg Med 2003;42:873–81.

[2] Ferrante FM. Principles of opioid pharmacotherapy: practical implications of basic mechanisms. J Pain Symptom Manage 1996;11(5):265–73.

[3] Bozarth MA, Wise RA. Anatomically distinct opiate receptor fields mediate reward and physical dependence. Science 1984;224(4648):516–7.

[4] McLellan AT, et al. Drug dependence, a chronic medical illness: implications for treatment, insurance, and outcomes evaluation. JAMA 2000;284(13):1689–95.

[5] Compton MA. Cold pressor pain tolerance in opiate and cocaine abusers: correlates of drug type and use status. J Pain Symptom Manage 1994;9(7):462–73.

[6] Jaffe J. Opiates: clinical aspects. In: Lowinson J, Ruiz P, Millman R, editors. Substance abuse: a comprehensive text. Baltimore (MD): Williams and Wilkens; 1997. p. 158–66.

[7] Taylor CB, et al. The effects of detoxification, relaxation, and brief supportive therapy on chronic pain. Pain 1980;8:319–29.

[8] Black RG. The chronic pain syndrome. Surg Clin North Am 1975;55:999–1012.

[9] Parran T. Prescription drug abuse. A question of balance. Med Clin North Am 1997;81(4): 967–78.

[10] Jetter A. The end of pain. Hippocrates 1996;Sep:43–8.
[11] Zednich AD, Hedges JR. Community-wide emergency department visits by patients suspected of drug-seeking behavior. Acad Emerg Med 1996;3(4):312–7.
[12] Wilford BB. Abuse of prescription drugs. West J Med 1990;152:609–12.
[13] Savage SR. Opioid use in the management of chronic pain. Med Clin North Am 1999;83(3): 761–86.
[14] Fishman SM, Wilsey B, et al. Adherence monitoring and drug surveillance in chronic opioid therapy. J Pain Symptom Manage 2000;20(4):293–307.
[15] Walker DJ, Zacny JP. Subjective, psychomotor, and physiological effects of cumulative doses of opioid mu agonists in heathy volunteers. J Pharmacol Exp Ther 1999;289(3): 1454–64.
[16] Brodner RA. Chronic pain exacerbated by long-term narcotic use in patients with nonmalignant disease: clinical syndrome and treatment. Mt Sinai J Med 1978;45(2): 233–7.
[17] McMillan DE. Effect of narcotic and narcotic antagonists on operant behavior. Adv Biochem Psychopharmacol 1974;8:345.
[18] Melzack R. The tragedy of needless pain. Sci Am 1990;262(2):19–25.
[19] Streltzer J. Chronic pain and addiction. In: Leigh H, editor. Consultation-liaison psychiatry: 1990 and beyond. New York: Plenum Press; 1994. p. 43–51.
[20] Schofferman J. Long-term use of opioid analgesics for the treatment of chronic pain of nonmalignant origin. J Pain Symptom Manage 1993;8(5):279–88.
[21] Savage SR. Long-term opioid therapy: assessment of consequences and risks. J Pain Symptom Manage 1996;11(5):274–86.
[22] Sternbach RA. Mastering pain. A twelve-step program for coping with chronic pain. New York: G.P. Putnam's Sons; 1987.
[23] Rinaldi RC, et al. Clarification and standardization of substance abuse terminology. JAMA 1988;259(4):555–7.
[24] Gallagher RM, et al. Chronic pain. Sources of late-life pain and risk factors for disability. Geriatrics 2000;55(9):40–4; 7.
[25] Scheck A. The burden of drugs. Emergency Medicine News 2001;23(6):38–9.
[26] Robinson RC, Gatchel RJ, et al. Screening for problematic prescription opioid use. Clin J Pain 2001;17(3):220–8.
[27] Gray CL, Kane CJ. Drug-seeking behavior in urolithiasis in the noncontrast computed tomography era: 2 cases. Urology 1999;54(4):744.
[28] Rockett IRH, Putnam SL, Jia H, et al. Assessing substance abuse treatment need: a statewide hospital emergency department study. Ann Emerg Med 2003;41(6):802–13.
[29] The National Clearinghouse for Alcohol and Drug Information. 1998 National Household Survey on Drug Abuse. Available at: http://health.org/govstudy/bkd331/default.aspx. Accessed March 9, 2005.
[30] Vastag B. Mixed message on prescription drug abuse. JAMA 2001;285(17):2183–4.
[31] D'Onofrio G. Treatment for alcohol and other drug problems: closing the gap. Ann Emerg Med 2003;41(6):814–7.
[32] Hoffmann NG, et al. Prevalence of abuse and dependency in chronic pain patients. Int J Addict 1995;30(8):919–27.
[33] Maruta T, et al. Drug abuse and dependency in patients with chronic pain. Mayo Clin Proc 1979;54:241–4.
[34] Chabal C, Erjavec MK, et al. Prescription opiate abuse in chronic pain patients: clinical criteria, incidence, and predictors. Clin J Pain 1997;13:150–5.
[35] Phillips DM. JCAHO pain management standards are unveiled. JAMA 2000;284(4):428–9.
[36] Ready LB, et al. Self-reported vs. actual use of medications in chronic pain patients. Pain 1982;12:285–94.
[37] Sharpe P, Smith G. Cannabis: time for scientific evaluation of this ancient remedy? Anesth Analg 2000;90(2):237–40.

[38] Kirsh KL, Whitcomb LA, Donaghy K, et al. Abuse and addiction issues in medically ill patients with pain: attempts at clarification of terms and empirical study. Clin J Pain 2002; 18(Suppl 4):S52–60.
[39] Brown RL, et al. Substance abuse among patients with chronic back pain. J Fam Pract 1996; 43(2):152–60.
[40] Joranson DE, et al. Trends in medical use and abuse of opioid analgesics. JAMA 2000; 283(13):1710.
[41] Zens M, et al. Long-term oral opioid therapy in patients with chronic nonmalignant pain. J Pain Symptom Manage 1992;7(2):69–77.
[42] Ytterberg SR, et al. Codeine and oxycodone use in patients with chronic rheumatic disease pain. Arthritis Rheum 1998;41:1603–12.
[43] Ducharme J. Acute pain and pain control: state of the art. Ann Emerg Med 2000;35(6): 592–603.
[44] Katon W, et al. Chronic pain: lifetime psychiatric diagnoses and family history. Am J Psychol 1985;142:1156–60.
[45] Ducharme J. Current approaches to pain control. Consultant 2001;Apr:618–23.
[46] Fordyce WE. Behavioral factors in pain. Neurosurg Clin N Am 1991;2(4):749–59.
[47] Bouckoms AJ, et al. Chronic nonmalignant pain treated with long-term oral narcotic analgesics. Ann Clin Psychiatry 1992;4:185–92.
[48] Marcus DA. Treatment of nonmalignant chronic pain. Am Fam Physician 2000;61:1331–8; 1345–6.
[49] Fishbain DA, et al. Validity of self-reported drug use in chronic pain patients. Clin J Pain 1999;15(3):184–91.
[50] Purucker M, Swann W. Potential for duragesic patch abuse. Ann Emerg Med 2000;35(3): 314.
[51] Arvanitis ML, Satonik RC. Transdermal fentanyl abuse and misuse. Am J Emerg Med 2002; 20(1):58–9.
[52] Ossipov MH, Lai J, Vanderah TW, et al. Induction of pain facilitation by sustained opioid exposure: relationship to opioid antinociceptive tolerance. Life Sci 2003;73(6):783–800.
[53] Weaver M, Schnoll S. Abuse liability in opioid therapy for pain treatment in patients with an addiction history. Clin J Pain 2002;18(Suppl 4):S61–9.
[54] Fishman SM, et al. The opioid contract in the management of chronic pain. J Pain Symptom Manage 1999;18(1):27–37.
[55] Wacker MS, Moniz CJ. Meperidine: second-line agent with first-line prescribing practices. Med Health R I 2001;84(1):10–4.
[56] Miller RR, Jick H. Clinical effects of meperidine in hospitalized medical patients. J Clin Pharmacol 1978;18:180–8.
[57] Clark RF, et al. Meperidine: therapeutic use and toxicity. J Emerg Med 1995;13(6):797–802.
[58] Harden RN, et al. The placebo effect in acute headache management: ketorolac, meperidine, and saline in the emergency department. Headache 1996;36(6):352–6.
[59] Larkin GL, et al. Efficacy of ketorolac tromethamine versus meperidine in the ED treatment of acute renal colic. Am J Emerg Med 1999;17(1):6–10.
[60] Mehl-Madrona LE. Comparison of ketorolac-chlorpromazine with meperidine-promethazine for treatment of exacerbations of chronic pain. J Am Board Fam Prac 1999;12(3): 188–94.
[61] Paris PM, Stewart R. Pain management. In: Rosen P, Barkin R, editors. Emergency medicine: concepts and clinical practice. 4th edition. St. Louis (MO): Mosby; 1998. p. 276–300.
[62] Plummer JL, et al. Morphine patient-controlled analgesia is superior to meperidine for postoperative pain. Anaesth Analg 1997;84(4):794–9.
[63] Ohqvist G, et al. A comparison between morphine, meperidine and ketobemidone in continuous intravenous infusion for postoperative relief. Acta Anaesthsiol Scand 1991; 35(1):44–8.

[64] Ordy JM. Comparisons of effects of morphine, meperidine, fentanyl, and fentanyl-droperidol. Clin Pharmacol Ther 1970;11(4):488–95.
[65] Hady S. Clinical evaluation of the most frequently used analgesics: morphine, pethidine, pentazocine, fentanyl and noramidopyrine (pyralgin). Anaesth Resusc Intensive Ther 1974; 2(1):3–40.
[66] Arner S, Meyerson BA. Lack of analgesic effect of opioids on neuropathic and idiopathic forms of pain. Pain 1988;3(1):11–23.
[67] Spiegel B. Meperidine or morphine in acute pancreatitis? Am Fam Physician 2001;64(2):219.
[68] Bowsher D. Paradoxical pain. When the metabolites of morphine are in the wrong ratio. BMJ 1993;306:473.
[69] Brown RL, et al. Chronic opioid analgesic therapy for chronic low back pain. J Am Board Fam Pract 1996;9(3):192–204.
[70] Compton P, Darakjian MA, Miotto K. Screening for addiction in patients with chronic pain and "problematic" substance use: evaluation of a pilot assessment tool. J Pain Symptom Manage 1998;16(6):355–63.
[71] Sees KL, Clark HW. Opioid use in the treatment of chronic pain: assessment of addiction. J Pain Symptom Manage 1993;8(5):257–64.
[72] Fishbain DA, et al. Drug abuse, dependence, and addiction in chronic pain patients. Clin J Pain 1992;8:77–85.
[73] Finlayson RD, et al. Substance dependence and chronic pain: profile of 50 patients treated in an alcohol and drug dependence unit. Pain 1986;26:167–74.
[74] American Academy of Pain Medicine. American Pain Society, American Society of Addiction Medicine. Consensus Statement. Definitions related to the use of opioids for the treatment of pain. Available at: http://www.painmed.org/productpub/statements/index.html. Accessed December 22, 2001.
[75] Jaffe J, Martin W. Opioid analgesics and antagonists. In: Gilman A, et al, editors. The pharmacologic basis of therapeutics. New York: Macillan; 1980. p. 491–531.
[76] De Craen AJM, Di Giulio G, et al. Analgesic efficacy and safety of paracetamol-codeine combinations versus paracetamol alone: a systematic review. BMJ 1996;313:321–5.
[77] Moulin DE, et al. Randomized trial of oral morphine for chronic non-cancer pain. Lancet 1996;347(8995):143–7.
[78] Passik SD, Weinreb HJ. Managing chronic nonmalignant pain: overcoming obstacles to the use of opioids. Adv Ther 2000;17(2):70–83.
[79] Porter J, Jick H. Addiction rare in patients treated with narcotics. N Engl J Med 1980;302(2): 123.
[80] Jick H, et al. Comprehensive drug surveillance. JAMA 1970;213(9):1455–60.
[81] Rosenberg D. Profits vs. pain relief. Does its maker push OxyContin too hard? Newsweek July 2, 2001;49.
[82] Martin WR, et al. Methadone—a reevaluation. Arch Gen Psychiatry 1973;28(2):286–95.
[83] Martin JE, Inglis J. Pain Tolerance and narcotic addiction. Br J Soc Clin Psychol 1965;4(3): 224–9.
[84] Ho A, Dole VP. Pain perception in drug-free and in methadone-maintained human ex-addicts. Proc Soc Exp Biol Med 1979;162(3):392–5.
[85] Finlayson RD, et al. Substance dependence and chronic pain: experience with treatment and follow-up results. Pain 1986;26:175–80.
[86] Sadeghi P, Zacny JP. Anesthesia is a risk factor for drug and alcohol craving and relapse in ex-abusers. Med Hypotheses 1999;53(6):490–6.
[87] MacLeod DB, Swanson R. A new approach to chronic pain in the ED. Am J Emerg Med 1996;14(3):323–6.
[88] Weissman DE, Haddox JD. Opioid pseudoaddiction—an iatrogenic syndrome. Pain 1989; 36(3):363–6.

[89] Cline DM. Management of patients with chronic pain. In: Tintinalli JE, Kelen GD, Stapczynski JS, editors. Emergency medicine, a comprehensive study guide. 5th edition. New York: McGraw-Hill; 1999. p. 274–80.
[90] Bernstein E, Bernstein JA, D'Onofrio G. Patients who abuse alcohol and other drugs: emergency department identification, intervention, and referral. In: Tintinalli JE, Kelen GD, Stapczynski JS, editors. Emergency medicine, a comprehensive study guide. 5th edition. New York: McGraw-Hill; 1999. p. 1938–43.
[91] Do you give poor care to patients in pain? ED Manag 2003;June:65–7.
[92] Pope D, et al. Frequent users of the emergency department: a program to improve care and reduce visits. Can Med Assoc J 2000;162(7):1017–20.
[93] Murphy TM. Chronic opioids for chronic low back pain—solution or problem? J Am Board Fam Pract 1996;9(3):225–7.

EMERGENCY MEDICINE CLINICS OF NORTH AMERICA

Emerg Med Clin N Am 23 (2005) 367–392

Painful Dilemmas: An Evidence-based Look at Challenging Clinical Scenarios

Derek R. Linklater, MD[a,b,*], Laurie Pemberton, DO[b], Steve Taylor, DO[c], Wesley Zeger, DO[c,d]

[a]*College of Medicine, Texas A & M University, College Station, TX 77843, USA*
[b]*Emergency Medicine Residency Program, Darnall Army Community Hospital, 36000 Darnall Loop, Fort Hood, TX 76544, USA*
[c]*Department of Emergency Medicine, Madigan Army Medical Center-University of Washington, Tacoma, WA 98431, USA*
[d]*Department of Emergency Medicine, University of Nebraska Medical Center, Omaha, NE 68198, USA*

Emergency medicine practitioners experience a wide variety of patient-care experiences, and although some of these cases are quite straightforward, it is common to encounter challenging cases that present therapeutic dilemmas. Our practice is replete with examples of cases requiring difficult medical judgments such as: "Should I give analgesics to a patient who has abdominal pain?"; "What is the best pharmaceutical treatment for a patient who has migraine headaches?"; and "Which drug regimen will maximize relief for a patient who has acute low back pain while minimizing side-effects?". These difficult clinical questions are further complicated by gaps in our collective medical knowledge, pre-existing attitudes regarding pharmaceutical selection, practice habits, and entrenched medical dogma. In this article, the authors present clinical strategies and current evidence that will enable the emergency practitioner to make informed therapeutic choices during these more challenging patient encounters.

Acute low back pain

Acute and chronic musculoskeletal low back pain are frequent complaints of patients presenting to the emergency room. These patients represent a particular challenge, because most come with predefined expectations

* Corresponding author. Department of Emergency Medicine, Darnall Army Community Hospital, 36000 Darnall Loop, Fort Hood, TX 76544.
E-mail address: derek.r.linklater@us.army.mil (D.R. Linklater).

doi:10.1016/j.emc.2004.12.007

regarding their emergency department visit. Although many of these expectations are appropriate (eg, respectful treatment, pain relief, and reassurance), patients occasionally present emergency practitioners with unrealistic presumptions regarding the course of their care. It is for this reason that knowledge of the natural history of low back pain and an understanding of the available therapeutic options can be invaluable in the care of these patients. In this section, the authors focus on low back pain that is not attributable to recognizable pathology, such as infections, fractures and tumors; or due to acute medical and surgical conditions, such as pancreatitis, pyelonephritis, or abdominal aortic aneurysm. We briefly outline the available treatment options and undertake to provide an evidence basis regarding their use. Finally, we provide a review of our current recommendations based on the available medical literature.

Natural history of acute low back pain

Back pain is extremely common in developed counties, with a lifetime incidence of 60% to 80% [1]. Low back pain represents a high dollar loss to society in terms of work absenteeism [2], medical expenses, and disability payments [3]. Despite the implication of these social trends, it is essential for emergency practitioners to begin their evaluation of patients who have low back pain secure in the knowledge that it is typically a benign and self-limited disease process. Most patients will improve in 6 to 12 weeks, although many patients suffer relapses within 1 year [4,5], and approximately 5% of patients go on to develop chronic pain. This expectation of eventual wellness is crucial to impart to the patient.

Expectation management

It is often beneficial to begin the patient encounter with a brief acknowledgment to the patient that low back pain is a frustrating illness, both for patients and clinicians. Patients are often upset because they can suffer significant pain after a seemingly trivial injury, or in some cases, may not even recognize the inciting event. Their pain can linger for weeks and can severely limit or even prevent activities of daily living and the ability to function at work. Many patients have already tried over-the-counter therapies and home remedies without success, and look to the emergency practitioner for help in managing their disease.

Clinicians are typically frustrated with back pain patients because of our perceived limited armamentarium of therapeutic options; the seeming inability of some patients to improve despite therapy; the desire to avoid being manipulated (either real or imagined) by patients into prescribing "inappropriate" types, dosages, or durations of medications; and the concerns regarding potential abuse of disability and worker's compensation payment.

Some patients are inappropriately demanding, and insist that the emergency department clinician perform tests or radiographs that are not indicated. Other patients have unrealistic expectations that their pain will be "cured" in the emergency department and will never return. These patients can be extremely challenging to deal with, because if their concerns are not addressed, they may file complaints with the hospital or group, seek care from other facilities, or become visibly angry and belligerent with the emergency department staff.

Often spending extra time with these patients during the initial part of the patient encounter and taking the following steps can pre-empt these problems:

1. Providing reassurance that their pain is being taken seriously
2. Performing a directed physical examination to exclude serious causes of low back pain
3. Providing prompt attempts at acute pain relief
4. Explaining which tests are (or are not) necessary, and the reasons
5. Communicating to the patient that he has a benign illness that will likely resolve within the next few weeks
6. Advising the patient that even with the best therapy, he may have some degree of continued pain, and will very likely have recurrent pain within the next 12 months
7. Conveying the need for primary care follow-up for continued evaluation and treatment
8. Assuring the patient that he can return to the emergency department at any time if the pain requires additional analgesia

Although these humane tactics may seem trivial, they can go a long way toward realigning the patient's expectations with the likely natural history of his disease.

Drug therapy

There is wide variation in practice patterns of treatment of low back pain. Most practitioners treat back pain patients with simple analgesics (eg, acetaminophen), nonsteroidal anti-inflammatory drugs (NSAIDS) (eg, ibuprofen or aspirin), opiates (eg, hydrocodone or oxycodone), or some combination. Additional oral medications that have been reported include muscle relaxants (eg, cyclobenzaprine or diazepam) and antidepressants (eg, imipramine or trazodone). There is substantial medical literature comparing many of the above agents to each other or to placebo, but there is a wide variety in methodological quality of the studies that makes the data difficulty to interpret. A summary of evidence-based recommendations regarding drug treatment follows.

Nonsteroidal anti-inflammatory drugs, analgesics, and opiates

Multiple randomized, controlled trails (RCTs) have evaluated the effectiveness of NSAIDS in the treatment of low back pain. These trials have examined the utility of NSAIDS compared with placebo, with other analgesics, and with each other. Due to various study designs and the quality of the studies' methodology, meta-analysis of pooled data is often used when evaluating efficacy and safety. The evidence suggests that patients using NSAIDS versus placebo are more likely to experience global improvement (odds ratio [OR] 2.0, 95% confidence interval [CI] 1.4–3.0) and less likely to need additional analgesics (OR 0.64, 95% CI 0.45–0.91) [6].

Although there are statistically significant differences in effectiveness noted in multiple RCTs, it must be stated that the clinical effect of drug treatment on low back pain is often small, and thus it is still unclear how much real benefit is obtained from drug use.

There is conflicting evidence as to whether NSAIDS are more effective than either acetaminophen or a combination of opiates and muscle relaxants in the treatment of low back pain [6,7]. RCTs noted a 50% incidence of adverse effects (primarily constipation and drowsiness) with opiates, and that the combination of acetaminophen and opiates increased the risk of adverse events over acetaminophen alone (OR 2.5, 95% CI 1.5–4.2) [6]. There is strong evidence to suggest that various types of NSAIDS are equally effective for acute low back pain [6,7], and thus no recommendation can be made to choose one over another based on efficacy. The NSAIDS' cost and safety profiles should be the overriding concerns when prescribing these agents for the treatment of low back pain.

Muscle relaxants

Many health care providers use muscle relaxants as a primary or adjuvant therapy for the treatment of low back pain. In a recent survey [8], it was reported that 13% of patients treated for low back pain received cyclobenzaprine. This information is best interpreted in light of the 1994 guideline recommendation by the Agency for Health Care Policy and Research (AHCPR, now the Agency for Health care Research and Quality [AHRQ]) that muscle relaxants not be used because they were no more effective than NSAIDS and adverse effects were common [9]. In the 2002 revision to these guidelines, the agency tempers this recommendation somewhat, and lists muscle relaxants as "sometimes helpful" [10]. Multiple RCTs have shown that muscle relaxants reduced pain and muscle tension and increased mobility more than placebos [6]. A recent study [11] indicated that patients treated with cyclobenzaprine were more likely to report symptom improvement by day 14 compared with those treated with placebo (OR 4.7, 95% CI 2.7–8.1), yielding a number needed to treat of 2.7. The magnitude of this effect was small, however, and came at the expense of increasing side effects. The available evidence seems to indicate that there is a modest improvement in patients treated with these agents, but that treatment must be individualized and side effects carefully monitored.

Adjuvant therapy

Pharmaceuticals have traditionally been the first line of therapy for low back pain, but given their modest benefit and side effects, interest is growing in adjuvant and alternative therapies. These therapeutic modalities may be used as a primary mode of treatment for back pain, or may be included in a more comprehensive back pain program that emphasizes multimodal therapy in an attempt to achieve optimum results.

Activity modifications

The traditional advice given to patients who have back pain was either to employ strict bed rest or to engage in minimal activity in hopes of preventing exacerbation of their injury. Two RCTs [12,13] have found that advising patients to stay active significantly increased rates of recovery, reduced pain, and reduced disability compared with patients given no advice. Six RCTs found that advising patients to stay active reduced sick leave and long-term disability compared with patients offered traditional therapy (analgesics and advice to rest and "let pain be your guide") [6]. No trials have yet reported on harm from activity recommendations; thus the current state of medical evidence seems to indicate that practitioners should recommend staying active to their patients who have back pain.

Temperature treatments

There are scant data regarding these modalities, including ice packs, heat packs, and warm or cool baths. Two recent RCTs looked at overnight and continuous low-level heat wrap therapy for acute nonspecific low back pain [1,14]. These studies, though of low methodological quality, indicate that modest improvement in pain scores, flexibility, and overall disability may be obtained through the use of these devices compared with placebo. More significantly, however, side effects were mild and infrequent. It is unclear if heat or cold are more effective than muscle relaxants, analgesics, or NSAIDS in the treatment of low back pain, but they are inexpensive, easy to use, and, if used carefully, are unlikely to injure the patient.

Spinal manipulation

The evidence regarding the efficacy of spinal manipulation for the treatment of low back pain is contradictory. Three of five RCTs examining the utility of spinal manipulation versus placebo reported slightly more relief after 3 weeks in the actively treated group, whereas the remaining two RCTs showed no benefit [6]. When compared with treatments such as drug therapy, the results are even more conflicting. The risk of serious harm is low when using trained chiropractors or osteopaths. Based on the available evidence, however, it is difficult to actively recommend this therapy to patients. What can be done is to involve the patient as an active member in formulating a treatment plan. Asking the patient about his beliefs regarding chiropractic or osteopathic manipulation can open the door to a discussion of the risks and benefits of these therapies, and the patient may well choose to try them in an attempt to obtain relief from pain.

Review of current recommendations

Treating back pain is challenging for clinicians, because even the best treatments show only modest improvements in patient outcomes. Changing patient expectations to reflect the natural history of the disease is key to a satisfying patient encounter. Patients must not leave the emergency department with unfulfilled expectations, and must be warned that not only will improvement take weeks rather than hours or days, but that they will likely relapse within the next 12 months. Drug treatment should begin with either an NSAID or acetaminophen, and absent any information proving improved efficacy, the choice should lie in minimizing adverse side effects or in patient preference. Simply asking patients which pain medications typically work well for them can give the clinician an idea of which types of analgesics a patient prefers. Muscle relaxants may be used as an alternative or supplement to the analgesic, but care must be taken to warn the patient of possible side effects, including drowsiness, disequilibrium, and nausea. Patients should be advised that one of the most important things they can do is to stay active, and that activity is more likely to offer beneficial outcomes than any other therapy. Adjuvant therapies such as warm or cool packs or spinal manipulation may be tried; the decision to do so should rest with the patient.

Migraine headaches

Approximately 18% of women and 6% of men experience migraine headaches [15]. Migraine headaches are a common complaint for which patients seek care in emergency departments [16], and there is significant variance in the practice patterns in the treatment of this disorder [17]. Although opiates are the most commonly used option, anti-emetics are reportedly used more that 15% of the time [17]. Of the anti-emetic medications used as initial treatment for migraines, prochlorperazine and droperidol were used 80% of the time [17]. Although they are efficacious [18–20] at a relatively low cost, the recent absence of intravenous prochlorperazine from hospital formularies and the black box warning given to droperidol [21] have likely impacted providers' therapeutic regimens. The goals of this section are to review some of current therapeutic options and to discuss current guidelines for the treatment of acute migraine headaches.

Anti-emetic medications

Metoclopramide and chlorpromazine are among the best-studied anti-emetic medications used as primary therapy. There have been no controlled trials using promethazine as monotherapy. Metoclopramide is a non-phenothiazine anti-emetic, whereas chlorpromazine is a phenothiazine. Both of these medications act centrally on the serotonergic system, are dopamine antagonists, and have effects on the chemoreceptor trigger zone [22,23].

Intravenous metoclopramide (10 mg) has been compared with prochlorperazine [20], chlorpromazine [24], ibuprofen [23], and placebo [23]. It's efficacy rate (defined as no rescue therapy) has ranged from 50% to 90% [20,23,25]. Metoclopramide has been reported as being superior to placebo and ibuprofen [23], and inferior to prochlorperazine [20]. When used orally (10 mg) for acute migraine relief, metoclopramide efficacy has ranged from 30% to 56% [26,27]. It has been shown to be better than ergotamine plus caffeine [27], and as good as oral sumatriptan [26] for pain relief at 2 hours.

Intravenous chlorpromazine has been compared with dihydroergotamine (DHE) [28], meperidine plus dimenhydrinate [25], and sumatriptan [29]. Dosing is weight-based (0.1 mg/kg/dose to total of 0.3 mg/kg) [24,25] or empiric (12.5 mg/dose to total 37.5 mg) [28,29]. Significant hypotension was not observed in any of these trials [25,28–30]. Efficacy rates have ranged from 81% to 95%. It is better at alleviating symptoms than meperidine plus dimenhydrinate and DHE alone, and it performed as well as sumatriptan and metoclopramide [25].

In general, metoclopramide and chlorpromazine are similarly efficacious as primary therapy in patients who have acute migraine headaches [15]. Although there were no significant side effects associated with these drugs, both can cause dystonia or akathisia. Concurrent administration of diphenhydramine may prevent these from occurring [31]. Furthermore, all of the patients who received chlorpromazine also received intravenous fluids, and that intervention may have been why orthostatic hypotension was not prevalent.

Nonsteroidal anti-inflammatory drugs

Of all the NSAIDS, ketorolac has been studied the most. Ibuprofen has been compared with metoclopramide (above), and performed similarly to placebo [23]. NSAIDS are thought to inhibit the migraine headaches through their anti-inflammatory properties as well as smooth muscle regulation [22]. Ketorolac has been compared with prochloperazine [32], meperidine plus promethazine [33], and nasal sumatriptan [34]. Dosing for ketorolac is 60 mg (intramuscularly) or 30 mg (intravenously). Overall efficacy was between 55% and 85%. Ketorolac did better than nasal sumatriptan, but was not as efficacious as prochlorperazine. It did appear to work as well as meperidine plus promethazine. Ketorolac (either intramuscularly or intravenously) may provide some relief to patients experiencing migraine headaches [15]. Other drugs should be considered first for monotherapy.

Ergot alkaloids

DHE is the best-studied medication in this class. An oral formulation (ergotamine tartrate plus caffeine) has been shown to be inferior to oral metoclopramide [27]. DHE is believed to work by binding to the serotonin receptors of blood vessels and inhibiting neurogenic inflammation [22]. DHE has been compared with meperidine plus promethazine [30], meperidine plus hydroxyzine [35], sumatriptan [36], and valproate [37]. Some studies combined DHE with an anti-emetic [30,35,37], whereas others used monotherapy [28,38]. Dosing is 1 mg (subcutaneously or intravenously), and may be repeated once if an adequate response is not achieved. Overall efficacy ranged from 23% to 93% [22], but it may have a slower onset of therapeutic effect [28,38]. There was no difference in relief of symptoms except when compared with chlorpromazine, where DHE was found to be inferior [28]. One of the reasons several of the trials may have combined DHE with an anti-emetic is secondary to its adverse gastrointestinal side-effect profile [28,37]. DHE may give some relief to patients who have migraine headaches, but adjunctive anti-emetic therapy is recommended [15].

Triptans

Triptans are a relatively new class of drugs that selectively target the serotonin receptor 5-hydroxytryptamine serotoin$_{1B/1D}$ (5-HT$_{1B/1D}$). Sumatriptan was the first drug in this class, and several have since followed. Sumatriptan is the only medication with both an oral and subcutaneous route of administration; other triptan drugs are only administered orally. Triptans are thought to act via three mechanisms: cranial vasoconstriction, peripheral trigeminal inhibition, and inhibition of the trigeminocervical complex [39]. Sumatriptan (6 mg) given subcutaneously has a consistent efficacy rate (defined as reduction of headache to "mild") of around 70% when compared with placebo [22,40], but this efficacy drops to 30% when efficacy is defined as "pain-free" [40]. Oral sumatriptan (50 mg or 100 mg) has an efficacy rate of 50% to 60% for reduction of headache to "mild," and efficacy of approximately 30% for a "pain-free" end point at 2 hours [39]. When compared with the other triptans in placebo-controlled trials, only rizatriptan and eletriptan performed significantly better. Rizatriptan (10 mg) and eletriptan (80 mg) had higher rates of reduction of headache to "mild" and "pain-free" at 2 hours [39]. Although the effects of these drugs were typically reported at 2 hours, the therapeutic response may reliably occur at 1 hour, making them more applicable to an emergency department setting [40].

Opiates

There is wide variation among hospitals in the prescription of opiate analgesics [16]. Of all the opiates, meperidine is the most commonly prescribed [17]. Although meperidine plus an anti-emetic has an efficacy similar to some of the migraine-abortive therapies [30,33,35], it is not superior [24]. Guidelines developed by the American Academy of Neurology (AAN) specifically recommend limiting opiate use and reserving this class of drugs as rescue medication. Some emergency department patients require frequent visits to control their chronic migraine symptoms, or may have failed multiple medication regimens. Strict adherence to the AAN guidelines for these patients may not be as appropriate.

Review of current recommendations

Current guidelines have been developed by the US Headache Consortium and are endorsed by the American College of Emergency Physicians [41]. These guidelines recommend triptan-class drugs as initial therapy for acute migraine headaches. The strength of these recommendations is based on the larger studies that yielded consistent results [15,41]; however, most of these trials have been conducted in the outpatient setting, with end points at 2 hours. Although a smaller number of patients have been studied, chlorpromazine has been shown to have equal efficacy in a number of studies, and may be considered an alternative first-line agent in the relief of acute migraine headaches, especially in the absence of prochloperazine availability and in view of the "black box warning" placed upon droperidol [15,21]. DHE and ketorolac may also have a role, but their improved efficacy rates were observed when primary end points were recorded at longer time intervals; metoclopramide may be a better option given its proven efficacy in the treatment of migraine headaches. Although opiates provide relief equivalent to the above medications for initial therapy, they should be considered as rescue therapy only. For patients frequently seeking emergency departments for opiate pain relief, these recommendations may not be as applicable.

Biliary and renal colic

Biliary colic

The axiom "Don't use morphine for biliary colic or pancreatitis because it increases pressure in the biliary tree" is one of medicine's most treasured and oft-repeated pieces of dogma. Medical students and allied health professionals are taught during their clerkships, usually by surgeons, to administer meperidine hydrochloride instead of morphine sulfate as an analgesic for patients who have pancreatitis and cholecystitis—the theory goes that morphine causes contraction of the sphincter of Oddi and may aggravate the patient's disease by diminishing biliary drainage and increasing pressure within the biliary tree. The *Washington Manual of Medical Therapeutics* [42] recommends meperidine for patients who have pancreatitis and cholecystitis because "it has no significant effect on the sphincter of Oddi." The accuracy of this concrete and specific recommendation must be questioned, however, because an extensive literature search fails to find the basis for this preference of meperidine over morphine in patients who have biliary colic. This idea of morphine being "bad" is probably based on old case reports [43] rather than any type of prospective, randomized, or placebo-controlled evidence. Human studies have shown that morphine causes increases in pressure at the sphincter of Oddi [44], but so do other opiates such as meperidine.

Radney et al [45] did a study comparing equianalgesic doses of morphine and meperidine in 40 patients undergoing cholecystectomy. These authors found that meperidine raised the common bile duct pressure 14% more than did morphine. A more recent review by Thompson [46] reported that "the sphincter of Oddi is exquisitely sensitive to all narcotics including meperidine ... " and that "No outcome-based studies have been performed ... ". There is no current clinical evidence linking morphine to increased risk over other opiates in causing or aggravating pancreatitis or cholecystitis. Morphine does, however, enjoy advantages over meperidine for patients who have all types of severe pain. A parental dose of meperidine can control pain for only 2 to 2.5 hours, whereas morphine's analgesic effect lasts for 3 to 4 hours. Meperidine also suffers the drawback of having potentially neurotoxic metabolites. Seizure risk increased significantly with prolonged, repeated administration of meperidine, due to accumulation of its metabolite normeperidine. The current state of medical evidence supports the use of morphine sulfate over meperidine hydrochloride for patients with cholecystitis or pancreatitis, regardless of what protestations dogmatists make.

Renal colic

Ureteral, commonly called renal, colic is a very common disorder, affecting up to 20% of the United States population [47]. Opiates are often given in the emergency department when these patients present in severe pain, but they are not the panacea. Opiates possess well-known side effects, including sedation, respiratory depression, nausea, hypotension, and over time, tolerance and possible addiction. NSAIDS are an alternative class of analgesics that have been used successfully in other countries to treat renal colic for over a decade [48]. Numerous studies in the United States have shown intramuscular ketorolac tromethamine, a parenteral NSAID, to be efficacious in the emergency treatment of renal colic and to cause few side effects [49,50]. More recently, studies have been published comparing ketorolac versus meperidine, and ketorolac has been shown to be more efficacious than meperidine in the treatment of renal colic [51,52].

The question of whether parenteral ketorolac is better than oral NSAIDS for the pain caused by renal colic has not yet been studied, but in the treatment of acute pain for emergency department patients, the literature demonstrates that there is no difference between intramuscular ketorolac and oral ibuprofen [53]. Additionally, evidence shows no difference between ketorolac and oral ibuprofen for acute musculoskeletal pain [54]. Although a direct comparison of oral ibuprofen versus parenteral ketorolac has not yet been performed, it can be postulated, after a review of current medical evidence, that we can expect oral ibuprofen to be as effective in the treatment of renal colic as ketorolac or meperidine. Given the significant difference in price (approximately $12 per dose for parenteral ketorolac [55] versus $0.20 per dose for ibuprofen [56]) between the two agents, we should consider using ibuprofen.

Review of current recommendations

The authors recommend the use of morphine for treating the pain of biliary colic when opioid analgesia is required to prevent patient suffering. There is no proven benefit of meperidine, and the potential for an increased incidence of side-effects makes its choice less optimal. Renal colic patients should definitely be treated with some form of prostaglandin-inhibiting pharmaceutical, such as an NSAID, and strong consideration should be given to using ibuprofen as a first-line drug. It is quite reasonable to use small, titrated doses of opiates to control severe pain in patients suffering from acute ureteral colic; NSAIDS typically take between 30 and 60 minutes to begin working, and this window of opportunity is a perfect occasion to use opiates in an attempt to smooth things out for the patient. It is recommended to discharge patients with clear return instructions, a stepped treatment plan, and a prescription for a small amount of rescue medication such as hydrocodone plus acetaminophen. Such a plan of care will minimize return visits for inadequate pain control, and may prevent unnecessary admissions for that purpose.

Sickle-cell disease

Sickle cell disease (SCD) is a common disease affecting more than 70,000 Americans [57], and is a frequent reason for emergency department visits. Pain from vaso-occlusive crises is the most common complaint among SCD patients presenting to the emergency department for care. SCD patients may be expected to have approximately one episode of pain each year [58], and these painful episodes are responsible for more than 75,000 hospitalizations annually [57]. The emergency care of these patients can be challenging because of the complex interplay of medical, social, economic, and social factors surrounding such care. Although in theory SCD may be treated in similar fashion to other painful conditions, the care of SCD patients often discomforts the emergency practitioner with concerns about opiate addiction, conscious fabrication of symptoms, and drug-seeking behavior. The care of these patients can be exceptionally difficult because of prior experiences, both the patients' and the providers', with cases that reflected inadequate treatment, therapeutic failures, differing attitudes and beliefs about pain, transference, counter-transference, and a host of other medical and psychosocial issues. There are many excellent reviews on SCD available in the medical literature, and the authors encourage readers to read some or all of them. In this section we attempt to distill some generally accepted management principles and provide insight into new therapeutic measures available for the treatment of these patients.

Care of the sickle-cell disease patient

Patients presenting to the emergency department with SCD have typically experienced several painful episodes during their lives, and have been treated by practitioners of varying levels of knowledge, experience, and skill. It is likely that they have encountered at least one, and likely several, occasions of latent or manifest hostility on the part of emergency practitioners. Medical practitioners' perceptions shape the care that they deliver. A recent paper [59] reported that a large majority (73%) of emergency physicians believe that more than 10% of SCD patients are addicted to opiates, and 44% of hematologists who the same belief. Most physicians feel a fiduciary responsibility to society to prevent expansion of opiate addiction; thus emergency practitioners are sometimes reluctant to treat patients with adequate doses of opiates. This phenomenon is extremely common in the treatment of SCD, in which many patients are viewed as exhibiting "drug-seeking behavior."

It is tempting for the emergency department practitioner to spend significant time and resources in attempting to determine if the patient is truly experiencing pain. This temptation can lead to inadequate treatment, or sometimes no treatment, in a desire to avoid "getting burned" by a patient who is not actually experiencing an acute painful crisis, but is in fact merely seeking narcotics for secondary gain. An approach more satisfying to the patient, and in keeping with generally accepted pain management principles (and new Joint Commission on the Accreditation of Hospital Organization [JCHAO] standards), is to simply accept that pain exists when the patient says it exists, and to devote maximum time to the relief of the patient's pain.

Conventional therapy

Conventional emergency department therapy in the treatment of vaso-occlusive SCD consists of the triad of oxygen, fluid resuscitation, and analgesia. Although these therapeutic interventions are commonly employed, prospective outcome-based evidence for some of them are lacking.

Oxygen

Several studies have examined the relationship of pulse oximetry and arterial blood gas analysis. One study [60] reported in 1996 that although pulse oximetry strongly correlated with oxygen saturation on ABG analysis ($r = 0.889$), it underestimated arterial oxygen saturation by 4.5%. A more recent study [61] placed this underestimation at a more conservative 1.6%. It seems clear from a review of this and similar literature that pulse oximetry can be safely used as a good estimate of arterial oxygen saturation.

Oxygen therapy in the treatment of acute vaso-occlusive crisis has been less well studied. The rationale behind oxygen therapy stems from the pathophysiology of the disease process. Erythrocytes containing abnormal hemoglobin within the context of SCD sickle under conditions of low oxygen tension. Theoretically, an increase in arterial oxygen saturation should reduce the amount of abnormal circulating erythrocytes by inducing them to de-sickle and, consequently should improve patient outcome. It must be noted, however, that some fraction of the abnormal erythrocytes are irreversibly sickled, and would not benefit from any amount of improved oxygenation. The prospective RCTs looking at this question found that in patients suffering from acute SCD pain crisis, 50% oxygen administration was associated with a significant reduction in reversibly sickled cells (RSCs), but not irreversibly sickled cells (ISCs), compared with patients who were treated with room air. This reduction in RSCs, however, was not associated with any significant change in the duration of severe pain, rates of opiate administration, or rates of hospitalization [62,63]. Although more research into this question is undoubtedly necessary, no evidence has yet been offered that administration of oxygen improves patient outcomes. Conversely, oxygen is inexpensive and readily available in almost every emergency department, and is unlikely to be harmful if given in proper doses for appropriate durations.

Intravenous fluids

Fluid therapy, typically with isotonic crystalloid, is another intervention commonly employed in the treatment of pain crises resulting from SCD. The theoretical benefit from fluid administration stems from the belief that euvolemia will help to reduce vascular sludging in the distal capillaries and may reduce pain. There are no good data available to recommend for or against fluid administration in acute sickle-cell pain crises. It must be noted, however, that patients who have SCD frequently have some degree of renal compromise because of their underlying condition, prior episodes of renal infarction, and use of medications that affect the renal axis, such as acetaminophen (potential for papillary necrosis) and NSAIDS (renal vasoconstriction). If fluids are to be given to patients who have SCD, it behooves clinicians to carefully monitor their hydration status and urinary output in order to ensure that overhydration does not complicate their therapy. Determination of serum creatinine and blood urea nitrogen (BUN) levels may be helpful in caring for patients who have SCD, and should be strongly considered.

Opiates

Opiate analgesia is indicated for the relief of pain due to SCD. One of the major pitfalls in the treatment of these patients is using inappropriate dosages or routes of administration. This can lead to suboptimal outcomes and therapeutic failures. Traditionally patients are treated with intermittent boluses of pure opiate agonists such as meperidine, morphine, and hydromorphone until pain control is achieved or an artificial threshold is reached beyond which the pain is declared refractory and admission is required. In academic emergency departments this threshold is typically two or three doses of parenteral opiates [64].

There are two problems with intermittent bolus administration: it can be challenging to administer just the right dose of medication; and when titrating dosages, it is imperative to frequently reassess the patient's need for additional pain control. Due to chronic nursing and staffing shortages in many emergency departments, patients may wait much longer than the 5 to 10 minutes recommended between reassessments when titrating opiate analgesia. Opiate titration, to be effective, must be rapid, or emergency practitioners may find themselves redosing patients after the initial medication has already been substantially cleared—unnecessary patient suffering usually ensues. Furthermore, patients who have experienced a number of such subtherapeutic dosing regimens may begin to request medications either in greater quantities or at inappropriately brief intervals, in an attempt to ensure that their pain is treated promptly and adequately; this can reinforce the inaccurate notion of drug-seeking behavior to clinicians.

Although meperidine has historically been used routinely in the care of patients who have SCD, it must be used with caution because of the potential for accumulation of the neurotoxic metabolite normeperidine. Patients who have prolonged painful conditions such as cancer-related pain or SCD are particularly at increased risk, because of the necessity of frequent and recurrent doses of meperidine during their hospitalization. A safer solution may be to substitute intravenous morphine or hydromorphone. It is reasonable to take patient preference into account when deciding on a management strategy; SCD patients usually have a history of pain crises and typically know what works best in their particular cases. If no such information from the patient is available, an initial dose of 5 to 10 mg of intravenous morphine with rapid reassessment and titration is usually a good starting point. Often the patient can assist emergency practitioners by relating the typical dosages and intervals for remedication that have been required during previous SCD pain episodes. Except in very specific circumstances, intramuscular administration of opiates to patients who have SCD is not as useful as intravenous dosing. Intramuscular administration is painful, rapid blood levels of the drug are less easily achieved, and titration to an appropriate level of pain relief is more difficult. Although it may be tempting for some practitioners to use intramuscular injection as a form of punishment for SCD patients who come to the emergency department, this practice is to be shunned.

The use of patient-controlled analgesia (PCA) pumps in the emergency department is a promising idea that offers some unique advantages over intermittent bolus injection. It allows patients to have some control over their pain relief, it decreases the need for frequent reassessments by nursing and physician staff, and it can provide a more even and steady flow of medication to the patient. The use of PCA pumps has been studied and found to be as effective as intermittent bolus injection of opiates in emergency department patients suffering from SCD [65]. Barriers to use of PCA include lack of easy availability in emergency departments, inexperience with dosage regimens among emergency department staff, unfamiliarity with the required medical equipment, and psychological resistance to embracing new practice habits. Use of PCA for treating SCD is a new twist on an old idea, and should be considered by emergency department practitioners who care for patients suffering from SCD.

Ketorolac

There is great interest among physicians who care for sickle-cell patients in reducing opiate use. One technique that is commonly employed is the use of alternative analgesics in an attempt to achieve a synergistic, or at least opiate-sparing, effect. Several small studies have examined the utility of adding intravenous or intramuscular ketorolac to various regimens of opiate treatment for acute SCD crisis. Two studies [66,67] report positive results and three [68–70] report no benefit. In counterpoint to the questionable benefit achieved with either single-dose or continuous infusions of ketorolac, a case study was published in 1999 [71] reporting irreversible renal failure in an SCD patient treated with ketorolac. Given the lack of overwhelming evidence to suggest efficacy of ketorolac in the treatment of acute painful SCD and the potential for significant renal side effects due to inhibition of vasodilatory prostaglandins, routine use is not recommended. If practitioners chose to use this drug for treatment of SCD patients, it is imperative to closely monitor renal function and to ensure pre- and post-treatment euvolemia.

Review of current recommendations

Care of patients who have acute crises due to SCD must begin with adopting the belief that these patients are truly in pain and will be honest with the emergency practitioner. Although there are undoubtedly SCD patients who will attempt to manipulate providers for secondary gain, it is inadvisable to begin therapeutic encounters with this assumption. Pharmaceuticals, predominantly opiates, should be given intravenously and in sufficient quantities to provide rapid relief of pain. Typically, the easiest way to achieve this goal is to rapidly and frequently titrate small to moderate doses of opiates until the patient feels comfortable. Patient-controlled analgesia should be considered, and may reduce nursing and physician workload if appropriate devices are readily available. Morphine should be used in place of meperidine, because of to the potential for neurotoxic metabolite accumulation, unless patients specifically state that morphine is ineffective for treating their pain. Ketorolac use is incompletely studied and cannot be routinely recommended, given the potential for adverse side-effects. Most emergency practitioners use two or three doses of parenteral opiates as their threshold for declaring the pain refractory to outpatient management, and thus requiring admission for continued care.

Corneal abrasions

Corneal abrasions are common throughout emergency departments and primary care facilities in the United States. In 1985, 2% of all patient visits to primary care offices were eye complaints; 8% were related to trauma or foreign bodies [72]. Eye injuries can also cause significant morbidity in the workplace. In 1998, Wong and associates [73] investigated the types of injuries that occurred at a major automotive corporation. They found that eye trauma comprised 6% of all injuries, and that corneal abrasions were the most common subtype at 87%.

Most corneal abrasions are small and heal spontaneously in less than 72 hours; however, one-third of eye injuries result in loss of work for at least 24 hours [74]. This loss of worker productivity has a cost measured in both sick days and wages. The goal for this section is to review some of the current pain treatment options available for corneal abrasions, in an attempt to provide strategies that will improve patient comfort and minimize morbidity.

Eye patching

Eye patching is a mechanical approach that has the potential to promote epithelial healing by applying light pressure and preventing eyelid movement. This approach has become controversial in recent years. Patients are often noncompliant with patching because of irritation or loss of depth perception and visual fields. Controlled studies have not found patching to improve outcome or comfort [75,76]. Furthermore, these studies have shown that unpatched abrasions healed faster and more comfortably than those with an eye patch [75,76]. Despite the results of these trials, eye patching is still suggested to relieve pain with abrasions that are larger than 10 mm in diameter [77].

Cycloplegics

Some of the pain associated with corneal abrasions can be attributed to pupillary constriction and ciliary spasm [78]. Thus the mainstays of treatment are topical pharmaceuticals that combat this response, such as parasympatholytics or cycloplegics. Cycloplegics work by dilation of the pupil and paralysis of the ciliary musculature. Short-acting cyclopentolate is preferred over topical scopolamine or atropine because of its shorter duration of action (36 hours versus 2 weeks) [77]. Cycloplegics, however, block accommodation, and can cause glare that may interfere with near work such as reading [77]. Patients who have relatively small, quick-healing abrasions may find that the side effects from cycloplegics are worse than the discomfort of the abrasion. The greatest benefit of cycloplegics may be in patients who have large abrasions or complaints of photophobia.

Oral opiates and topical nonsteroidal anti-inflammatory drugs

Opiates have long been the foundation of pain control in patients who have corneal abrasions. Although most corneal abrasions heal overnight without treatment, opiates help to relieve pain and suffering. Administration of opiates alleviates continued irritation, and may allow a comfortable night's sleep. The sedating side effects of opiates can, however, impair the cognitive and physical abilities required to carry out occupational responsibilities. In attempting to mitigate these potential side effects, much interest has been shown in using nonsedating alternatives such as NSAIDS to treat this painful condition.

Recent studies have evaluated the usefulness of NSAID ophthalmic solutions such as diclofenac and ketorolac in the care of patients who have corneal abrasions. A review of five blinded RCTs suggests improvements in patient's pain perceptions with administration of topical NSAIDS versus placebo [79–83]. A meta-analysis by Weaver and Terrell in 2003 [84] reviewed these same five studies, and concluded that administration of ophthalmic NSAIDS may reduce the need for sedating analgesics and appears to benefit those who cannot tolerate the sedative side-effects of opioids. Caution should be exercised in extrapolating these findings to all clinical scenarios, however. Although topical NSAIDS appear to reduce the pain of corneal abrasions compared with placebo, no trials have yet been conducted that compare the usefulness of topical NSAIDS to oral administration of NSAIDS or opiates.

Topical anesthetics

Topical anesthetics such as proparacaine and tetracaine are used by physicians during the examination of the painful eye. One or two drops of either medication renders the corneal surface insensate, allowing cooperation with a full examination that otherwise might be difficult because of pain. They are not currently recommended for repeated use, secondary to the prospect of corneal epithelium toxicity. This toxicity can result in inhibition of healing and promotion of ulceration, and carries the potential for permanent scarring [77,85].

Summary of current recommendations

Because most abrasions will spontaneously heal within 72 hours, the goal of management is to provide analgesia and comfort to the patient. This helps to prevent irritation or mechanical trauma due to eye rubbing and pressure. Systemic narcotics have long been the mainstay of therapy, and cycloplegics are recommended for large corneal abrasions. Topical NSAIDS may offer pain relief for patients who cannot tolerate the side effects of narcotics, but their use should be correlated with the expectation of clinical benefit and the experience of providers. Topical anesthetics should not be prescribed or used on long-term basis because of concerns stemming from their potential for corneal toxicity.

Acute abdominal pain

A discussion on painful dilemmas would not be complete without mention of the use of analgesics in patients who have a potential surgical abdomen. Sir Zachary Cope, in his successful and influential book, *Early Diagnosis of the Acute Abdomen* [86], set a standard in the 1920s that is still followed by many practitioners today. In his earlier editions, Cope states "though it may appear cruel, it is really kind to withhold morphine until one is certain or not that surgical interference is necessary, ie, until a reasonable diagnosis has been made." Because the book was considered a clinical reference, there was no citation or bibliography. Although this idea was not based on any documented medical evidence, physicians everywhere took Dr. Cope's opinion as their own.

Dr. William Silen, who took over for Cope and has revised the latest editions of the book, now supports the use of early analgesia; however, despite almost 20 years of studies supporting the use of early analgesia, a recent survey showed that 80% of US emergency medicine physicians still withhold opiate analgesia until a surgical assessment has been made [87]. The goal of this section is to present the studies that specifically address this issue, so that practitioners may make evidence-based decisions pertaining to their own practice.

The current state of the medical literature

The literature specifically looking at the use of early analgesics in patients who have undifferentiated abdominal pain dates back only to the 1980s. Before 1986, no prospective trials on the use of opiate analgesia in patients who have acute abdominal pain existed. Zoltie and Cust of the United Kingdom published the first trial [88]. They administered two different doses of sublingual buprenorphine (200 mcg and 400 mcg—approximately equivalent to 3.3 mg and 6.6 mg of morphine, respectively)—versus placebo in over 200 adults admitted for acute abdominal pain, and reported that the diagnosis was never altered by a change in physical signs after the administration of the opioid. The placebo group had more pain relief than the sublingual buprenorphine group, however, which renders the usefulness of these data questionable. Sublingual buprenorphine is not a popular analgesic today.

Attard and coworkers, also from the United Kingdom, published the next prospective study in 1992 [89]. In their trial, 100 consecutive patients who presented to the emergency department with acute abdominal pain of less than 48 hours duration received an injection of either intramuscular papaveretum or saline. All patients were then admitted to the hospital. Forty-seven of the 50 patients (94%) who received analgesia had at least 20% improvement in the pain score, compared with only 7 of the 50 (14%) receiving saline. The initial diagnosis and the decision to operate or observe were incorrect in 2 analgesia-treated patients and 9 saline-treated patients. Six of the patients treated with placebo had unnecessary operations. The length of hospital stay was similar in both groups, and no side effects or deaths occurred in either group.

A study by Pace and Burke, published in 1996 [90], also provides evidence that early pain relief was not associated with detrimental effects on diagnostic accuracy. These two US physicians administered morphine versus placebo to 75 patients who had acute abdominal pain and presented to the emergency department. Pain was improved in the morphine group, with no difference between groups in the accuracy of the provisional diagnosis.

In 1997, LoVecchio and colleagues [91] specifically looked at whether or not the administration of analgesia would change physical examination findings. Their study enrolled 49 adults who had acute abdominal pain and peritoneal signs. All patients had a surgical evaluation and a definitive plan before receiving either intravenous morphine or placebo. The pain was significantly improved in the group receiving morphine. Of the 32 patients receiving morphine, 16 had changes in their tenderness and localization, versus 1 of the 16 from the placebo group. The usefulness of the study is limited for emergency practitioners because these patients had a definitive treatment plan before administration of analgesics, and therefore neither changes in outcome nor time to treatment could be assessed.

In 1999 Vermeulen and associates from Switzerland [92] published a prospective, randomized, double-blind, placebo-controlled trial designed to determine the influence of early pain relief in patients who presented to the emergency department with right lower quadrant pain. The study authors specifically looked at the diagnostic performance of ultrasonography and at the appropriateness of the surgical decision when morphine was given. Three hundred and forty patients aged 16 and older were enrolled in the study. The results again showed a significant reduction in pain for those given morphine. Analgesia improved the positive predictive value, but worsened the negative predictive value of ultrasonography in those who received morphine, although the results were not statistically significant. The appropriateness to discharge patients without surgery was 100% in all groups.

In 2000, Mahadevan and Graff [93] published an RCT looking at whether administration of an analgesic to patients who had right lower quadrant pain caused greater alteration of abdominal signs predictive of appendicitis than placebo. Sixty-eight patients aged 12 and older received either tramadol or placebo. Their study concluded that the analgesic group had less normalization of signs, as measured by physical findings and proven appendicitis. There were no adverse effects or untoward patient outcomes associated with analgesic administration.

In 2002 Kim et al [94] published an RCT assessing the effects of intravenous morphine on the physical examination in pediatric patients aged 5 to 18. In this study, 60 patients were enrolled and received either intravenous morphine or placebo. Diagnostic impression and physical examination findings by both pediatric emergency physicians and surgeons were recording before treatment and 15 and 30 minutes after treatment. Children who received morphine had a reduction in pain without a reduction in diagnostic accuracy.

In 2003, Thomas and coauthors [95] published a prospective RCT looking at the effects of intravenous morphine analgesia on diagnostic accuracy in emergency department adult patients who had abdominal pain. Seventy-four patients were enrolled and received either intravenous morphine or placebo. The results revealed, through correlation with clinical course and final diagnosis, no instance of masked physical examination findings.

The above-cited studies illustrate that early use of analgesia is appropriate in patients who present with undifferentiated abdominal pain, and will not mask physical examination findings or miss potential life-threatening causes of abdominal pain. Unfortunately, these studies are not flawless. Many of the studies were severely limited by inappropriately small sample sizes. Experts recommend at least 1000 patients to validate a practice guideline for the use of analgesics in patients who have undifferentiated abdominal pain. Additionally, most of the studies focused on adults and did not specifically examine the elderly and pediatric populations.

None of the above trials was able to identify a patient in whom giving early analgesia led to a poor outcome. In fact, a literature search failed to reveal any report of a misdiagnosis attributed to the administration of analgesia. The lack of evidence may result from lack of analgesic use by physicians, reporting bias, or fear of litigation following the reporting of adverse events.

Review of current recommendations

1. Establish a broad differential diagnosis after a thorough history and physical examination.
2. Administer opiate analgesia early in the patient's diagnostic course. The authors recommend intravenous fentanyl or morphine in small doses. Fentanyl has the advantage of a brief onset of action, which makes it easier to titrate. Fentanyl also enjoys a shorter half-life than drugs such as morphine, which tends to further reduce any chance of prolonged

masking of signs or symptoms. The goal is not to make the pain go completely away, but to make the pain tolerable for the patient while further studies and observation occur.

3. Order appropriate laboratory and imaging studies.
4. Consult with a surgeon early. If the consultant is irate about a patient receiving an opiate before a final diagnosis is made, the use of naloxone can be offered for the surgeon to administer to the patient. No trial has addressed this issue to date, and care must be taken to explain the reasoning behind this course of action to the patient.
5. Perform serial abdominal examinations and include a period of observation in the emergency department before dispositioning the patient home. Even with the advent of spiral computerized tomography and ultrasound, the clinical examination remains extremely important in making the correct diagnosis and disposition.
6. If the patient is to be discharged home, strict discharge instructions must be provided, including clear guidelines illustrating why a return to the emergency department may be necessary.
7. Arrange close follow-up with the patient's primary care physician or an emergency department within 8 to 24 hours. This practice reiterates to the patient the fact that the emergency provider has not made a specific diagnosis, and that time may be needed to make the final diagnosis clear.

Summary

Difficult clinical decisions are a part of every emergency practitioner's life. Dealing with difficult patients and recalcitrant consultants is seldom enjoyable, but can be made more palatable through the use of some of the clinical strategies contained in this article. Knowledge of the current best evidence and a willingness to discard outdated practice ideas will help ensure that emergency practitioners continue to provide state-of-the-art medical care. Expressions of care, concern, and respect for patients' problems, and development of a therapeutic alliance with these patients will maximize patient, and ultimately physician, satisfaction.

References

[1] Nadler SF, Steiner DJ, Petty SR, et al. Overnight use of continuous low-level heatwrap therapy for relief of low back pain. Arch Phys Med Rehabil 2003;84:335–42.

[2] Freymoyer JW. Back pain and sciatica. N Engl J Med 1988;318:291–300.

[3] Kelsey JL, Holbrook TL, Grazier KL. The frequency of occurrence, impact and cost of selected musculoskeletal conditions in the United States. Park Ridge (IL): American Academy of Orthopedic Surgeons; 1984. p. 154–6.

[4] Wahlgren DR, Atkinson JH, Epping-Jordan JE, et al. One year follow up of first onset low back pain. Pain 1997;73:213–21.

[5] Van den Hoogen HJ, Koes BW, van Eijk JT, et al. On the course of low back pain in general practice: one year follow up study. Ann Rheum Dis 1998;57:13–9.
[6] Van Tulder MW, Scholten RJ, Koes BW, et al. Nonsteroidal anti-inflammatory drugs for low back pain; a systematic review within the framework of the Cochrane Collaberation Back Review Group. Spine 2000;19(25):2501–13.
[7] Low back pain and sciatica. Clin Evid 2001. BMJ Publishing Group;(6):864–83.
[8] Jackson JL, Browning R. The impact of national low back pain guidelines on clinical practice [abstract]. J Gen Intern Med 2001;16(Suppl 1):142.
[9] Bigos SJ, Bowyer OR, Braen GR, et al. Clinical practice guideline number 14: acute low back problems in adults: assessment and treatment. ACHPR Publication 95–0642. Rockville (MD): Agency for Health Care Policy and Research, Public Health Service, US Dept of Health and Human Services; 1994.
[10] Adult low back pain. Available at: http://www.guideline.gov/summary/summary.aspx?doc_id=5883&nbr=3869&string=low+AND+back+AND+pain. Accessed March 15, 2005.
[11] Browning R, Jackson JL, O'Malley PG. Cyclobenzaprine and back pain, a meta-analysis. Arch Intern Med 2001;161:1613–20.
[12] Waddell G, Feder G, Lewis M. Systematic reviews of bed rest and advice to stay active for acute low back pain. Br J Gen Pract 1997;47:647–52.
[13] Hagen EM, Eroksen HR, Ursin H. Does early intervention with a light mobilization program reduce long-term sick leave for low back pain? Spine 2000;25:1973–6.
[14] Nadler SF, Steiner DJ, Erasala GN, et al. Continuous low-level heatwrap thearapy for treating acute nonspecific low back pain. Arch Phys Med Rehabil 2003;84:329–34.
[15] Silberstein SD. Practice parameter: evidence-based guidelines for migraine heachache (an evidence-based review). Quality Standards Subcommittee of the American Academy of Neurology. Available at: http://www.aan.com/professionals/practice/guideline/index.cfm?fuseaction=home.view&guideline=67. Accessed March 15, 2005.
[16] Vinson DR, Hurtado TR, Vandenberg JT, et al. Variations among emergency departments in the treatment of benign headache. Ann Emerg Med 2003;41(1):90–7.
[17] Vinson DR. Treatment patterns of isolated benign headache in US emergency departments. Ann Emerg Med 2002;39(3):215–22.
[18] Richman PB, Allegra J, Eskin B, et al. A randomized clinical trial to assess the efficacy of intramuscular droperidol for the treatment of acute migraine headache. Am J Emerg Med 2002;20(1):39–42.
[19] Richman PB, Reischel U, Ostrow A, et al. Droperidol for acute migraine headache. Am J Emerg Med 1999;17(4):398–400.
[20] Coppola M, Yealy DM, Leibold RA. Randomized, placebo-controlled evaluation of prochlorperazine versus metoclopramide for emergency department treatment of migraine headache. Ann Emerg Med 1995;26(5):541–6.
[21] Horowitz BZ, Bizovi K, Moreno R. Droperidol—behind the black box warning. Acad Emerg Med 2002;9(6):615–8.
[22] Kelly AM. Migraine: pharmacotherapy in the emergency department. J Accid Emerg Med 2000;17(4):241–5.
[23] Ellis GL, Delaney J, DeHart DA, et al. The efficacy of metoclopramide in the treatment of migraine headache. Ann Emerg Med 1993;22(2):191–5.
[24] Lane PL, McLellan BA, Baggoley CJ. Comparative efficacy of chlorpromazine and meperidine with dimenhydrinate in migraine headache. Ann Emerg Med 1989;18(4):360–5.
[25] Cameron JD, Lane PL, Speechley M. Intravenous chlorpromazine vs intravenous metoclopramide in acute migraine headache. Acad Emerg Med 1995;2(7):597–602.
[26] Tfelt-Hansen P, Henry P, Mulder LJ, et al. The effectiveness of combined oral lysine acetylsalicylate and metoclopramide compared with oral sumatriptan for migraine. Lancet 1995;346(8980):923–6.

[27] Le Jeunne C, Gomez JP, Pradalier A, et al. Comparative efficacy and safety of calcium carbasalate plus metoclopramide versus ergotamine tartrate plus caffeine in the treatment of acute migraine attacks. Eur Neurol 1999;41(1):37–43.
[28] Bell R, Montoya D, Shuaib A, et al. A comparative trial of three agents in the treatment of acute migraine headache. Ann Emerg Med 1990;19(10):1079–82.
[29] Kelly AM, Ardagh M, Curry C, et al. Intravenous chlorpromazine versus intramuscular sumatriptan for acute migraine. J Accid Emerg Med 1997;14(4):209–11.
[30] Scherl ER, Wilson JF. Comparison of dihydroergotamine with metoclopramide versus meperidine with promethazine in the treatment of acute migraine. Headache 1995;35(5): 256–9.
[31] Vinson DR, Drotts DL. Diphenhydramine for the prevention of akathisia induced by prochlorperazine: a randomized, controlled trial. Ann Emerg Med 2001;37(2):125–31.
[32] Seim MB, March JA, Dunn KA. Intravenous ketorolac vs intravenous prochlorperazine for the treatment of migraine headaches. Acad Emerg Med 1998;5(6):573–6.
[33] Davis CP, Torre PR, Williams C, et al. Ketorolac versus meperidine-plus-promethazine treatment of migraine headache: evaluations by patients. Am J Emerg Med 1995;13(2): 146–50.
[34] Meredith JT, Wait S, Brewer KL. A prospective double-blind study of nasal sumatriptan versus IV ketorolac in migraine. Am J Emerg Med 2003;21(3):173–5.
[35] Carleton SC, Shesser RF, Pietrzak MP, et al. Double-blind, multicenter trial to compare the efficacy of intramuscular dihydroergotamine plus hydroxyzine versus intramuscular meperidine plus hydroxyzine for the emergency department treatment of acute migraine headache. Ann Emerg Med 1998;32(2):129–38.
[36] Touchon J, Bertin L, Pilgrim AJ, et al. A comparison of subcutaneous sumatriptan and dihydroergotamine nasal spray in the acute treatment of migraine. Neurology 1996;47(2): 361–5.
[37] Edwards KR, Norton J, Behnke M. Comparison of intravenous valproate versus intramuscular dihydroergotamine and metoclopramide for acute treatment of migraine headache. Headache 2001;41(10):976–80.
[38] Winner P, Ricalde O, Le Force B, et al. A double-blind study of subcutaneous dihydroergotamine vs subcutaneous sumatriptan in the treatment of acute migraine. Arch Neurol 1996;53(2):180–4.
[39] Ferrari MD, Roon KI, Lipton RB, et al. Oral triptans (serotonin 5-HT(1B/1D) agonists) in acute migraine treatment: a meta-analysis of 53 trials. Lancet 17 2001;358(9294): 1668–75.
[40] Akpunonu BE, Mutgi AB, Federman DJ, et al. Subcutaneous sumatriptan for treatment of acute migraine in patients admitted to the emergency department: a multicenter study. Ann Emerg Med 1995;25(4):464–9.
[41] Machter DB, Young WB, Rosenberg JH, et al. Evidence-based guidelines for migraine headache in the primary care setting: pharmacological management of acute attacks. American Academy of Neurology US Headache Consortium. Available at: http://www.aan.com/professionals/practice/guideline/index.cfm?fuseaction=home.view&guideline=67. Accessed March 15, 2005.
[42] Willis J. Gastrointestinal disease. In: Carey CF, Lee HH, Woeltje KF, et al, editors. The Washington manual of medical therapeutics. 29th edition. Philadelphia: Lippincott-Raven; 1998. p. 302–28.
[43] Walters W, McGowan JM, Butsch WL, et al. The pathologic physiology of the common bile duct. JAMA 1937;109:1591–7.
[44] Helm JF, Venu RP, Geenen JE, et al. Effects of morphine on the human sphincter of Oddi. Gut 1988;29:1402–7.
[45] Radnay PA, Brodman E, Mankikar D, et al. The effects of equi-analgesic doses of fentanyl, morphine, meperidine and pentazocine on common bile duct pressure. Anaesthesist 1980;29: 26–9.

[46] Thompson DR. Narcotic analgesic effects on the sphincter of Oddi: a review of the data and therapeutic implications in treating pancreatitis. Am J Gastroenterol 2001;96(4):1266–72.
[47] Lingeman JE, Steidle CP, Adams MC. Calculous disease of the kidney and bladder. In: Harwood-Nuss A, editor. The clinical practice of emergency medicine. Philadelphia: JB Lippincott; 1991. p. 214–20.
[48] Holmlund D, Sjodin JG. Treatment of ureteral colic with intravenous indomethacin. J Urol 1978;120:676–7.
[49] Sandhu DP, Iacovou JW, Fletcher MS, et al. A comparison of intramuscular ketorolac and pethidine in the alleviation of renal colic. Br J Urol 1994;74:690–3.
[50] Larsen LS, Miller A, Allegra JR. The use of intravenous ketorolac for the treatment of renal colic in the emergency department. Am J Emerg Med 1993;11:197–9.
[51] Larkin GL, Peacock WF 4th, Pearl SM, et al. Efficacy of ketorolac tromethamine versus meperidine in the ED treatment of acute renal colic. Am J Emerg Med 1999;17:6–10.
[52] Cordell WH, Wright SW, Wolfson AB, et al. Comparison of intravenous ketorolac, meperidine, and both (balanced analgesia) for renal colic. Ann Emerg Med 1996;28: 151–8.
[53] Wright JM, Price SD, Watson SA. NSAID use and efficacy in the emergency department: single doses of oral ibuprofen versus intramuscular ketorolac. Ann Pharmacother 1994;28: 309–12.
[54] Turturro MA, Paris PM, Seaberg DC. Intramuscular ketorolac versus oral ibuprofen in acute musculoskeletal pain. Ann Emerg Med 1995;26:117–21.
[55] Available at: http://www.walgreens.com/library/finddrug/druginfo.jhtml?particularDrug= Toradol. Accessed January 14, 2004.
[56] Available at: http://www.walgreens.com/library/finddrug/druginfo.jhtml?particularDrug= Ibuprofen. Accessed January 14, 2004.
[57] Marlowe KF, Chicella MF. Treatment of sickle cell pain. Pharmacotherapy 2002;22(4): 484–91.
[58] Platt OS, Thorington BD, Brambilla DJ, et al. Pain in sickle cell disease. Rates and risk factors. N Engl J Med 1991;325(1):11–6.
[59] Shapiro BS, Benjamin LJ, Payne R, et al. Sickle cell-related pain: perceptions of medical practitioners. J Pain Symptom Manage 1997;14(3):168–74.
[60] Comber JT, Lopez BL. Evaluation of pulse oximetry in sickle cell anemia patients presenting to the emergency department in acute vasooclusive crisis. Am J Emerg Med 1996;14(1):16–8.
[61] Fitzgerald RK, Johnson A. Pulse oximetery in sickle cell anemia. Crit Care Med 2001;29(9): 1803–6.
[62] Zipursky A, Robieux IC, Brown EJ, et al. Oxygen therapy in sickle cell disease. Am J Pediatr Hematol Oncol 1992;14:22–8.
[63] Robieux IC, Kellner JD, Coppes MJ, et al. Analgesia in children with sickle cell crisis: comparison of intermittent opioids vs. continuous intravenous infusion of morphine and placebo-controlled study of oxygen inhalation. Pediatr Hematol Oncol 1992;9(4):317–26.
[64] Silbergleit R, Jancis MO, McNamara RM. Management of sickle cell pain crisis in the emergency department at teaching hospitals. J Emerg Med 1999;17(4):625–30.
[65] Gonzalez ER, Bahal N, Hansen LA, et al. Intermittent injection vs patient-controlled analgesia for sickle cell crisis pain. Comparison in patients in the emergency department. Arch Intern Med 1991;151(7):1373–8.
[66] Perlin E, Finke H, Castro O, et al. Enhancement of pain control with ketorolac tromethamine in patients with sickle cell vaso-occlusive crisis. Am J Hematol 1994;46(1): 43–7.
[67] Beiter JL Jr, Simon HK, Chambliss CR, et al. Intravenous ketorolac in the emergency department management of sickle cell pain and predictors of its effectiveness. Arch Pediatr Adolesc Med 2001;155(4):496–500.
[68] Hardwick WE Jr, Givens TG, Monroe KW, et al. Effect of ketorolac in pediatric sickle cell vaso-occlusive pain crisis. Pediatr Emerg Care 1999;15(3):179–82.

[69] Richardson P, Steingart R. Meperidine and ketorolac in the treatment of painful sickle cell crisis. Ann Emerg Med 1993;22(10):1639–40.
[70] Wright SW, Norris RL, Mitchell TR. Ketorolac for sickle cell vaso-occlusive crisis pain in the emergency department: lack of a narcotic-sparing effect. Ann Emerg Med 1992;21(8): 925–8.
[71] Simckes AM, Chen SS, Osorio AV, et al. Ketorolac-induced irreversible renal failure in sickle cell disease: a case report. Pediatr Nephrol 1999;13(1):63–7.
[72] Shields T, Sloane PD. A comparison of eye problems in primary care and ophthalmology practices. Fam Med 1991;23(7):544–6.
[73] Wong TY, Lincoln A, Tielsch JM, et al. The epidemiology of ocular injury in a major US automobile corporation. Eye 1998;12(Pt 5):870–4.
[74] Alexander MM, MacLeod JD, Hall NF, et al. More than meets the eye: a study of the time lost from work by patients who incurred injuries from corneal foreign bodies. Br J Ophthalmol 1991;75(12):740–2.
[75] Arbour JD, Brunette I, Boisjoly HM, et al. Should we patch corneal erosions? Arch Ophthalmol 1997;115(3):313–7.
[76] Flynn CA, D'Amico F, Smith G. Should we patch corneal abrasions? A meta-analysis. J Fam Pract 1998;47(4):264–70.
[77] Bradford C, Chamblee D, Hunnewell J, et al. Basic ophthamology. 7th edition. San Francisco (CA): American Academy of Ophthamology; 1999.
[78] Peak D, Chisholm C, Knoop K. Ophthalmic trauma. In: Knoop KJ, Stack LB, Storrow AB, editors. Atlas of emergency medicine. 2nd edition. Mc-Graw-Hill Companies; Printed in Spain; 2002.
[79] Alberti MM, Bouat CG, Allaire CM, et al. Combined indomethacin/gentamicin eyedrops to reduce pain after traumatic corneal abrasion. Eur J Ophthalmol 2001;11(3): 233–9.
[80] Goyal R, Shankar J, Fone DL, et al. Randomised controlled trial of ketorolac in the management of corneal abrasions. Acta Ophthalmol Scand 2001;79(2):177–9.
[81] Kaiser PK, Pineda R 2nd. A study of topical nonsteroidal anti-inflammatory drops and no pressure patching in the treatment of corneal abrasions. Corneal Abrasion Patching Study Group. Ophthalmology 1997;104(8):1353–9.
[82] Szucs PA, Nashed AH, Allegra JR, et al. Safety and efficacy of diclofenac ophthalmic solution in the treatment of corneal abrasions. Ann Emerg Med 2000;35(2):131–7.
[83] Jayamanne DG, Fitt AW, Dayan M, et al. The effectiveness of topical diclofenac in relieving discomfort following traumatic corneal abrasions. Eye 1997;11(Part 1):79–83.
[84] Weaver CS, Terrell KM. Evidence-based emergency medicine. Update: do ophthalmic nonsteroidal anti-inflammatory drugs reduce the pain associated with simple corneal abrasion without delaying healing? Ann Emerg Med 2003;41(1):134–40.
[85] Peyman GA, Rahimy MH, Fernandes ML. Effects of morphine on corneal sensitivity and epithelial wound healing: implications for topical ophthalmic analgesia. Br J Ophthalmol 1994;78(2):138–41.
[86] Cope Z. The early diagnosis of the acute abdomen. New York: Oxford University Press; 1921.
[87] Wolfe JM, Lien D, Lenkoski C, et al. Analgesic administration to patients with acute abdomens: a survey of emergency physicians. Acad Emerg Med 1998;5:528.
[88] Zoltie N, Cust MP. Analgesia and the acute abdomen. Ann R Coll Surg Engl 1986;68: 209–10.
[89] Attard AR, Corlett MJ, Kidner NJ, et al. Safety of early pain relief for acute abdominal pain. BMJ 1992;305:554–6.
[90] Pace S, Burke TF. Intravenous morphine for early pain relief in patients with acute abdominal pain. Acad Emerg Med 1996;3:1086–92.
[91] LoVecchio F, Oster N, Sturmann K, et al. The use of analgesics in patients with acute abdominal pain. J Emerg Med 1997;15:775–9.

[92] Vermeulen B, Morabia A, Unger PF, et al. Acute appendicitis: influence of early pain relief on the accuracy of clinical and US findings in the decision to operate—a randomized trial. Radiology 1999;210:639–43.
[93] Mahadevan M, Graff L. Prospective randomized study of analgesic use for ED patients with right lower quadrant pain. Am J Emerg Med 2000;18:753–6.
[94] Kim MK, Strait RT, Sato TT, et al. A randomized clinical trial of analgesia in children with acute abdominal pain. Acad Emerg Med 2002;9:281–7.
[95] Thomas SH, Silen W, Cheema F, et al. Effects of morphine analgesia on diagnostic accuracy in emergency department patients with abdominal pain: a prospective randomized trial. J Am Coll Surg 2003;196:18–31.

ELSEVIER
SAUNDERS

Emerg Med Clin N Am 23 (2005) 393–414

EMERGENCY
MEDICINE
CLINICS OF
NORTH AMERICA

Pediatric Pain Management in the Emergency Department

Beverly H. Bauman, MD[a,b,*], John G. McManus, Jr, MD, FACEP[a]

[a]*Department of Emergency Medicine, Oregon Health & Sciences University, CDW-EM, 3181 SW Sam Jackson Park Road, Portland, OR 97239, USA*
[b]*Department of Pediatrics, Oregon Health & Sciences University, DC10S, 3181 SW Sam Jackson Park Road, Portland, OR 97239, USA*

Emergency care for children and adolescent patients accounts for about one third of the nation's emergency department (ED) visits each year [1]. Many of these pediatric visits are related to painful injuries from trauma and accidents. Children also frequently present to emergency departments having painful medical and surgical conditions that are not related to trauma. Therefore, emergency physicians and the entire emergency care team should be proficient in the assessment and safe management of pain in children. Yet effective, compassionate pediatric pain management can be challenging, because there are many special considerations when providing pediatric analgesia. Choosing the most appropriate method in a given patient and situation entails assessment of the child's acute medical condition, emotional and cognitive capabilities, and an understanding of his or her baseline chronic anatomic and physiologic state related to chronic medical conditions and age. Because the provision of effective pain relief in children also often requires a team effort to provide anxiolysis or sedation, emergency physicians need to understand their resources and ensure that the ED staff is adequately trained, and that the ED is appropriately equipped for the team effort of close monitoring during sedation with analgesia.

Over the past 25 years, pediatric emergency medicine research and literature have progressively augmented our knowledge of safe and effective pediatric pain management strategies. Yet there is still much more we need to do to understand the painful experiences of children and to develop

* Corresponding author. Department of Emergency Medicine, Oregon Health & Sciences University, CDW-EM, 3181 SW Sam Jackson Park Road, Portland, OR 97239.
E-mail address: baumanb@ohsu.edu (B.H. Bauman).

doi:10.1016/j.emc.2004.12.008 ***emed.theclinics.com***

optimal safe ways of addressing those needs within the system and context of a busy pediatric ED. In this article, the authors review the history of ED pediatric pain management and sedation, discuss special considerations in pediatric pain assessment and management, review various pharmacologic and nonpharmacologic methods of alleviating pain and anxiety, and present ideas to improve the culture of the pediatric ED, so that it can achieve the goal of becoming pain-free.

History of pediatric pain management and procedural sedation

Fortunately, pediatric analgesia and sedation practices have advanced dramatically in the past 25 years. In response to the need to prevent complications and deaths from unsafe sedation practices, the American Academy of Pediatrics (AAP) published The Sedation Guidelines in 1985 [2]. At that time, undertreatment of pain and anxiety was very common, and many children were simply immobilized for procedures. Those patients who were administered some medications commonly received choral hydrate or an intramuscular injection of a combination of meperidine, promethazine, and chlorpromazine (demerol, phenergan and thorazine, or the "DPT lytic cocktail"). In 1990, Selbst and Clark [3] showed that children who presented to an emergency department were much less likely than adults to receive pain medications for the painful conditions of sickle cell crisis, lower extremity fractures, or second- to third-degree burns.

The results of a survey on emergency sedation practices published in 1990 [4] for pediatric laceration repair showed that over 10% of emergency departments never provided pediatric sedation, that meperidine was the most commonly used drug in emergency departments for pediatric sedation and analgesia, and that only a small minority of institutions had formal discharge criteria after sedation. The safety profile and efficacy of the DPT lytic cocktail was described by Terndrup et al in 1991 [5]. In that study, there were no serious complications, but 29% of the patients were insufficiently sedated, and patients remained affected by the drugs for extended time periods, long after the procedure was over. Now the use of that drug combination is no longer recommended, because we have safer and more effective drug alternatives for pediatric analgesia and sedation [6].

It became apparent that the 1985 AAP guidelines were not being widely used to assure safe practices, so in 1992 the AAP published "The Guidelines for Monitoring and Management of Pediatric Patients During and After Sedation of Diagnostic and Therapeutic Procedures" [7]. This document was written by the AAP Committee on Drugs and established guidelines for which patients should be sedated and when they should be sedated, medical personnel and training, availability of equipment and medication, documentation, monitoring, and safe discharge practices.

The American Academy of Emergency Physicians Pediatric Committee published its own statement on pediatric sedation and analgesia in 1994 [8] and stated that "sedation and analgesia are essential components of the ED management of pediatric patients." The statement provided a practice guideline, including documentation and patient selection and discharge criteria as well as a summary of medication choices.

By 2000, there had been numerous advances and widespread increase in the use of agents to improve pediatric painful conditions, such as the use of topical agents such as Lidocaine, Epinephrine, Tetracaine (LET) and Eutectic Mixture of Local Anesthetics (EMLA), improvement in the techniques of the use of local agents, and greater use of a variety of analgesics, sedatives, and anxiolytics. Many emergency departments are now actively expanding the use of nonpharmacologic adjuncts such as distractions (toys, music, games), child life therapists, imagery, and increased parental involvement in order to improve the experience of children during their emergency department care. The pain-free pediatric ED is a laudable goal, which many departments now strive to attain through comprehensive efforts that start from the moment a child presents to triage with a painful condition. Standard curricula that many hospitals require for pediatric and emergency medicine credentialing emphasize pediatric sedation and pain management. The 2002 Pediatric Advanced Life Support (PALS) Provider Course contains an educational module on pediatric sedation [9]. The 2004 edition of the Advanced Pediatric Life Support (APLS) text [10] likewise includes a chapter on pediatric analgesia and sedation.

Thus it is clear that there have been dramatic improvements in and increased acceptance of the use of analgesia and sedation in emergency medical care of children over the past 2 decades. Future directions include more widespread use of technical advances such as capnography during sedation [11,12], increased awareness of systems issues that could lead to risk with analgesia and sedation, expanded use of some drugs, and increased education and regulations for the entire emergency health care team when providing pediatric analgesia and sedation.

How children differ from adults with respect to pain management

There are numerous reasons why the management of pediatric pain in the ED can differ dramatically from pain management in adults. One of the most striking differences is related to the cognitive abilities and developmental status of the child. Respiratory mechanics and airway anatomy are also different in infants and children in comparison with adults. Likewise, children metabolize some medications differently than adults. Due to their small body size, drug toxicities with agents such as local anesthetics may be a greater risk. To safely and effectively manage pediatric pain, emergency physicians need a practical understanding of these differences.

The hospital environment and medical personnel can be terribly frightening to some children, which has the potential to increase their perception of pain. Parents may also be anxious about their child's condition, which can augment the fear in a child. Yet if children are separated from their parents, the child will likely become even more frightened. Because of their cognitive immaturity, children can have difficulty understanding the need for and nature of particular treatments. This can increase their lack of cooperation and make any treatments or procedures more difficult. These barriers can be greatest in children who have developmental delays or in very young children. Emergency physicians and the entire ED staff should take these issues into consideration when working with children, and attempt to maximize nonpharmacologic interventions in order to reduce anxiety and gain the cooperation of the child. When nonpharmacologic interventions are inadequate to overcome the patient's apprehension, sedation is often needed to proceed with a necessary procedure or to obtain imaging studies.

Respiratory physiology and airway anatomy in small children have many differences in comparison with adolescents and adults. These differences should be considered when planning parenteral analgesia and sedation. Small children have a relatively high oxygen consumption and low alveolar volume with respect to weight. Therefore, they will desaturate more rapidly with periods of apnea in comparison with adults [13]. Upper respiratory tract infections are very common in toddlers, which can increase the risk of sedation by increasing the frequency of mild desaturations during the sedation or in the recovery period [14]. The tongue is relatively larger in the oropharynx, and it can easily fall back into the airway during moderate or deep sedation. The large occiput means that extra attention is needed to position the head during sedation and ensure optimal airway position. Appropriately sized airway equipment should be immediately available during any sedation.

The absorption and metabolism of some drugs changes as neonates mature to infants and toddlers. Choosing the correct dose of drugs, including analgesics and sedatives, will not always be as straightforward as dosing on a milligram per kilogram basis. As the body grows, there are changes in body composition. This alters the physiologic spaces into which a drug may be distributed. Hepatic enzyme systems, protein binding of drugs related to plasma concentration of proteins, renal filtration and excretion of drugs and their metabolites, metabolic rate, and respiratory physiology all mature and change as infant develops. Therefore, clinicians should have easy access to references when choosing the doses of medications such as analgesics and sedatives [15].

Pain assessment in children

There are many published guidelines for the assessment and management for pediatric pain [16–20]; however, guidelines and continuing medical education do not necessarily alter health care provider behavior [21,22]. It is important to realize that appropriate pediatric pain assessment must begin with educating our providers and supervisors about not only the measurement of pediatric pain, but also the specific factors involved in the evaluation of pain.

To be adequate, assessment of pediatric pain should be individualized, comprehensive, measured, continuous, monitored, and documented [23–25]. Pain is an inherently subjective multifactorial experience, and should be assessed as such. Pain is unique to each individual, and is influenced by several factors, including age [26], race [27], gender [28,29], culture [17,30], emotions, cognitive ability [20,31], expectations, and prior experience [17,20,32]. Despite this, current evidence has shown lack of assessment and treatment of pain by health care providers in many settings [23,31,33,34]. Even when pain is assessed, it is often underestimated by health care providers [35–37]. Although the focus on assessment has resulted in possibly better documentation of patients' pain, it has not resulted in better treatment of pain [20,38,39].

Patient self-reporting is considered the "most reliable indicator of the existence and intensity of pain" [39,40]. The lack of objective measurement in self-reporting of pain can be frustrating, and makes direct quantitative assessment difficult. Children as young as 2 can give providers some information about their degree of pain, and should be believed [20]; however, parents and providers often do not believe a child's self-report of pain and believe that children may exaggerate their suffering to obtain secondary gain [41]. It has been documented that care providers often diminish pediatric suffering and alleviate their own assessment frustration by accusing children of protesting too much [42].

So, how does one remain unbiased and measure self-reporting of pain? As other authors in this issue describe, pain is complex and multidimensional, and cannot be easily quantified by one-dimensional parameters such as blood pressure or pulse rate. Pain involves psychological, behavioral, physiological, and emotional components [33,39,42]. The interactions of these components explain why there is variation in patients' response to pain and perception of pain. Also, the degree of injury or tissue damage alone is an inefficient method for determining a patient's appropriate pain intensity [43]. Finally, many pediatric patients are unable to self-report pain level [39,42], making it necessary to rely on behavioral and physiological observations and knowledge of the specific pathophysiologic processes involved.

The ideal tool for pain measurement and assessment should include the acknowledgment, intensity, and continued measurement of the pain in regards to therapy and time. This multidimensional tool should also account for all the factors that influence pain perception and intensity. Also, the tool should remain unbiased with regards to culture, age, cognitive state, ethnicity, gender, and previous pain experiences. Because of the complexity required for the ideal multidimensional measurement tool, one-dimensional pain scales have been developed for use in the acute pain setting in children above the age of 3. These scales rely on the ability of the child to self-report and his or her appropriate cognitive ability. Some one-dimensional scales that have been validated and used in the school aged pediatric population to measure and assess pain include: (1) the modified Visual Analog Scale (VAS) [44,45], (2) the Oucher Scale [46,47], (3) the Colored Analog Scale

Box 1. One-dimensional pain scales

Visual analog scale (VAS)—no pain to worst pain
A 100 mm line on which patients place a mark to estimate their pain and the distance from the origin (no pain) is measured.

Oucher Scale
A vertical numerical scale from 10 to 100 for children who can count to 100, with a corresponding vertical photographic scale of expressions of no hurt to worse hurt. Pictures are available in different races.

Colored Analog Scale (CAS)
Colors are assigned (markers or crayons) for "most or worst hurt," "a little less hurt," and "no hurt." A numeric value can also be placed on each color.

Faces Pain Scale
Six cartoon faces ranging from very happy (smiling face) to very sad (sad face).

Body Outline Tool
The child marks an X or colors the painful area on a non gender-specific line drawing of a child's body. Different colors can be used to quantify the pain.

Poker Chip Tool
Four poker chips are used; one chip represents a little hurt and four chips is the most hurt the child could experience.

(CAS) [48], (4) the Faces Pain Scale [49,50], (5) the Body Outline Tool [51,52], and (6) the Poker Chip Tool [39]. These are described in Box 1.

There are also several multidimensional tools available for pediatric pain assessment that incorporate behavioral patterns and physiologic signs for children who are nonverbal or who have decreased cognitive ability [39]. These are listed in Box 2.

Use of these scales to assess pediatric pain has been shown to be inferior to self-report [51]; however, younger children and neonates who lack verbal communication skills and children who have limited cognitive ability necessitate the use of these pain assessment tools that rely solely on physiologic and behavioral indictors. These scales have not been well studied in the ED, but have been used and validated in other settings such as the intensive care unit and the operating room [39,52,55,60].

Because of the paucity of validated pain assessment research in the ED setting, no specific scale or measurement tool can be endorsed. Until such research is available, the use of one-dimensional tools in the acute pain

Box 2. Multidimensional pain scales that incorporate behavioral patterns and physiologic signs, showing appropriate age range of patients

Postoperative pain

Postoperative Pain Score (POPS); 0–3 years [53]
Liverpool Infant Distress Scale (LIDS); neonates [54]
Neonatal Facial Coding System (NFCS); neonates <4 months [55]
FLACC (face, legs, activity, cry, consolability); 2 months–7 years [56]
Toddler-Preschooler Postoperative Pain Scale (TPPS); 1–5 years [56]
COMFORT ; 0–3 years [56]
Children's Hospital of Eastern Ontario Pain Scale (CHEOPS); 1–7 years [57]

Procedural pain

Crying, Requires oxygen to maintain saturation greater than 95%, Increased vital signs, Expression, Sleepless (CRIES); neonates [58]
Pain Assessment Tool (PAT); neonates [39]
Neonatal Infant Pain Scale (NIPS); neonates [52]
Modified Behavioral Pain Scale (MBPS); 4–6 months [59]
Neonatal Assessment of Pain Inventory (NAPI); 0–3 years [60]

Decreased cognitive ability

Noncommunicating Child's Pain Checklist—Postoperative Version (NCCPC-PV) [56]

Modified from Ref [39].

setting is recommended for appropriate children. The Oucher Scale [46,47] for assessment in children above 3 years of age is recommended for the prehospital setting [61]. For the noncommunicative child and children who have decreased cognitive ability, scales that incorporate behavioral and physiologic markers must be used to guide therapy [30,31,39]. The American Pain Society, in conjunction with the American Academy of Pediatrics, states that "Observation of behavior should be used to complement self-report and can be an acceptable alternative when valid self-report is not available" [31]. Until further research is done to validate assessment tools that rely on physiologic and behavioral markers, it is best to use a multidisciplinary team to decide which assessment tool is most appropriate in a setting [39]. Finally, pain management does not end with proper assessment. Focus on provider education should be on the adequate treatment and relief from unnecessary suffering for the patient, not just on the initial assessment and documentation of pain.

Nonpharmacologic interventions

Appropriate therapy for pediatric patients in pain should not be limited to analgesia or anesthesia. Although appropriate use of analgesia is important, there are many nonpharmacologic interventions recommended to improve pain management [62–64]. Nonpharmacologic therapy can be assigned to three broad categories: (1) cognitive (2) behavioral, and (3) physical. Nonpharmacological therapeutic interventions include

Cognitive
Music, guided imagery, distraction, positive reinforcement, decentralization, hypnosis
Behavioral
Relaxation techniques, biofeedback exercises, breathing control
Physical
Heat and cold application, massage or touch, position and comfort, temperature regulation, transcutaneous electrical nerve stimulation, acupuncture, chiropractic, immobilization

Several cognitive, behavioral, and physical interventions have been shown to be effective [39,62,63]. To understand the possible mechanism of action for these nonpharmacologic therapies, a basic understanding of the gate control hypothesis is necessary. The gate control hypothesis has been one proposed mechanism for the effectiveness of these nonpharmacologic interventions [64]. This hypothesis postulates the presence of blocking or gating mechanisms along the pain pathway, prohibiting pain from reaching the brain through stimulation of inhibitory neurons. These neurons can be stimulated and close the "pain gates" through stimulation of nonpainful receptors or excitatory messages from the brain itself [65]. A more thorough discussion of the pathophysiology of pain and this hypothesis can be found in the articles on pathophysiology by Fink and on chronic pain by Hansen elsewhere in this issue.

Cognitive

Music [66], guided imagery [64], distraction [67], and hypnosis [68–71] are examples of cognitive therapies that have been shown to be effective in reducing patient's pain. The use of cognitive interventions may help distract the patient and improve control over pain, and may even contribute to endorphin release [65]. In the United Kingdom, the Royal College of Pediatrics and Child Health [72] recommends a dedicated play therapist in accident and emergency (A & E) departments who treat more than 18,000 pediatric patients per year. Patient cooperation and provider education are necessary for cognitive interventions to be successful.

Behavioral

Behavioral techniques have also been used with success in pain management. Some of the interventions include: relaxation techniques, biofeedback exercises, and breathing control [73–76]. These techniques also aid in distracting the patient and shifting the focus from pain; however, these interventions also require education for the provider and patient to be effective.

Physical

Most providers probably provide physical interventions as part of their routine management to pediatric patients in pain; however, there are several techniques that are probably neglected or are not fully used. Some of the physical strategies that have been proven to be useful include heat and cold application [77,78], massage or touch [77], position and comfort (splinting) [79], temperature regulation, acupuncture [80,81], and transcutaneous electrical nerve stimulation [82].

Pharmacologic methods of treating pain in pediatric patients

There are numerous factors that impact the appropriate choice of an analgesic when a child presents too the ED with a painful condition. The severity of pain or nature of the underlying illness or injury will dictate whether an intravenous catheter is indicated. Intravenous access may then change the approach to pain management. Clinicians need to understand that analgesics and sedatives can have some overlapping properties, because some analgesics also partially sedate. Reducing anxiety will help a child's perception of the situation and help him cope with the pain; however, pure sedatives do not have analgesic properties, and analgesics are much less effective as a sedative than a pure sedative is. Therefore, when choosing drugs to treat pain, it is important to choose the agent or combination of agents that will achieve your desired goals [59].

Specific techniques and therapies to address common painful conditions in the ED and reduce the pain of specific common ED procedures are discussed in a subsequent section. Local and topical anesthetics will be discussed there.

Tables 1 and 2 show commonly used systemic analgesics for pediatric patients in the emergency department. Meperidine doses are not listed because its use is not recommended, due to its unfavorable effect of lowering of the seizure threshold from the accumulation of its metabolite, normeperidine.

Table 1
Mild to moderate pain—NSAIDS and weak analgesics

Drug	Route	Mg/Kg and interval
Acetaminophen	PO	10–15 mg/kg every 4 hours Maximum total dose: 75 mg/kg/day Adult dose: 4 grams/day
	PR	10–15 mg/kg every 4–6 hours (25–40 mg/kg first dose)
Ibuprofen	PO	4–10 mg/kg every 6 hours
Ketorolac (approved for children 2–16 years)	IV	0.5 mg/kg to a maximum of 15 mg as a single dose Adult maximum: 30 mg
	IM	1 mg/kg to a maximum of 30 mg as a single dose Adult maximum: 60 mg

Abbreviations: IM, intramuscular; IV, intravenous; PO, by mouth; PR, per rectum.
Data from Refs [83,84].

If the patient experiences mild respiratory depression due to narcotics, mild verbal stimulation can be tried to encourage deeper breathing. Naloxone should be immediately available in the emergency department for respiratory depression related to narcotic use that cannot be resolved with verbal stimulation. If the respiratory situation is not too urgent, very small doses of naloxone can be titrated to effect while trying to avoid extreme pain or withdrawal symptoms. The dose of naloxone will be determined by the urgency of the situation and degree of respiratory depression. If the situation is not too urgent, 2 microgram/kg doses can be given incrementally over several minutes while following respiratory effort. If the situation is more urgent, a 10–20 microgram/kg dose may be needed while providing assisted ventilation [85].

One special consideration is for neonates receiving opiates. Narcotic clearance is slower in neonates, and it increases over the first 2 to 6 months of life to mature clearance rates. It is recommended that neonates who receive narcotics be placed on continuous pulse oximetry monitoring and be observed in an area where rapid airway intervention can be provided, due to the risk of apnea [85].

Table 2
Moderate to severe pain—initial doses opiod analgesics

Drug	Route	Dose for child < 50 kg	Dose for child > 50 kg
Codeine	PO	0.5–1.0 mg/kg every 3–4 hr	30–60 mg every 3–4 hr
Oxycodone	PO	0.1–0.2 mg/kg every 3–4 hr	5–10 mg every 3–4 hr
Hydrocodone (combined with acetaminophen)	PO	0.05–0.2 mg/kg every 4–6 hr	5–10 mg every 4–6 hr
Morphine	IV/sq	0.1 mg/kg every 2–4 hr	5–8 mg every 2–4 hr
Fentanyl	IV/sq	0.5–1.0 microgram/kg every 1–2 hr	25–50 microgram every 1–2 hr
Hydromophone (dilaudid)	IV/sq	0.02 mg/kg every 2–4 hr	1 mg every 2–4 hr

Data from Refs [10,85,86].

Pediatric procedural sedation

Children who arrive in the ED having a painful condition are often anxious and agitated about the pain they are experiencing. The environment of the ED may also be quite frightening to a child. When procedures are performed that increase discomfort, children's anxiety can escalate even further. To adequately manage their condition in a humane fashion, nonpharmacologic interventions should be tried to calm patients. Frequently, however, this is not adequate to allow the child to relax and cooperate with therapy. Emergency physicians need the knowledge and clinical skills to safely and effectively provide sedation that can be combined with analgesia for the pediatric patient who has a painful condition or who will undergo a painful procedure in the ED. A comprehensive review of the details of the pharmacology of all sedative options is beyond the scope of this article, but important features of sedatives which are particularly useful in children in the emergency department are summarized.

Pediatric sedation is similar to adult sedation in many aspects. As in adult patients, the pediatric patient should have a history and physical examination before sedation. The American Society of Anesthesiologists (ASA) physical status classification system should be used to give the patient an ASA class. Typically, only those pediatric patients in Class I (normally healthy person) or Class II (mild systemic disease) receive monitored sedation by emergency physicians in the ED. Timing of the last oral intake is an important piece of history, because it will affect the plans for sedation. Clinicians should weigh the issue of the urgency of the patient's physical condition with the information about the timing of last oral intake when planning the timing of the monitored sedation [87]. Each ED should have a protocol for documentation of sedation, and all the necessary airway equipment and reversal agents should be at the bedside before administration of the sedative. The physician should anticipate the desired goal of the depth of sedation, whether it be minimal (anxiolysis), moderate, or deep sedation [10]. In addition to continuous pulse oximetry, continuous capnography is a newer technology that is adding a greater dimension of safety for sedation [11]. These issues apply to all patients, children or adults.

Procedural sedation for pediatrics is a group of skills and body of knowledge for which hospitals require specific credentialing. To ensure that their medical staff members are adequately trained before credentialing, some hospitals will require certain courses and documentation of prior experience. The anesthesia group at Dartmouth Hitchcock Medical Center in Lebanon, New Hampshire has taken a lead nationally with its educational efforts on safe procedural sedation in children. The Dartmouth Hitchcock Medical Center Pediatric Sedation Course material can be downloaded from the internet [88]. This course is one example of a method to improve the understanding of sedation amongst all the team involved in emergency pediatric sedation.

There are numerous appropriate choices of sedatives that can be combined with analgesics to provide procedural sedation for children. The drug or combination of drugs chosen for a particular patient will depend on many factors, including the acute medical or surgical condition of the child, chronic medical conditions, timing of last oral intake, experience of the emergency team with particular drugs, the desired depth of sedation, and the anticipated length of time the child will require sedation. Listed below are some of the important features of commonly used sedatives in the emergency care of children.

Ketamine

Ketamine produces a state of trancelike dissociation and the effects of sedation, analgesia, and amnesia. One reason why it is very popular for pediatric sedation in the ED is its safety profile and the preservation of airway reflexes. It is most commonly administered by the intravenous (IV) or intramuscular route, but may also be given orally or rectally. When given IV, care should be taken that it be administered over 1 to 2 minutes to avoid laryngospasm, which is a rare complication. Ketamine may increase oral secretions, so the concomitant administration of atropine or glycopyrolate will reduce that effect. Emergence reactions are common in adults, but uncommon in children, and can be treated with benzodiazepines if they occur. Contraindications to the use of ketamine include head injury or concern of increased intracranial pressure, increased intraocular pressure, and psychosis. Initial intravenous dose is 0.05 to 1.0 mg/kg with titration to effect. Generally, 2 mg/kg will be the maximum needed for initial sedation, but further doses may be administered if the procedure is lengthy. The usual intramuscular dose is 4 to 5 mg/kg [89,90].

Benzodiazepines

Midazolam is the benzodiazepine that is used most commonly for procedural sedation, because it is short acting. It causes sedation and amnesia and anxiolysis, although some children have paradoxical disinhibition and increased agitation with low doses. It can be given orally at 0.3 to 0.7 mg/kg, or by the IV or intramuscular route at 0.05 to 0.2 mg/kg. The intranasal route is irritating to the nasal mucosa and is less preferred. The benzodiazepines have no analgesic properties and are frequently combined with opiates for painful procedures. Diazepam and lorazepam are other benzodiazepines, but due to their longer action, they are less popular for procedural sedation in the emergency department. Flumazenil is the reversal agent for benzodiapines, and its dose is 0.01 mg/kg to a maximum of 0.2 mg/kg. It should be immediately available for monitored sedation performed with benzodiazepines to reverse respiratory depression which cannot be improved with stimulation [10,90].

Barbiturates

Barbiturates are another class of pure sedatives with no analgesic properties. They work on the gamma-aminobutyric acid (GABA) receptors in the brain. They can produce respiratory depression and hypotension, and are contraindicated in people with porphyria. Pentobarbital and methohexital are the two commonly used barbiturates for pediatric procedural sedation. Pentobarbital is a short-acting agent that may be administered by the IV, intramuscular, or rectal route. Administering this drug by the intravenous route allows smooth titration when giving an initial dose of 2.5 mg/kg followed by subsequent doses of 1.25 mg/kg. Methohexital is a very rapid-acting barbiturate that is frequently administered rectally in a dose of 18 to 25 mg/kg, but can also be given intravenously as a 0.5 to 1 mg/kg dose [10,90].

Propofol

Propofol is a disubstituted phenol. It rapidly reaches high concentrations in the brain for quick sedation, and it also has a rapid recovery time. These pharmacokinetic features are desirable for short procedures in the ED. Experts in sedation recommend capnography in addition to continuous pulse oximetry while administering propofol, because of this drug's potential to cause significant respiratory depression. Hypotension is another potential side effect. It has anticonvulsant and amnestic properties, but it is not an analgesic, so many physicians give a dose of fentanyl before administration of propofol for painful procedures. Propofol is commonly dosed as a 1 mg/kg bolus followed by incremental 0.05 mg/kg doses. When a longer procedure is planned, a propofol drip or intermittent small supplemental doses will be needed because of the rapid recovery [91–93].

Etomidate

Although not currently approved for children younger than 12, this drug is gaining in popularity for pediatric sedation because physicians have gained comfort in its use for rapid sequence induction before intubation. The dose of etomidate will depend on the intended purpose. When used for sedation, the etomidate dose is 0.1–0.2 mg/kg IV. When used as an induction agent prior to intubation, the dose is 0.2–0.6 mg/kg IV. It is a pure sedative with no analgesic properties. Etomidate can cause myoclonic jerks, which may limit its use if the patient needs to be fairly motionless for imaging studies [8,10].

Nitrous oxide

Nitrous oxide is an odorless, tasteless gas that is used in combination with oxygen as an inhalational sedative-hypnotic. It is administered to cooperative children by a demand-flow mask. It is contraindicated in pregnancy and pregnant personnel should not assist in its administration. One advantage is that an intravenous line is not needed to provide sedation. Most EDs do not have the delivery device and scavenger apparatus, which limits its popularity as a sedative [8,94,95].

Reducing pain with common painful emergency department procedures

Many children are frightened with the prospect of getting a "shot" when they see medical personnel; however, the pain of needle sticks for blood draws and intravenous line placement, intramuscular injections, spinal taps, and laceration repair can all be reduced with the application of the following techniques.

Techniques for blood draws and intravenous lines

EMLA (AstraZeneca, Wilmington, Delaware) is a combination of lidocaine and prilocaine, which comes in both a cream and a disc formulation. The cream must be used with an occlusive dressing, but the disc has the advantage of being more convenient, and the occlusive dressing is not needed. EMLA results in anesthesia down to 3 to 4 mm, but one disadvantage is that it takes 60 minutes to achieve maximal effect. EMLA can cause vasoconstriction, which can make vein cannulation more difficult. It is available by prescription only. A newer topical anesthetic is ElaMax (Ferndale Laboratories, Ferndale, Michigan), which is 4% lidocaine. It works more rapidly, achieving its maximal effect in 30 minutes. Because ElaMax can be purchased over the counter without a prescription, parents of children who have chronic illnesses can purchase it and apply this medication even before arrival to the emergency department if they anticipate the need for blood work or an intravenous line [96,97].

Lidocaine iotonphoresis, Numby Stuff (Iomed, Salt Lake City, Utah), is an alternative to topical anesthetics for line placements. The iontophoresis device drives a solution of 2% lidocaine with epinephrine into the intact skin under the influence of an electric current. Within 10 to 20 minutes, it can anesthetize to a greater depth (8–9 mm) than EMLA or ElaMax, but the device may cause discomfort during the time of the electric current [98].

Another method to reduce the discomfort of line placement is through the use of a small injection with a 30 gauge needle of warmed lidocaine buffered with sodium bicarbonate. Using a simple otoscope light to transilluminate the palm has also been shown to increase the success of intravenous placement, which will reduce the number of sticks a child experiences [99].

Intramuscular injections

There are several methods that can be used to reduce the pain with intramuscular injections. Ethyl Chloride, Fluori-Methane, and Fluro-Ethyl (Gebauer, Cleveland, Ohio) are vapocoolant sprays that cause a temporary freezing of the skin surface and can be applied by either a spray or with a cotton ball that has been sprayed with the liquid. This anesthesia effect begins almost immediately and lasts less than 1 minute. These vapocoolant sprays should only be applied to intact skin. Ethyl Chloride is flammable, which may limit its availability in the ED [96,100].

A new device called the ShotBlocker (Bionix Medical Technologies, Toledo, Ohio) is able to reduce the pain of intramuscular injections. The ShotBlocker is a flexible plastic device, which has multiple small raised bumps on the surface that touches the skin surrounding the planned location of the injection. The mechanism of pain reduction is felt to be through stimulation of nearby skin afferent nerve fibers, which reduces the sensation of the needle. Unpublished results show reduction of severity of pain with intramuscular injections in children and adults (Brett Smith, Bionix Medical Technologies, personal communication, December 2003).

One commonly administered medication in the pediatric emergency department is ceftriaxone. This antibiotic may be mixed with 1% lidocaine without epinephrine as an acceptable diluent when given by the intramuscular route [101]. Ceftazidime may also be mixed with 1% lidocaine as a diluent [102]. To reduce the pain of intramuscular injections, checking a standard drug reference text for the compatibility of the drug with lidocaine can reduce the pain of the injection.

Lumbar puncture

Febrile neonates and other small children who require a spinal tap can have EMLA or ElaMax applied to their lower back soon after arrival in the ED, in order to reduce the pain of the needle stick. The use of 1% local lidocaine into the skin overlying the interspace is important for neonates as well as older children and adults, to reduce the pain of the spinal tap. Allowing a neonate to suck on a sugar-coated pacifier during procedures can also help sooth the small infant [10].

Wounds requiring suture repair

LET is a combination of lidocaine, epinephrine, and tetracaine, which is compounded into a gel or viscous solution or liquid by the local hospital pharmacy. The application of LET to an open wound with a cotton ball will anesthetize a superficial wound. If further anesthesia is needed for deeper effect, lidocaine can be injected with a fine gauge needle into the area where LET has already initiated anesthesia. TAC is a combination of tetracaine, adrenaline, and cocaine, which can also be used for similar wounds. Due to the expense, toxicity, and risk of a controlled substance with the use of TAC, it has been largely replaced by the safer and less expensive LET [95].

When injecting children's wounds with a local anesthetic, care should be taken not to exceed the maximum safe recommended doses. The maximum safe dose of lidocaine without epinephrine is 4 mg/kg, but the quantity increases to 5 to 7 mg/kg if lidocaine with epinephrine is used. The maximum recommended dose of bupivocaine, with or without epinephrine, is 2.0 mg/kg in neonates and 2.5 mg/kg in children. Injectable diphenhydramine also has local anesthetic properties, and can be injected when the maximum amount of other local anesthetics has already been reached.

Scalp lacerations

One technique that has received recent attention in the literature is the hair appositon technique (HAT) for scalp lacerations. This method reduces the pain associated with scalp laceration repair and also reduces the time required for the repair in comparison with sutures. After cleaning the wound and achieving hemostasis, small clumps of hair on either side of the wound edges are gently pulled together to reapproximate the wound edges. Then the two small clumps of hair are twisted together with a single twist. A cyanoacrylate tissue glue is placed on the top of the twisted hair to secure the hair and the wound in place. This method avoids cutting hair and knotting hair. Patients also do not have to experience the discomfort of suture removal, because the glue will fall out after a few weeks of normal hair washing. This technique is not appropriate for wounds that have ongoing bleeding, because it does not result in hemostasis. The study achieved success in scalp lacerations that were linear, nonstellate wounds less than 10 cm in length [103,104].

Creating the pain-free pediatric emergency department

Eliminating every bit of pain in every pediatric patient throughout his or her entire ED stay may be impossible; however, it is a humane goal for clinicians to continually strive for a systematic approach to reducing pain and anxiety in all children who present to the emergency department. To achieve the greatest improvements, a department needs the commitment of all the physicians, nurses, and ancillary care providers to create a culture in which the prevention and treatment of pain is given a high priority. We now know about many ways to decrease pain in children, but using these methods in a coordinated fashion requires an organized approach and a staff that is committed to recognition and treatment of pain.

From the moment a patient comes to the attention of the triage nurse, children can be screened for their degree of pain as a "fifth vital sign." The triage area can be equipped with various pediatric pain assessment tools to help the nurse. A policy can be written to allow the triage nurse to administer appropriate doses of oral medication for those children in mild to moderate pain for conditions such as ear pain or musculoskeletal injuries. Children in severe pain should be brought to the attention of a physician immediately for guidance in treatment of pain. The triage nurse can also screen for conditions that might require an intravenous line, blood draws, or spinal tap. Then EMLA or ELA-Max can be placed on two appropriate extremity sites when the patient first arrives for care. A febrile neonate could also immediately have EMLA or ELA-Max placed on the lower back in anticipation of a spinal tap. Likewise, topical LET could be applied by the triage nurse under the guidance of a protocol for small lacerations that will later need irrigation and repair.

The waiting room and each examination room can be child-friendly with games, decorations, and videos that help a child relax while awaiting evaluation and management. Even the radiology suite can be made child-friendly with decorations on the walls. Staff could all be trained in distraction and imagery techniques to help children cope with their anxiety.

Once the patient is awaiting care in an examination room, additional techniques can be employed. When the ED is stocked with iontophoresis equipment and its specific lidocaine preparation, that can be an additional method to help with more rapid intravenous placements. For intramuscular injections, topical vapocoolant spray could be quickly available in the ED. Alternatively, a ShotBlocker can be used to distract the pain of an intramuscular injection. If the drug is compatible with lidocaine, it can be mixed in lidocaine to further reduce the pain of the injection. Ceftriaxone is one commonly used drug in pediatric emergency care that is compatible with lidocaine.

Pacifiers and sucrose can also be stocked in the emergency department and given to small infants who are undergoing procedures such as intravenous lines, spinal taps, or urinary catheterization. For infants needing a spinal tap, local lidocaine should be injected with a fine gauge needle before insertion of the spinal needle.

Patient controlled analgesia (PCA) flow sheets and order forms can be available and the staff trained in their use for conditions characterized by chronic pain exacerbations, such as sickle cell disease [105]. The patient may then guide his or her own effective analgesia after the initial bolus of a narcotic while awaiting transfer to an inpatient bed.

For those patients who are discharged to home from the ED, pain management should continue with the appropriate analgesic prescriptions at discharge. Discharge instructions regarding home management of pain and information about any sedation medications that were administered in the emergency department should be given. Follow-up should be ensured if it is anticipated that the condition could result in ongoing pain [106].

There have been impressive advances in our ability to address pediatric pain and anxiety in the ED over the past few decades. With ongoing investigations into better nonpharmacologic and pharmacologic methods to prevent and treat pain, we can anticipate further improvements in the decades to come. Changing our attitudes about the priority of pediatric pain management has the potential to yield enormous benefits for our patients with the use of our present technologies, drugs, and knowledge.

References

[1] Tamariz VP, Fuchs S, Baren JM, et al. Pediatric emergency medicine education in emergency medicine training programs. Acad Emerg Med 2000;7:774–8.

[2] Committee on Drugs. American Academy of Pediatrics. Guidelines for the elective use of conscious sedation, deep sedation, and general anesthesia in pediatric patients. Pediatrics 1985;76:317–21.

[3] Selbst SM, Clark M. Analgesic use in the emergency department. Ann Emerg Med 1990;19: 1010–3.

[4] Hawk W, Crockett RK, Ochsenschlager DW, et al. Conscious sedation of the pediatric patient for suturing: a survey. Pediatr Emerg Care 1990;6:84–8.

[5] Terndrup TE, Dire DJ, Madden CM, et al. A prospective analysis of intramuscular meperidine, promethazine, and chlorpromazine in pediatric emergency department patients. Ann Emerg Med 1991;20:31–5.

[6] Johnson AM. Opiates. Clin Ped Emerg Med 2000;1:328–33.

[7] Committee on Drugs. AAP Guidelines for monitoring and management of pediatric patients during and after sedation for diagnostic and therapeutic procedures. Pediatrics 1992;89:1110–5.

[8] Sacchetti A, Schafermeyer R, Gerardi M, et al. Pediatric analgesia and sedation. Ann Emerg Med 1994;23:237–50.

[9] Hazinski MF, Zaritsky AL, Nadkarni VN, et al, editors. PALS provider manual. Dallas (TX): American Heart Association; 2002. p. 379–96.

[10] Sacchetti A. Procedural sedation and analgesia. In: Gausche-Hill M, Fuchs S, Yamamoto L, editors. APLS the pediatric emergency medicine resource. 4th edition. Sudbury (MA): Jones and Bartlett; 2004. p. 498–523.

[11] McQuillen KK, Steele DW. Capnography during sedation/analgesia in the pediatric emergency department. Pediatr Emerg Care 2000;16:401–4.

[12] Yildizdas D, Yapicioglu H, Yilmaz HL. The value of capnography during sedation/ analgesia in pediatric minor procedures. Pediatr Emerg Care 2004;20:162–5.

[13] Benumof JL, Dagg R, Benumof R. Critical hemoglobin desaturation will occur before return to an unparalyzed state following 1 mg/kg intravenous succinylchoine. Anesthesiology 1997;87:979–82.

[14] Holzman RS. Risk and outcome in pediatric anesthesia. In: Yemen TA, editor. Pediatric anesthesia handbook. New York: McGraw-Hill; 2002. p. 1–12.

[15] Kearns GL, Abdel-Rahman SM, Alander SW, et al. Developmental pharmacology—drug disposition, action, and therapy in infants and children. N Engl J Med 2003;349:1157–67.

[16] Berde C, Albin A, Glazer J, et al. American Academy of Pediatrics Report of the Subcommittee on Disease-Related Pain in Childhood Cancer. Pediatrics 1990;86: S818–25.

[17] Zeltzer LK, Altman A, Cohen D, et al. American Academy of Pediatrics Report of the Subcommittee on the Management of Pain Associated with Procedures in Children with Cancer. Pediatrics 1990;86:S826–31.
[18] Principles of analgesic use in the treatment of acute pain and cancer pain. 4th edition. Glenview (IL): American Pain Society; 1999. p. 1–64.
[19] McManus J. Acute pain management: operative or medical procedures and trauma. Clinical practice guideline no. 1. Rockville (MD): Agency for Health Care Policy and Research; 1992.
[20] American Academy of Pediatrics. The assessment and management of acute pain in infants, children, and adolescents. Pediatrics 2001;108:793–7.
[21] Lomas J, Anderson GM, Domnick-Pierre K, et al. Do practice guidelines guide practice? The effect of a consensus statement on the practice of physicians. N Engl J Med 1989;321: 1306–11.
[22] Haynes RB, Davis DA, McKibbon A, et al. A critical appraisal of the efficacy of continuing medical education. JAMA 1984;251:61–4.
[23] Schechter NL, Berde CB, Yaster M. Pain in infants, children, and adolescents: an overview. In: Schechter NL, Berde CB, Yaster M, editors. Pain in infants, children, and adolescents. Baltimore (MD): Williams & Wilkins; 1993. p. 3–9.
[24] Ilowite NT, Walco GA, Pochaczevsky R. Assessment of pain in patients with juvenile rheumatoid arthritis: relation between pain intensity and degree of joint inflammation. Ann Rheum Dis 1992;51:343–6.
[25] Petrie A. Individuality in pain and suffering. Chicago: University of Chicago Press; 1967.
[26] Jones JS, Johnson K, McNinch M. Age as a risk factor for inadequate emergency department analgesia. Am J Emerg Med 1996;14:157–60.
[27] Todd KH, Deaton C, D'Adamo AP, et al. Ethnicity and analgesic practice. Ann Emerg Med 2000;35(1):11–6.
[28] Carr TD, Lemank KL, Armstrong FD. Pain and fear ratings: clinical implications of age and gender differences. J Pain Symptom Manage 1998;15:305–13.
[29] Kelly AM. Does the clinically significant difference in visual analog scale pain scores vary with gender, age or cause of pain? Acad Emerg Med 1998;5:1086–90.
[30] Abu-Saad H. Cultural group indicators of pain in children. Matern Child Nurs J 1984;13: 187–96.
[31] Breau LM, Finley GA, McGrath PJ, et al. Validation of the non-communicating children's pain checklist—postoperative version. Anesthesiology 2002;96:528–35.
[32] The Assessment and management of acute pain in infants, children and adolescents: a position statement from the American Academy of Pediatrics Committee on Psychosocial Aspects of Child and Family Health and American Pain Society Task Force on Pain in Infants, Children, and Adolescents. Glenview (IL): American Pain Society; 2001.
[33] Cordell WH, Keen KK, Giles BK, et al. The high prevalence of pain in emergency care. Am J Emerg Med 2002;20(3):165–9.
[34] Schecter NI. The under treatment of pain in children: an overview. Pediatr Clin North Am 1989;36:781–94.
[35] Nolan K. Ethical issues in pediatric pain management. In: Schechter NL, Berde CB, Yaster M, editors. Pain in infants, children, and adolescents. Baltimore (MD): Williams & Wilkins; 1993. p. 123–32.
[36] Hammond D. Unnecessary suffering: pain and the doctor-patient relationship. Perspect Biol Med 1979;23:152–60.
[37] Jylli L, Olsson GL. Procedureal pain in a paediatric surgical emergency unit. Acta Paediatr 1995;84:1403.
[38] Ricard-Hibon A, Chollet C, Belpomme V, et al. Epidemiology of adverse effects of prehospital sedation analgesia. Am J Emerg Med 2003;21(6):461–6.
[39] Franck LS, Greenberg CS, Stevens B. Pain assessment in infants and children. Pediatr Clin North Am 2000;47(3):487–512.

[40] Acute Pain Management Guideline Panel. Acute pain management: operative or medical procedures and trauma: clinical practice guideline. Washington (DC): US Department of Health and Human Services; 1992.
[41] Hammond D. Unnecessary suffering: pain and the doctor-patient relationship. Perspect Biol Med 1979;23:152–60.
[42] McGrath PJ, Craig KD. Developmental and psychological factors in children's pain. Pediatr Clin North Am 1989;36:823–36.
[43] Walker J. Taking pains. Nurs Times 1992;88:38–40.
[44] Huskisson E. Visual analogue scales. In: Melzack R, editor. Pain measurement and assessment. New York: Raven Press; 1983. p. 33–7.
[45] McCormack HM, Horne DJ, Sheather S. Clinical applications of visual analogue scales: a critical review. Psychol Med 1988;18:1007–19.
[46] Beyer JE, Knott CB. Construct validity estimation for the African-American and Hispanic versions of the Oucher Scale. J Pediatr Nurs 1998;13:20.
[47] Beyer JE, Denyes MJ, Villaruel AM. The creation, validation and continuing development of the Oucher: a measure of pain intensity in children. J Pediatr Nurs 1992;7:335.
[48] McGrath PA, Seifert CE, Speechley KN, et al. A new analogue scale for assessing children's pain: an initial validation study. Pain 1996;64:435.
[49] Wong DL, Baker CM. Pain in children: comparison of assessment scales. J Pediatr Nurs 1988;14:9.
[50] Bieri D, Reeve RA, Champion GD, et al. The Face Pain Scale for the self assessment of the severity of pain experienced by children: development, initial validation, and preliminary investigation for the ratio scale properties. Pain 1990;41:139.
[51] Beyer JE, McGrath PJ, Berde CB. Discordance between self-report and behavioral pain measures in children age 3–7 years after surgery. J Pain Symptom Manage 1990;5: 350–6.
[52] Hudson-Barr D. Validation of the Pain Assessment in Neonates (PAIN) scale with the Neonatal Infant Pain Scale (NIPS). Neonatal Netw 2002;21(6):15–21.
[53] Barrier G, Attia J, Mayer MN, et al. Measurement of post-operative pain and narcotic administration in infants using a new clinical scoring system. Intensive Care Med 1989; 15(Suppl):37–9.
[54] Horgan MF. Further development of the Liverpool Infant Distress Scale. J Child Health Care 2002;6(2):96–106.
[55] Peters JW. Neonatal Facial Coding System for assessing postoperative pain in infants: item reduction is valid and feasible. Clin J Pain 2003;19(6):353–63.
[56] Hartrick CT, Kovan JP. Pain assessment following general anesthesia using the toddler preschooler postoperative pain scale: a comparative study. J Clin Anesth 2002;14(6):411–5.
[57] Terndrup TE. Pediatric pain control. Ann Emerg Med 1996;27(4):466–70.
[58] Krechel SW, Bildner J. CRIES: a new neonatal postoperative pain measurement score: initial testing of validity and reliability. Paediatr Anaesth 1995;5:53.
[59] Taddio A, Nulman I, Koren BS, et al. A revised measure of acute pain in infants. J Pain Symptom Manage 1995;10:456–63.
[60] Schade JG, Joyce BA, Gerkensmeyer J. Comparison of three preverbal scales for postoperative pain assessment in a diverse pediatric sample. J Pain Symptom Manage 1996; 12:348.
[61] Maio RF, Garrison HG, Spaite DW, et al. Emergency Medical Services Outcomes Project (EMSOP) IV: pain measurement in out-of-hospital outcomes research. Ann Emerg Med 2002;40(2):172–9.
[62] Golden BA. A multidisciplinary approach to nonpharmacological pain management. J Am Osteopath Assoc 2002;102(Suppl):S1–5.
[63] Kennedy RM, Luhmann JD. The "ouchless emergency department." Getting closer: advances in decreasing distress during painful procedures in the emergency department. Pediatr Clin North Am 1999;46(6):1215–47.

[64] Doody SB, Smith C, Webb J. Nonpharmacologic interventions for pain management: pain and post anesthesia management. Crit Care Nurs Clin North Am 1991;3(1): 69–75.
[65] Fields H. Pain. New York: McGraw-Hill; 1987.
[66] Standley JM, Hanser SB. Music therapy research and applications in pediatric oncology. J Pediatr Oncol Nurs 1995;12:3–8.
[67] McCaffery M. Nursing approaches to nonpharmacological pain control. Int J Nurs Stud 1990;27:1–5.
[68] Jonas D, Day A, Binns F. Management of paediatric pain 1: non-drug approaches. Nurse Prescriber/Community Nurse 1998;4(2):44–5.
[69] Ellittson J. Numerous cases of surgical operations without pain in the mesmeric state. Philadelphia: Lea and Blanchard; 1843.
[70] Goldie L. Hypnosis in the casualty department. BMJ 1956;2:1340–2.
[71] Chaves J. Recent advances in the application of hypnosis to pain management. Am J Clin Hypn 1994;37(2):117–29.
[72] Royal College of Paediatrics and Child Health. Accident and emergency services for children. London: Royal College of Paediatrics and Child Health; 1999.
[73] Alcock DS, Feldman W, Goodman JT. Evaluation of child life intervention in emergency department suturing. Pediatr Emerg Care 1985;1:111–5.
[74] Manne SL, Backerman R, Jacobsen PB. An analysis of behavioral intervention for children undergoing venipuncture. Health Psychol 1994;13:556–66.
[75] French GM, Painter EC, Coury DL. Blowing away a shot pain: a technique for pain management during immunization. Pediatrics 1994;93:384–8.
[76] Jacobsen E. Progressive relaxation. Chicago: Chicago University press, Midway Reprint; 1974.
[77] McCaffery M, Pasero C, editors. Pain clinic manual. 2nd edition. St. Louis (MO): Mosby; 1999.
[78] Albrecht S. Cryotherapy as analgesic technique in direct, postoperative treatment following elective joint replacement. Z Orthop Ihre Grenzgeb 1997;135(1):45–51.
[79] O'Donnell J, Ferguson LP, Beattie TF. The use of analgesia in the paediatric accident and emergency department. Emerg Med J 2002;19:195–7.
[80] NHI Consensus Conference. Acupuncture. JAMA 1998;280(17):1518–24.
[81] Frank BL. Medical acupuncture enhances standard wilderness medical care: a case study from the Inca trail, Machu Picchu, Peru, April 2, 1997. Wilderness Environ Med 1997;8(3): 161–3.
[82] Royal College of Paediatrics and Child Health. Prevention and control of pain in children. London: BMJ Publishing Group; 1997.
[83] Yaster M. Nonsteroidal anti-inflammatory drugs. In: Yaster M, Krane EJ, Kaplan RF, et al, editors. Pediatric pain management and sedation handbook. St. Louis (MO): Mosby; 1997. p. 18–27.
[84] Physician's Desk Reference. 58th edition. Montvale (NJ): Thomson PDR; 2004. p. 2966–70.
[85] Berde CB, Sethna NF. Drug therapy: analgesics for the treatment of pain in children. N Engl J Med 2002;347(14):1094–103.
[86] Yaster M, Kost-Byerly S, Maxwell LG. Opiod agonists and antagonists. In: Schechter NL, Berde CB, Yaster M, editors. Pain in infants, children, and adolescents. 2nd edition. Philadelphia: Lippincott Williams & Wilkins; 2003. p. 181–224.
[87] Linzer JF. Conscious sedation: what you should know before and after. Clin Ped Emerg Med 2000;1:306–10.
[88] Dartmouth Hitchcock Medical Center Pediatric Sedation Course. Version 1.0. Available at: http://an.hitchcock.org/PediSedation/. Accessed April 2004.
[89] Petrack EM. Ketamine. Clin Ped Emerg Med 2000;1:281–4.

[90] Krauss B, Green SM. Sedation and analgesia for procedures in children. N Engl J Med 2000;13:938–45.
[91] Hennes H, Havel CJ. Propofol for procedural sedation in children. Clin Ped Emerg Med 2000;1:324–7.
[92] Green SM, Krauss B. Propofol in emergency medicine: pushing the sedation frontier. Ann Emerg Med 2003;42:792–7.
[93] Guenther E, Pribble CG, Junkins EP, et al. Propofol sedation by emergency physicians for elective pediatric outpatient procedures. Ann Emerg Med 2003;42:783–91.
[94] Luhmann JD, Kennedy RM. Nitrous oxide in the pediatric emergency department. Clin Ped Emerg Med 2000;1:285–9.
[95] Flood RG, Krauss B. Procedural sedation and analgesia for children in the emergency department. Emerg Med Clin North Am 2003;21:121–39.
[96] Zempsky WT, Schechter NL. What's new in the management of pain in children. Pediatr Rev 2003;24(10):337–48.
[97] Kleiber C, Sorenson M, Whiteside K, et al. Topical anesthetics for intravenous insertion in children: a randomized equivalency study. Pediatrics 2002;110(4):758–61.
[98] Zempsky WT, Anand KF, Sullivan KM, et al. Lidocaine iontophoresis for topical anesthesia before intravenous line placement in children. J Pediatr 1998;132(6):1061–3.
[99] Goren A, Laufer J, Yativ N, et al. Transillumination of the palm for venipuncture in infants. Pediatr Emerg Care 2001;17(2):130–1.
[100] Reis EC, Holubkov R. Vapocoolant spray is equally effective as EMLA cream in reducing immunization pain in school-aged children. Pediatrics 1997;100(6). Also available at: http://www.pediatrics.org/cgi/content/full/100/6/e5. Accessed January 7, 2005.
[101] Physician's Desk Reference. 58th edition. Montvale (NJ): Thomson PDR; 2004. p. 2937–41.
[102] Physician's Desk Reference. 58th edition. Montvale (NJ): Thomson PDR; 2004. p. 1510–3.
[103] Ong Eng Hock M, Ooi SBS, Saw SM, et al. A randomized controlled trial comparing the hair apposition technique with tissue glue to standard suturing in scalp lacerations (HAT study). Ann Emerg Med 2002;40(1):19–26.
[104] Singer AJ. Hair apposition for scalp lacerations. Ann Emerg Med 2002;40(1):27–9.
[105] Melzer-Lange MD, Walsh-Kelly CM, Lea G, et al. Patient-controlled analgesia for sickle cell pain crisis in a pediatric emergency department. Pediatr Emerg Care 20(1):2–16.
[106] Zempsky WT. Developing the painless emergency department: a systematic approach to change. Clin Ped Emerg Med 2000;1:253–9.

ELSEVIER
SAUNDERS

Emerg Med Clin N Am 23 (2005) 415–431

EMERGENCY
MEDICINE
CLINICS OF
NORTH AMERICA

Pain Management in the Prehospital Environment

John G. McManus Jr, MD, FACEP[a,b,c,d,*], Donald R. Sallee Jr, MD, FAAEM[e]

[a]*Army Institute of Surgical Research, Brooke Army Medical Center, San Antonio, TX 78201, USA*
[b]*Department of Emergency Medicine, Oregon Health and Science University, Portland, OR 97239, USA*
[c]*Department of Military and Emergency Medicine, Uniformed Services University of the Health Sciences, Fort Sam Houston, TX 77002, USA*
[d]*Emergency Medical Services, Fort Sam Houston, TX 77002, USA*
[e]*Emergency Medical Services, Naval Medical Center, San Diego, CA 92134, USA*

> "Care more for the individual patient than for the special features of the disease."
>
> William Osler, 1899

Pain is the leading complaint among individuals presenting to emergency departments, with up to 70% of emergency department patients having pain as part of their chief complaint [1]. Therefore, pain is also a major reason why individuals seek care from prehospital providers. In fact, McLean et al [2] found that at least 20% of prehospital patients reported moderate or severe pain. Multiple other studies [3–7] have also demonstrated that prehospital providers and emergency physicians fail to adequately recognize, assess, and treat pain. These inadequacies in prehospital pain management have resulted in recommendations to incorporate assessment scales and treatment protocols, and to undertake further pain research [6–9]. Despite these recommendations, many emergency medical services (EMS) systems still lack protocols that adequately address and treat pain in the prehospital setting.

The opinions or assertions contained herein are the private ones of the authors and are not to be construed as official or as reflecting the views of the Department of Defense, Department of the Army, Department of the Navy, or Oregon Health and Sciences University.

* Corresponding author. CDW-EM, 3181 SW Sam Jackson Park Road, Portland, OR 97239.

E-mail address: mcmanujo@ohsu.edu (J.G. McManus).

0733-8627/05/$ - see front matter
doi:10.1016/j.emc.2004.12.009

In addition to inadequate protocols, there are many obstacles to adequate pain assessment and management in the unique prehospital environment. Some of these obstacles are agent availability, provider education level, controlled substance regulation, transport time, possible delay in transport, and lack of education and research [6,9,10]. This article presents a review of the current literature addressing some of these pain assessment and management obstacles in the prehospital setting, and provides possible suggestions and solutions for future directions in pain education, assessment, and management in the prehospital arena.

History

The introduction of an ambulance service into the United States Army in the early 1860s led to the first uses of prehospital analgesia. Many of these early ambulances carried "medicinal" brandy or other liquors for pain management. Civilian ambulances saw their first use of analgesia practice after the Civil War. In addition to providing liquors, these civilian ambulances carried rudimentary splints. Although not fully recognized as doing so at the time, these rudimentary splints also provided a measure of pain relief for the patient. In fact, most protocols during the early period of prehospital care involved only on-scene treatment, with transportation back to the patient's home. As medical care continued to evolve and hospital-based care gained more prominence, little attention was given to the prehospital medical care of the patient throughout most of the twentieth century. This unfortunate trend in of prehospital medical treatment is exemplified by the fact that even in the 1960s at least half of these "ambulances" in the United States were hearses [6]. During this time, the acceptable protocols were to transport the patient to the hospital without providing on-scene or in-route medical care.

The recognition, assessment and treatment of patients' pain has recently gained much focus and importance in the management of prehospital patients [6,9]. Pain has been termed "the fifth vital sign" after receiving increased attention from the Joint Commission on Accreditation of Health Care Organizations (JCAHO) [11]. The National Association of EMS Physicians (NAEMSP) has also issued a position paper on prehospital pain management, addressing the importance of the recognition, assessment, and treatment of prehospital pain [6].

Protocols

One area that will help improve pain assessment and treatment in the prehospital setting is the development of pain protocols. Currently, many systems require that the paramedic contact a base hospital physician before administering any pharmacological analgesia. This can lead to a delay in the delivery of analgesia to the patient in pain.

In one study [8], a protocol allowing paramedics to administer morphine sulfate to patients who have extremity injuries without on-line medical control led to patients receiving their first dose of pain medication several minutes earlier. On many occasions, the patient received the pain medications before transport. Interestingly, the total amount of morphine sulfate given per patient and the number of patients receiving prehospital medication did not change when compared before and after implementation of the protocol. Also, there were no adverse events noted in this study.

Many factors need to be included in the development and implementation of these prehospital pain protocols. Protocol components are listed in Box 1.

During the development of pain protocols, it is best to have a multidisciplinary approach. Use of local medical expertise, not only during the development of pain protocols, but also during ongoing assessment, will help improve and standardize pain assessment and treatment, especially in unique populations such as pediatric, chronic, obstetric, elderly, and trauma pain patients [6,9].

Once established, pain protocols should address assessment, indications for medications, and complications associated with analgesia administration. Some potential complications from treatment include respiratory depression, apnea, hypotension, nausea, vomiting, and allergic reactions. Pain management protocols should also require adequate documentation and monitoring of patients who receive prehospital analgesia. Ongoing

Box 1. Prehospital pain management protocol components

Assessment and documentation of patient's pain
Valid and reliable measurement tools for assessment
Treatment indications and contraindications for pain
Possible pharmacological and nonpharmacological recommendations
Possible complications from medications and the treatment recommendations for complications
Adequate patient monitoring and ongoing assessment during transport
Use of local expert input for special situations; ie, pediatric pain, chronic pain, trauma pain, and so on
Communication of information to receiving medical personnel
Adequate quality improvement tools to ensure protocols are appropriate, effective, and followed

Modified from Alonso-Serra, Wesley K. Position paper: Prehospital pain management. Prehosp Emerg Care 2003;7:482; with permission.

patient assessment of pain and therapy is another necessary component of a successful protocol. Communication to the receiving medical provider of the patient's pain assessment, treatment, and response to treatment needs to be addressed as well. Finally, pain management protocols and outcomes should be part of the EMS quality improvement and assurance process.

Myths

There are many assumptions or "myths" held by medical providers that have served as barriers to effective prehospital pain management [12,13]. Some of these are listed in Box 2.

One common myth is the belief that providers already do a good job of providing adequate pain control; however, as cited above, there are many studies to the contrary. Another belief is that administration of pain medications before arriving at a definitive diagnosis may alter presenting signs and symptoms or mask a serious underlying disorder [12]. Pain medications do not affect peritoneal signs or cause fractures to heal before further evaluation. Effective pain management also alleviates some of the patient's duress and anxiety, allowing for a more accurate evaluation [14–16].

Another belief is that any amount of narcotic administered should provide adequate analgesia. If analgesia is provided, often the doses used are inadequate [1,5,6,12,17]; giving 2 mg of morphine to a healthy adult provides little relief. The normal dose can start at 0.1 mg/kg as a bolus and be titrated up to effect. Accompanying this myth is the belief that administering any narcotic can lead to chronic dependence. One study has shown that only 4 patients out of almost 12,000 developed possible opioid dependence patients [13]. Providers also believe that use of any agent is effective for adequate pain relief. These beliefs are more prevalent in the pain management of the elderly or pediatric population [4,18–20].

Box 2. Common provider "myths" about patients' pain

Care providers currently do a good job providing adequate assessment and treatment of pain.
Pain medications may mask serious underlying disorders.
Two mg of morphine provides adequate analgesia in all healthy adults.
Pain affects all people in the same manner.
Use of narcotics in acute pain leads to increase in addiction.
Use of pain medications increases adverse events.
Patients often exaggerate or over-report pain.
Prior interactions do not effect care provider's ability to remain objective.

The myth that all people experience pain in the same manner is also detrimental. The meaning and treatment of pain can be affected by the culture, age, ethnicity, and gender of the patient [6]. Culture has a powerful effect on the beliefs about, behavior under, and meaning of pain [21]. Studies have also shown that there is provider bias and undertreatment of pain in patients of different culture, gender, age, and ethnicity [22–28].

Another belief held by health care providers is that increased adverse effects will occur with analgesia use. It is true that care providers require close monitoring and additional training in analgesia use to prevent adverse events [8]; however, many studies have reported few to no complications in prehospital analgesia administration [8,29,30].

Finally, the patient's and care provider's perception of current pain also affects the adequate management of pain. When the patient says that his pain is a 15 on a scale of 1 to 10, is he exaggerating to get medication or is his pain that severe? The lack of a concrete measurement and the reliance on patient self-reporting of pain level often leads to disbelief by the provider. The myth that patients are unable to adequately self-assess their pain must be overcome through provider education [6,8,9].

Pain assessment

After protocol development, adequate pain management in the prehospital setting begins with effective assessment of pain. Articles in this issue by Todd on the measurement of pain and by Bauman et al on pediatric pain discuss the assessment and measurement tools available for pain in depth; however, the unique and often challenging prehospital environment requires some discussion and recommendations.

To be adequate, assessment of patient's pain should be individualized, comprehensive, continuous, measured, monitored, and documented [9]. Pain is unique to each individual, and is influenced by several factors, including age [28], race [24,27], gender [22,25,26], culture [21], emotions, cognitive state, expectations, and prior experience [6,9]. Despite this knowledge, current evidence has shown lack of assessment and treatment of pain by prehospital providers in regards to those factors [3–6,9]. Also, the focus on assessment has resulted in better documentation of patients' pain without better treatment of pain [29].

Determining the ideal measurement tool used to properly assess pain also presents a challenge for the prehospital health care provider. The lack of objective measurement can be frustrating for the health care provider. Patient self-reporting is considered the "most reliable indicator of the existence and intensity of pain" [31]. So how does one measure such self-reporting? As other authors in this issue have stated, pain is complex and multidimensional, and cannot be as easily quantified as one-dimensional parameters such as blood pressure or pulse rate. Pain involves psychological, behavioral, physiological, and emotional components [1,6,9]. The interactions of these components explain why there is variation in patients' response to pain and perception of pain. Also, the degree of injury or tissue damage alone is an inefficient method for determining a patient's appropriate pain intensity [32]. Finally, many patients in the prehospital setting are unable to self-report pain level [29].

The ideal tool for pain measurement and assessment should include the acknowledgment, intensity, and continued measurement of the pain in regards to therapy and time. This multidimensional tool should also account for all the factors that influence a patient's pain perception and intensity. Also, the tool should remain unbiased with regards to culture, age, cognitive state, ethnicity, gender, and previous pain experiences. Because of the complexity required for the ideal multidimensional measurement tool, one-dimensional pain scales were developed for use in the acute pain setting [9,33]. The three common one-dimensional adult pain scales are the visual analog scale (VAS) [34,35], the numeric rating scale (NRS) [36] and the verbal or adjective rating scale (VRS/ARS) [37–39]. These are briefly described below:

- Visual analog scale (VAS): a 100 mm line with "no pain" at the beginning, and "worst pain" at the end. Patients place a mark to estimate their pain, and the distance from the origin (no pain) is measured.
- Numeric rating scale (NRS): patients rate their pain with numbers, from no pain (0) to worst pain (10 or 100).
- Verbal or adjective rating scale (VRS/ARS): patients chose the best adjective that describes their pain—none, mild, moderate, severe, or unbearable.

There are also unidimensional scales used in the pediatric population to measure and assess pain [40–43]. Children have limited cognitive ability to use most of the adult scales; however the VAS has been used with success in children older than 5. Children under 5 have used modified VAS scales, color scales, and the Faces Pain Scale with some success [44,45]. These scales may also be helpful in adult patients who lack the cognitive ability to communicate. The article on pediatric pain by Bauman et al in this issue describes other one-dimensional pediatric scales and neonatal pain scales that may be used to assess children's pain. No studies have been conducted in the prehospital setting to evaluate pediatric pain scales.

There are also several multidimensional tools available for pain assessment that incorporate some of the factors listed above associated with pain [6,9]; however, these tools are time-consuming and require extensive education to administer and evaluate. The role of multidimensional tools in the prehospital environment may be limited to EMS systems that require lengthy or specialized transport. The use of these tools would require much education and a dedicated multidisciplinary approach.

Although not ideal, the use of one-dimensional tools in the prehospital environment is usually recommended for pain assessment because of their ease of use and logistic feasibility [6,9,33]. For adult patients, the ARS and NRS are recommended for prehospital pain assessment [6,9]. Because literature is lacking regarding out-of-hospital assessment for pediatric pain, medical directors must decide which instrument may work best in his environment. Emergency Medical Services Outcomes Project (EMSOP) IV: pain measurement in out-of-hospital outcomes research [42] tentatively recommends the Oucher Scale for assessment in children above 3 years of age, while awaiting further research [9]. It is also important that the medical director consider including a pain assessment tool in the protocol for other special populations such as the elderly and trauma, obstetric, and chronic pain patients. Another goal, if possible, is to incorporate the same pain measurement tool used by receiving providers and facilities. Also, one must remember that it is important to assess all pain, despite the level of ability to communicate with the patient. As described, there may be behavioral and physiological changes that accompany pain and could be used to aid in therapy [46]. Although observational measures may be inferior to self-report, this may be the only means of assessment in some patients. Finally, pain management does not end with proper assessment. Focus for provider education should be on the adequate treatment and relief from unnecessary suffering for the patient, not just on the initial assessment.

Pharmacologic interventions

There are few studies available that look at the safety and efficacy of prehospital analgesia. Most analgesia studies are retrospective and are considered Class III or IV levels of evidence [47]. One study [48] revealed only 38 randomized control trials relating to prehospital care since 1989, and none were related to pain assessment or management. The available literature does, however, report many options for prehospital analgesic use, and reports few adverse events [29,30]. One French observational prehospital study [29] did report a 2% cardiac-arrest-without-death rate and a 12% arrythmia rate in critically ill, intubated patients; however, because these patients underwent rapid sequence intubation (sedation) and were critically ill, these side effects cannot be linked directly to analgesia use alone.

The appropriate analgesic in the prehospital environment would be one that is safe, easily administered, and that possess rapid onset, short duration, and low abuse potential. The following agents are some of the more commonly used analgesics found in the prehospital environment.

Morphine sulfate

Morphine sulfate is advocated in many prehospital protocols for cardiac chest pain not relieved with nitrates. Also, morphine is finding increasing acceptance in managing hip and long bone fractures [2,5]. Morphine should be administered intravenously, and its effect can be titrated. The onset of action is in minutes, with a half-life of 2 to 3 hours. It can also be given intramuscularly to patients whose situation precludes the immediate placement of an intravenous (IV) feed; however, this route of administration has a delayed onset of action of about 5 minutes, and is more difficult to titrate. When administered intramuscularly, the effects will last for 3 to 5 hours. The dose for both routes is 0.05 to 0.3 mg/kg. An added benefit of morphine sulfate is the fact that undesired effects such as respiratory depression and apnea can be reversed with naloxone. Naloxone has proven to be safe in the prehospital environment and is readily available for many providers [49].

Fentanyl

Another opioid that is used in the prehospital environment is fentanyl. Its rapid onset and potency are major advantages. It is given intravenously in doses of 1 to 4 mcg/kg. An onset of action of 30 seconds to 2 minutes provides faster potential relief than morphine sulfate. Its duration is 30 minutes to 1 hour, requiring more frequent dosing by the prehospital provider. A small study in Australia [50] noted that intranasal fentanyl can provide significant pain relief in children; however, this study involved a small number of patients and was conducted in an emergency department. Oral fentanyl has also been used with success with few side effects [51,52]. Respiratory depression may be seen in fentanyl use, but is a less common when compared with morphine sulfate; however, a rare side effect of fentanyl, chest wall rigidity, may not be relieved by naloxone, and may require paralysis to ventilate a patient. Some organizations may be reluctant to use opioid medications, because these medications present administrative difficulties. Also, federal and state regulations may limit certain systems' and providers' type, route, dose, or use of these controlled substances.

Nalbuphine

Nalbuphine has been shown to be safe and effective for use in the prehospital environment [53–55]. Nalbuphine is a mixed narcotic agonist-antagonist with minimal respiratory and hemodynamic side effects. Naloxone can be used to reverse any adverse side effects. One retrospective case review of 10 patients [56] did show an increased opiate requirement in patients admitted to the emergency department. Because nalbuphine is not regulated by the Controlled Substances Act and may have a lower abuse potential than pure opioids, it may be another option for the prehospital provider.

Nonsteroidal anti-inflammatory drugs

Although nonsteroidal anti-inflammatory drugs (NSAIDS) are a group of medications that can be readily available to the pre-hospital provider, few systems use them. Certain NSAIDS, such as ketorolac, can provide meaningful pain relief for certain conditions, including renal colic. Ketoralac can be administered intravenously and intramuscularly. Although many types of NSAIDS are available over the counter and therefore assumed safe by many people, these medications can have serious side effects when used chronically.

Nitrous oxide

Nitrous oxide can be inhaled to produce sedation and analgesia, and was first used in the prehospital setting in 1970 [57]. It has been safely used in the prehospital environment with excellent results [58]. Advantages include self-administration and an onset and duration of action of 3 to 5 minutes. Supplemental oxygen should be administered while a patient is receiving this intervention. Additionally, the mask used to administer this medication should be equipped with a demand valve, and the mask should not be secured to the patient's face. As adequate analgesia is obtained, the mask will fall from the patient's face, preventing oversedation and possible hypoxia. Minor side effects such as nausea and vomiting have been reported [47,57]. Also, because nitrous oxide is a gas, it should not be used in patients who have suspected pneumothorax or bowel obstruction. Some limitations of nitrous oxide use include regulations concerning use of a gas in an enclosed space, and it's high abuse potential by providers.

Tramadol

Tramadol has been looked at in the prehospital setting as an alternative to morphine, and has been compared with nitrous oxide [59,60]. Tramadol is a centrally acting analgesic that has been shown to be useful in the treatment of many pain disorders [61,62]. Tramadol has a unique mechanism of action that combines mu-opioid activity with inhibition of serotonin/norepinephrine reuptake. A few prehospital studies that involved pain management in trauma patients [59,60] found that tramadol's analgesia and physiological effects were similar to those of other opioids, with a 30% nausea rate.

Other medications

Additional pharmacological agents that have been used in the prehospital environment include ketamine, midazolam, lorazepam, and valium. Ketamine is commonly used in emergency departments for pediatric sedation. Currently, there are no published articles on its routine use in the prehospital environment. Benzodiazepines such as midazolam, lorazepam, and valium are not analgesics, but sedatives or anxiolytics. These medications can treat the anxiety or agitation that often accompanies pain. Great care should be used when giving a patient one of these medications, because anxiety or agitation could be an indication of a more ominous condition, such as hypoxia. Also, these medications should not be used in lieu of pain medication, because benzodiazepines do not provide pain relief. Finally, caution should be used when combining benzodiazepines with opiates, due to their synergistic effect of lowering patient's blood pressure and producing respiratory depression and apnea [63].

Local and regional anesthesia

There are limited data on the use of local and topical anesthetics in the prehospital setting. The use of local or topical anesthesia may be a consideration in special populations or in populations requiring long transport. Other articles in this issue describe the use and techniques of local and topical anesthetics for pain management.

The use of regional anesthesia or "blocks" is also described in detail in other articles in this issue. Regional anesthesia has been used with success in the wilderness and austere environments [64,65]. With the proper training and education, these techniques used in the right environment may improve pain management for these select patients.

Nonpharmacological Interventions

Appropriate therapy for patients in pain should not be limited to analgesia or anesthesia. Although pharmacologic approaches are important, there are many nonpharmacological interventions recommended to enhance pain management [6,66–68]. Also, because of provider level, medication allergies, medication availability, and possible access issues, pharmacological therapy may not be available. Nonpharmacological therapy can be assigned to three broad categories:

- Cognitive: music, guided imagery, distraction, positive reinforcement, decentralization, hypnosis
- Behavioral: relaxation techniques, biofeedback exercises, breathing control
- Physical: heat and cold application, massage or touch, position and comfort, temperature regulation, transcutaneous electrical nerve stimulation, acupuncture, chiropractic, immobilization

Although not scientifically proven, several cognitive, behavioral, and physical interventions have been shown to be effective [68]. To understand the possible mechanism of action for these nonpharmacological therapies, a basic understanding of the gate-control hypothesis is necessary. The gate-control hypothesis has been one proposed mechanism for the effectiveness of these nonpharmacological interventions [66]. This hypothesis postulates the presence of blocking or gating mechanisms along the pain pathway that prohibit pain from reaching the brain through stimulation of inhibitory neurons. These neurons can be stimulated and close the "pain gates" through stimulation of nonpainful receptors or excitatory messages from the brain itself [69]. A more thorough discussion of the pathophysiology of pain and this hypothesis can be found in the chapters on pathophysiology by Hansen and on chronic pain also by Hansen, elsewhere in this issue.

Cognitive

Music, guided imagery [66], distraction [70], and hypnosis [71–74] are examples of cognitive therapies that have been shown to be effective in reducing patient's pain. The use of cognitive interventions may help distract the patient and improve control over his pain, and may even contribute to endorphin release [69]. For cognitive interventions to be successful, they require patient cooperation and provider education.

Behavioral

Behavioral techniques have also been used with success in pain management. Some of the interventions include: relaxation techniques, biofeedback exercises, and breathing control [75–78]. These techniques also aid in distracting the patient and shifting the focus from his pain; however, these interventions also require education for the provider and patient to be effective.

Physical

Most prehospital providers probably provide physical interventions as part of their routine management to patients in pain; however, there are several techniques that are probably neglected or are not fully used. Some of the physical strategies that have been proven to be useful include heat and cold application [79,80], massage or touch [79], position and comfort (splinting) [81], temperature regulation, acupuncture [82–85], and trans-cutaneous electrical nerve stimulation [86,87].

Monitoring and continued assessment

After undertaking a pain management strategy, it is important to continually reassess the patient. The prehospital patient treatment form should document any clinical or subjective improvement of the patient. In addition, any clinical or technical problems encountered when administering the medication should be accurately documented. Monitoring a patient's level of sedation and pain control, particularly when using pharmacological agents that can cause physiologic change, is important for patient safety [61]. Many of the medications used for pain management can produce respiratory or hemodynamic changes.

Simple manual observation is not enough, however. Noninvasive methods already employed to monitor prehospital patients also need to be used. Following the effects of pain control interventions on parameters such as blood pressure and pulse oximetry are essential. If available, noninvasive end tidal CO2 monitoring is another potentially important parameter to follow. All physiologic changes as well as response to therapy need to be documented and investigated by the prehospital provider.

Ongoing education for prehospital providers will improve their ability to use interventions, and to interpret, monitor, and respond to changes in the patient's condition. Prehospital pain management education should be accomplished using a multidiscipline approach incorporating not only appropriate assessment and treatment of pain techniques, but also continued assessment for changes in patients' pain and physiology.

Quality improvement

Once a prehospital pain management protocol is established, it has to be continually evaluated. Quality improvement measurement in pain management is complex and is constantly evolving. A thorough evaluation of the quality of pain care in the prehospital setting should include the measurement of practice patterns and patient outcomes [88]. Quality control programs can increase provider awareness in pain management and improve compliance to pain protocols [29]. Box 3 lists quality assessment markers.

Provider practice pattern evaluation begins with proper education and training, with attention to identification, assessment, treatment, reassessment, documentation, and reporting of pain. Specific end points and benchmarks need to be established and communicated on a regular basis to the providers, with continued flexibility for improvement [6,88]. All forms of therapy, pharmacologic and nonpharmacologic, need to be reviewed and evaluated for effectiveness and incidence of adverse events. Provider documentation needs to be reviewed to ensure protocol compliance and appropriate treatment. Open communication among providers and institutions should occur on a regular basis to assess appropriateness and adequacy of pain control in the prehospital setting.

Measurements of patient's outcomes are also essential for quality improvement. Gordon and associates [88] review several studies that have looked at pain management outcomes in hospitalized patients as a means to measure and improve quality pain control. Some of the outcome measures applicable to the prehospital setting are: adequate assessment of pain is documented, pain is reassessed at regular and frequent intervals, pain is treated with analgesia and other modalities when appropriate, complications and prevalence of side effects associated with pain management are documented and addressed, patients are informed about pain management, and patient satisfaction with pain treatment and the quality of pain management across points of care transition are evaluated.

Box 3. Quality improvement markers for prehospital pain management

Provider practice pattern

1. Education and training in identification, assessment, treatment, reassessment, documentation, and reporting of pain
2. Pain end points and benchmarks need to be established and known.
3. Frequent review of pain modality effectiveness
4. Chart review for documentation and protocol compliance
5. Need for continued patient assessment and identification of adverse events
6. Open communication with providers and institutions about pain management

Patient outcomes

1. Adequate assessment of pain
2. Reassessment of pain at frequent and regular intervals
3. Effectiveness of pain management with pharmacologic and nonpharmacologic modalities
4. Prevalence and adverse events associated with pain management therapy
5. Patient satisfaction with treatment of pain
6. Evaluation of the quality of pain management at transition points of care

Modified from Gordon DB, Pellino TA, Miaskowski C, et al. A 10-year review of quality improvement monitoring in pain management: recommendations for standardized outcome measures. Pain Manag Nurs 2002;3(4):116–30; with permission.

Summary

Pain measurement and relief is complex, and should be a priority for prehospital providers and supervisors. The available literature continues to prove that we are poor pain relievers, despite the high prevalence of pain in the out-of-hospital patient population. Lack of education and research, along with agent availability, controlled substance regulation, and many myths given credence by health care providers, hinder our ability to achieve adequate pain assessment and treatment in the prehospital setting. Protocols must be established to help guide providers through proper acknowledgment, measurement, and treatment for prehospital pain. Nonpharmacologic therapies must also be taught and reinforced as important adjuncts to pain management. Finally, formation of quality improvement pain programs that evaluate patient outcomes and provider practice patterns will help EMS systems understand the pain management process and provide areas for improvement. Only through emphasis on pain education, research, protocol, and program monitoring development will the quality of pain assessment and management in the prehospital setting improve.

References

[1] Cordell WH, Keen KK, Giles BK. The high prevalence of pain in emergency care. Am J Emerg Med 2002;20(3):165–9.
[2] McLean SA, Maio RF, Domeier RM. The epidemiology of pain in the prehospital setting. Prehosp Emerg Care 2002;6(4):402–5.
[3] DeVellis P, Thomas SH, Wedel SK. Prehospital and emergency department analgesia for air-transported patients with fractures. Prehosp Emerg Care 1998;2:293–6.
[4] Basket PJ. Acute pain management in the field. Ann Emerg Med 1999;34(6):784–5.
[5] McEachin DD, McDermott JT, Swor R. Few emergency medical service patients with lower extremity fractures receive prehospital analgesia. Prehosp Emerg Care 2002;6:406–10.
[6] Alonso-Serra HM, Wesley K. National Association of EMS Physicians position paper: prehospital pain management. Prehosp Emerg Care 2003;7(4):482–8.
[7] Abbuhl FB, Reed DB. Time to analgesia for patients with painful extremity injuries transported to the emergency department by ambulance. Prehosp Emerg Care 2003;7(4): 445–7.
[8] Fullerton-Gleason L, Crandall C, Sklar DP. Prehospital administration of morphine for isolated extremity injuries: a change in protocol reduces time to medication. Prehosp Emerg Care 2002;6(4):411–6.
[9] Maio RF, Garrison HG, Spaite DW, et al. Emergency Medical Services Outcomes Project (EMSOP) IV: pain measurement in out-of-hospital outcomes research. Ann Emerg Med 2002;40(2):172–9.
[10] Yealy DM. Prehospital pain research. Ann Emerg Med 1996;27(4):471–3.
[11] Joint Commission on Accrediatition of Healthcare Organizations. Comprehensive accreditation manual for hospitals, the official handbook. Chicago: JCAHO Publication; 1998.
[12] Rodenberg H. Myths of prehospital analgesia. JEMS 2003;28(6):72–3.
[13] Dachs R. Eleven common myths about pain control. Available at: http://www.emedmag.com/html/pre/fea/features/121501.asp. Accessed February 1, 2005.
[14] Vermeulen B, Morabia A, Unger PF, et al. Acute appendicitis: influence of early pain relief on the accuracy of clinical and US findings in the decision to operate-a randomized trial. Radiology 1999;210:639–43.
[15] LoVecchio F, Oster N, Sturmann K, et al. The use of analgesics in patients with acute abdominal pain. J Emerg Med 1997;15:775–9.
[16] Pace S, Burke TF. Intravenous morphine for early pain relief in patients with acute abdominal pain. Acad Emerg Med 1996;3:1086–92.
[17] White LJ, Cooper JD, Chambers RM, et al. Prehospital use of analgesia for suspected extremity fractures. Prehospital Emerg Care 2000;4:205–8.
[18] Schecter NI. The under treatment of pain in children: an overview. Pediatr Clin North Am 1989;36:781–94.
[19] O'Donnell JJ, Maurice SC, Beattie TF. Emergency analgesia in the pediatric population. Part III. Nonpharmacological measures of pain relief and anxiolysis. Emerg Med J 2002;19: 195–7.

[20] Hauswald M, Anison C. Prescribing analgesia: the effect of patient age and physician specialty. Pediatr Emerg Care 1997;13:262–3.
[21] Walker AC, Tan L, George S. Impact of culture on pain management: an Australian nursing perspective. Holist Nurs Pract 1995;9(2):48–57.
[22] Unruh AM. Gender variations in clinical pain experience. Pain 1996;65:123–67.
[23] Raferty KA, Smith-Coggins R, Chen AHM. Gender associated differences in emergency department pain management. Ann Emerg Med 1995;26:414–21.
[24] Todd KH, Deaton C, D'Adamo AP, et al. Ethnicity and analgesic practice. Ann Emerg Med 2000;35(1):11–6.
[25] Carr TD, Lemank KL, Armstrong FD. Pain and fear ratings: clinical implications of age and gender differences. J Pain Symptom Manage 1998;15:305–13.
[26] Kelly AM. Does the clinically significant difference in visual analog scale pain scores vary with gender, age or cause of pain? Acad Emerg Med 1998;5:1086–90.
[27] Hostetler MA, Auinger P, Szilagyi PG. Parenteral analgesic and sedative use among ED patients in the United States: combined results from the National Hospital Ambulatory Medical Care Survey 1992–1997. Am J Emerg Med 2002;20(3):139–43.
[28] Jones JS, Johnson K, McNinch M. Age as a risk factor for inadequate emergency department analgesia. Am J Emerg Med 1996;14:157–60.
[29] Ricard-Hibon A, Chollet C, Belpomme V, et al. Epidemiology of adverse effects of prehospital sedation analgesia. Am J Emerg Med 2003;21(6):461–6.
[30] Pena BM, Krauss B. Adverse events of procedural sedation and analgesia in a pediatric emergency department. Ann Emerg Med 1999;34:483–91.
[31] Acute Pain Management Guideline Panel. Acute pain management: operative or medical procedures and trauma: clinical practice guideline. Washington (DC): US Department of Health and Human Services; 1992.
[32] Walker J. Taking pains. Nurs Times 1992;88:38–40.
[33] Ho K, Spence J, Murphy MF. Review of pain-measurement tools. Ann Emerg Med 1996;27: 427–32.
[34] McCormack HM, Horne DJ, Sheather S. Clinical applications of visual analogue scales: a critical review. Psychol Med 1988;18:1007–19.
[35] Huskisson EC. Visual analogue scales. In: Melzack R, editor. Pain management and assessment. New York: Raven Press; 1983. p. 33–7.
[36] Downie WW, Leatham PA, Rhind VM. Studies with pain rating scales. Ann Rheum Dis 1978;37:378–81.
[37] Keele KD. The pain chart. Lancet 1958;2:6–8.
[38] Jensen MP, Karoly P, Braver S. The measurement of clinical pain intensity: a comparison of methods. Pain 1986;27:117–26.
[39] Woodforde JM, Merskey H. Some relationships between subjective measures of pain. J Psychosom Res 1972;16:173–8.
[40] Wong DL, Baker CM. Pain in children: comparison of assessment scales. Paediatr Nurs 1988;14:9–17.
[41] Beyer JE, Knott CB. Construct validity estimation for the African-American and Hispanic versions of the Oucher Scale. J Pediatr Nurs 1998;13:20–31.
[42] Beyer JE, Denyes MJ, Villaruel AM. The creation, validation and continuing development of the Oucher: a measure of pain intensity in children. J Pediatr Nurs 1992;7: 335–46.
[43] Kuttner L, LePage T. Faces scales for the assessment of pediatric pain: a critical review. Can J Behav Sci 1989;21:198–209.
[44] Tyler DC, Tu A, Douthit J. Toward validation of pain measurement tools for children: a pilot study. Pain 1993;52:301–9.
[45] McGrath PA. An assessment of children's pain: a review of behavioral, physiological and direct scaling techniques. Pain 1987;31:147–76.

[46] McGrath PJ, Johnson G, Goodman JT, et al. The Children's Hospital of Eastern Ontario Pain Scale (CHEOPS): a behavioral scale for rating postoperative pain in children. In: Fields H, Dubner R, Crevero L, editors. Advances in pain research and therapy, vol. 9. New York: Raven Press; 1985. p. 387–93.
[47] Borland ML, Jacobs I, Rogers I. Options in prehospital analgesia. Emerg Med 2002;14: 77–84.
[48] Brazier H, Murphy AW, Lynch C, et al. Searching for the evidence in pre-hospital care: a review of randomised controlled trials. J Accid Emerg Med 1999;16(1):18–23.
[49] Yealy DM. The safety of prehospital naloxone administration by paramedics. Ann Emerg Med 1990;19(8):902–5.
[50] Borland ML, Jacobs I, Geelhoed G. Intranasal fentanyl reduces acute pain in children in the emergency department: a safety and efficacy study. Emerg Med 2002;14(3):275–80.
[51] Schutzman SA, Burg J, Liebelt E, et al. Oral transmucosal fentanyl citrate for premedication of children undergoing laceration repair. Ann Emerg Med 1994;24:1059–64.
[52] Lind GH, Marcus MA, Mears SL, et al. Oral transmucosal fentanyl citrate for analgesia and sedation in the emergency department. Ann Emerg Med 1991;20:1117–20.
[53] Stene JK, Stofberg L, MacDonald G, et al. Nalbuphine analgesia in the prehospital setting. Am J Emerg Med 1988;6(6):634–9.
[54] Hyland-McGuire P, Guly HR. Effects on patient care of introducing prehospital intravenous nalbuphine hydrochloride. J Accid Emerg Med 1998;15(2):99–101.
[55] Chambers JA, Guly HR. Prehospital intravenous nalbuphine administered by paramedics. Resusitation 1994;27:153–8.
[56] Houlihan KPG, Mitchell RG, Flapan AD, et al. Excessive morphine requirements after prehospital nalbuphine analgesia. J Accid Emerg Med 1999;16(1):29–31.
[57] Basket PJ, Withnell A. use of entonox in the ambulance service. BMJ 1970;2:41–3.
[58] Johnson JC, Atherton GL. Effectiveness of nitrous oxide in a rural EMS system. J Emerg Med 1991;9:45–53.
[59] Vergnion M, Degesves S, Garlet L, et al. Tramadol, an alternative to morphine for treating posttraumatic pain in the prehospital situation. Anesth Analg 2001;92(6):1543–6.
[60] Ward ME, Radburn J, Morant S. Evaluation of intravenous tramadol for use in the prehospital situation by ambulance paramedics. Prehospital Disaster Med 1997;12(2): 158–62.
[61] Grond S, Radbruch L, Meuser T, et al. High-dose tramadol in comparison to low-dose morphine for cancer pain relief. J Pain Symptom Manage 1999;18:174–9.
[62] Schnitzer TJ, Gray WL, Paster RZ, et al. Efficacy of tramadol in treatment of chronic low back pain. J Rheumatol 2000;27:772–8.
[63] Reves JG, Croughwell N. Valium-fentanyl interaction. In: Reves JG, Hall K, editors. Common problems in cardiac anaesthesia. Chicago: Churchill; 1987. p. 356.
[64] Calkins MD, Kuzma PJ, Larkin TM, Green DL. Pain management in the special operations environment: regional anesthetics. Mil Med 2001;166:211–6.
[65] Dickison AE. Pain management in the field. Wilderness Medical Society summer conference & annual meeting compendium. Colorado Springs (CO): Wilderness Medical Society; 2001. p. 189–211.
[66] Doody SB, Smith C, Webb J. Nonpharmacologic interventions for pain management: pain and post anesthesia management. Crit Care Nurs Clin North Am 1991;3(1):69–75.
[67] Kennedy RM, Luhmann JD. The "ouchless emergench department": getting closer: advances in decreasing distress during painful procedures in the emergency department. Pediatr Clin North Am 1999;46(6):1215–47.
[68] Golden BA. A multidisciplinary approach to nonpharmacological pain management. J Am Osteopath Assoc 2002;102(Suppl):S1–5.
[69] Fields H. Pain. New York: McGraw-Hill; 1987.
[70] McCaffery M. Nursing approaches to nonpharmacological pain control. Int J Nurs Stud 1990;27:1–5.

[71] Jonas D, Day A, Binns F. Management of paediatric pain 1: non-drug approaches. Community Nurse 1998;4(2):44–5.

[72] Ellittson J. Numerous cases of surgical operations without pain in the mesmeric state. Philadelphia: Lea and Blanchard; 1843.

[73] Goldie L. Hypnosis in the casualty department. BMJ 1956;2:1340–2.

[74] Chaves J. Recent advances in the application of hypnosis to pain management. Am J Clin Hypn 1994;37(2):117–29.

[75] Alcock DS, Feldman W, Goodman JT. Evaluation of child life intervention in emergency department suturing. Pediatr Emerg Care 1985;1:111–5.

[76] Manne SL, Backerman R, Jacobsen PB. An analysis of behavioral intervention for children undergoing venipuncture. Health Psychol 1994;13:556–66.

[77] French GM, Painter EC, Coury DL. Blowing away a shot pain: a technique for pain management during immunization. Pediatrics 1994;93:384–8.

[78] Jacobsen E. Progressive relaxation. Chicago: Chicago University Press, Midway Reprint; 1974.

[79] McCaffery M, Pasero C, editors. Pain clinic manual. 2nd edition. St. Louis (MO): Mosby; 1999.

[80] Albrecht S. Cryotherapy as analgesic technique in direct, postoperative treatment following elective joint replacement. Z Orthop Ihre Grenzgeb 1997;135(1):45–51.

[81] O'Donnell J, Ferguson LP, Beattie TF. The use of analgesia in the paediatric accident and emergency department. Emerg Med J 2002;19:195–7.

[82] NHI Consensus Conference. Acupuncture. JAMA 1998;280(17):1518–24.

[83] Frank BL. Medical acupuncture enhances standard wilderness medical care: a case study from the Inca trail, Machu Picchu, Peru, April 2, 1997. Wilderness Environ Med 1997;8(3): 161–3.

[84] Weiner DK, Ernst E. Complementary and alternative approaches to the treatment of persistent musculoskeletal pain. Clin J Pain 2004;20(4):244–55.

[85] Kober A, Scheck T, et al. Prehospital analgesia with acupressure in victims of minor trauma: a prospective, randomized, double-blinded trial. Anesth Analg 2002;95(3):723–7.

[86] Royal College of Paediatrics and Child Health. Prevention and control of pain in children. London: BMJ Publishing Group; 1997.

[87] Solomon RA, Vierstein MC, Long DM. Reductions of post-operative pain and narcotic use by transcutaneous electrical nerve stimulation. Surgery 1980;87:142.

[88] Gordon DB, Pellino TA, Miaskowski C, et al. A 10-year review of quality improvement monitoring in pain management: recommendations for standardized outcome measures. Pain Manag Nurs 2002;3(4):116–30.

ELSEVIER
SAUNDERS

Emerg Med Clin N Am 23 (2005) 433–465

EMERGENCY MEDICINE CLINICS OF NORTH AMERICA

Basic Pharmacology and Advances in Emergency Medicine

Grant D. Innes, MD, FRCP(C)[a,b,*], Peter J. Zed, BSc, BSc(Pharm), PharmD[b,c,d]

[a]*Department of Emergency Medicine, Providence Health Care and St. Paul's Hospital, 1081 Burrard Street, Vancouver, BC, Canada, V6Z 1Y6*
[b]*Departments of Surgery and Emergency Medicine, University of British Columbia, Vancouver, BC, Canada*
[c]*CSU Pharmaceutical Sciences, Vancouver General Hospital, 855 West 12th Avenue, Vancouver, BC, Canada, V5Z 1M9*
[d]*Faculty of Pharmaceutical Sciences, University of British Columbia, Vancouver, BC, Canada*

Pain is the most common reason patients seek care in emergency departments (ED), and emergency physicians treat many patients who have severe pain, ranging from shingles to long bone fractures to myocardial infarction. The volume and severity of pain-related problems make pain management a core skill in emergency medicine, yet there is ongoing evidence that pain is inadequately treated in the ED [1].

When pain is mild, simple analgesics alone may suffice. But the neurophysiology of pain is complex, involving the central and peripheral nervous system at biochemical, neural, cognitive and emotional levels [2,3]. Given the multiple processes, mediators, and receptors responsible for initiating and modulating pain, it is clear that no single agent will provide optimal analgesia in all cases. For more severe pain, it is often necessary to use potent analgesics and analgesic combinations, and it is logical to combine different drugs to capitalize on their complementary mechanisms of action.

Multimodal analgesia is a critical concept in pain management, and a practice that emergency physicians use on an hourly basis. Multimodal analgesia may involve diverse methods of pain control (eg, regional block, transcutaneous nerve stimulation, and analgesics) or diverse drug combinations. Acetaminophen, anti-inflammatories, opioids and other adjunctive

* Corresponding author. Department of Emergency Medicine, St. Paul's Hospital, 1081 Burrard Street, Vancouver, BC, Canada, V6Z 1Y6.
E-mail address: ginnes@interchange.ubc.ca (G.D. Innes).

doi:10.1016/j.emc.2004.12.010 ***emed.theclinics.com***

agents (eg, tricyclics, anticonvulsants, sedating drugs) can be combined in fixed or variable combinations to provide additive or synergistic pain relief without additive side effects. Evidence suggests that multimodal drug combinations enhance analgesic activity, minimize adverse effects, and enable the use of lower doses of component analgesics (ie, opioid sparing strategy) [4]. Alternatively, a sustained-release analgesic can be used to manage baseline pain levels in conjunction with an as-needed analgesic for breakthrough attacks.

Fixed-dose combinations like acetaminophen (Tylenol #3) or acetaminophen and oxycodone (Percocet) are widely used and convenient, but offer limited flexibility and may preclude the optimal dosing of component drugs to meet patient needs. Wherever possible, clinicians should tailor the pharmaceutical cocktail to the nature of the pain and the patient's specific needs, rather than adopting a "one size fits all" approach.

To provide optimal pain control for their patients, emergency physicians should have an in-depth understanding of analgesic drugs and how to use and combine them effectively. The purpose of this article is to describe the pharmacology and use of analgesic agents that are most useful in the management of acute pain in the ED.

Acetaminophen

Description

Acetaminophen is a synthetic nonopiate derivative of p-aminophenol that has analgesic and antipyretic effects, but no anti-inflammatory properties [5]. It is effective, alone or in combination with other agents (eg, acetylsalicylic acid [ASA], opioids), for the treatment of musculoskeletal injuries, headache, earache, back pain, and dysmenorrhea, and is considered the drug of choice for pain associated with osteoarthritis [6–9]. Acetaminophen is also considered the drug of choice for the management of fever in both children and adults.

Pharmacology

Acetaminophen's analgesic mechanism is poorly understood, but though to be related to inhibition of prostaglandin synthetase. Its antipyretic effects are through actions on the hypothalamic heat-regulating center.

Dosing

Acetaminophen can be administered by the oral or rectal route. For adults and children older than 12, the usual dose is 325 to 1000 mg every 4 to 6 hours as necessary, not to exceed 4 g daily. Children under 12 years of age should take 10 to 15 mg/kg every 4 to 6 hours as necessary, not to exceed 75 mg/kg per day.

Contraindications

Acetaminophen should be avoided in patients who have a known hypersensitivity to acetaminophen.

Precautions

There is some evidence that chronic, excessive alcohol consumption may increase the risk of hepatotoxicity. Chronic alcoholics should avoid regular or excessive use of acetaminophen.

Adverse effects

Acetaminophen is well-tolerated when used at recommended doses. Minor dermatological reactions including pruritic maculopapular rash and urticaria have been reported. Neutropenia, thrombocytopenia, and, rarely, agranulocytosis have also been reported. Hepatoxicity is rare at therapeutic doses, but can result from ingestion of a single toxic dose or multiple excessive doses of acetaminophen [5].

Important drug interactions

Anticonvulsants

Anticonvulsants that induce hepatic microbial enzymes, including phenytoin, barbiturates, and carbamazepine, may aggravate acetaminophen-induced hepatotoxicity because of increased conversion of the drug to hepatotoxic metabolites. Usually, no dosage reduction is required in patients taking concomitant therapeutic doses of acetaminophen and anticonvulsants; however, patients should limit acetaminophen use while receiving anticonvulsants.

Oral anticoagulants

Conflicting results have been reported regarding the likelihood of a drug interaction between acetaminophen and warfarin. In a case-control study of 289 patients [10], Hylek et al reported that in patients receiving warfarin, acetaminophen ingestion was independently associated in a dose-dependent manner with significant elevation of International Normalized Radio (INR) greater than 6. For those in the highest acetaminophen dose category (>9100 mg/week), the odds of having an INR greater than 6 were increased 10 fold (95% confidence interval [CI] 2.6–37.9). These authors concluded that acetaminophen is an unrecognized cause of overanticoagulation, but the trial was limited by the possible presence of other confounding risk factors for overcoagulation and lack of causality assessment.

The mechanism of acetaminophen-warfarin interaction is not known, but may relate to acetaminophen inhibition of the cytochrome P-450 microsomal enzyme system, with a resulting increase in warfarin blood concentration.

Until the magnitude of this interaction is defined, acetaminophen remains preferable to nonsteroidal anti-inflammatories (NSAIDS) as a mild analgesic and antipyretic in patients receiving warfarin, because of the potential for serious bleeding complications when warfarin and NSAIDS are used concomitantly. It is recommended that patients receiving acetaminophen and warfarin receive more frequent INR monitoring until values have stabilized.

Comments and controversies

Acetaminophen is equipotent as an analgesic and antipyretic. It is the safest therapeutic option for mild to moderate pain in children and adults, and the agent of first choice for the management of fever. Its efficacy, favorable adverse effect profile, and lack of significant drug interactions relative to salicylates make acetaminophen an attractive choice for pain management in a variety of patients with and without comorbid medical conditions.

Nonsteroidal anti-inflammatories

Description

NSAIDS are one of the most commonly prescribed drug classes worldwide [11]. By inhibiting cyclooxygenase (COX), the enzyme responsible for prostaglandin biosynthesis, NSAIDS provide anti-inflammatory, analgesic and antipyretic properties. This makes them valuable agents for the ED treatment of acute headache, renal and biliary colic, gout, and other musculoskeletal complaints; however, although they are effective for inflammation, pain and fever, NSAIDS are associated with potentially limiting adverse effects.

Pharmacology

There are two types of COX enzymes—COX-1 and COX-2—that mediate prostaglandin generation [12]. COX-1 is present in all cells, producing prostaglandins that have important homeostatic functions. COX-2 has an insignificant presence in most tissues until induced by injury or inflammation. Once induced, it generates prostaglandins that mediate ongoing inflammation and pain [12]. NSAIDS inhibit both forms of COX enzyme, which explains their effect on inflammation, pain and fever. Unfortunately, this nonspecific COX inhibition contributes to undesirable adverse effects.

In the gastrointestinal tract, COX-1 mediates the generation of endothelial cell-derived prostacyclin, a vasodilator that enhances mucosal perfusion and integrity. In the stomach, COX-1 enhances mucosal perfusion, bicarbonate production, and mucus production, key gastric defense mechanisms. COX-1 inhibition compromises gastrointestinal (GI) mucosal integrity, predisposing to erosions and ulceration, and antiplatelet effects increase bleeding risk.

In the cardiovascular system, COX-1 generates platelet thromboxane A_2, which has prothrombotic and vasoconstrictive effects to facilitate thrombosis and hemostasis. COX-1 and COX-2 produce endothelial prostacyclin, which has balancing vasodilatory and antiplatelet effects that are protective during states of abnormal platelet activation. Consequently, anti-inflammatory agents that inhibit primarily COX-1 (eg, NSAIDS) have antiplatelet effects that may be cardioprotective, whereas agents that inhibit prostacyclin more than thromboxane (ie, COX-2 inhibitors) might have prothrombotic effects that increase the risk of cardiovascular events [13–15].

In the kidney, COX-1 produces vasodilatory prostaglandins that maintain renal blood flow and glomerular filtration rate, especially in volume-depleted patients. NSAIDS block this COX-1 protective effect, causing renal ischemia and functional damage in some people. As a result, NSAIDS may cause renal sodium retention, edema, weight gain, hypertension, congestive heart failure, hyperkalemia, and rarely, acute renal failure [13]. Acute renal failure occurs at a rate of 2 per 100,000 person-years in the general population and 5 to 10 times more often in NSAIDS users. The risk of NSAID-related nephrotoxicity is dose-dependent, age- and comorbidity-related, and likely to occur during the first month of therapy [16].

Dosing

Table 1 outlines the usual and maximum daily doses of NSAIDS [5,17]. Although some agents have been advocated for specific indications (eg, indomethacin for gout), there is no compelling evidence that any one NSAID is superior to any other—for any indication. Consequently, NSAIDS should be selected based on convenience, cost, and availability rather than on theoretical efficacy advantages.

Ketorolac, unique as the only parenteral NSAID available in North America [18], has proven effective in the emergency department treatment of various acute pain states [19–26]. Parenteral administration results in a faster onset of action than oral or rectally-administered agents, offers an advantage in patients unable to tolerate oral medications, and in some cases reduces the need for opioids [27]; however, in patients able to tolerate oral agents, ketorolac has little advantage over orally or rectally administered NSAIDS [28–30].

Contraindications

NSAIDS are contraindicated in patients who have known hypersensitivity to NSAIDS.

Precautions

Conditions associated with dehydration increase the risk of renal toxicity, and may impair cardiac function in some patients. All NSAIDS should be

Table 1
Common nonsteroidal anti-inflammatory formulations

Drug	Usual dose	Maximum daily dose
Acetylsalicylic acid	325–650 po/pr every 4–6 hours	650 mg po every 4 hours (max 5 g/day)
Diclofenac	IR: 50–75 po/pr every 6–8 hours SR: 75–100 po every 8–12 hours	IR: 50 mg po/pr every 6 hours SR: 75 mg po every 8 hours (max 225 mg/day)
Diflunisal	250–500 mg po every 8–12 hours	500 mg po every 8 hours (max 1.5 g/day)
Etodolac	200–400 mg po every 6–8 hours	400 mg po every 8 hours (max 1.2 g/day)
Flurbiprofen	50–100 mg po every 12 hours	100 mg po every 12 hours (max 300 mg/day)
Ibuprofen	200–800 mg po every 6–8 hours	800 mg po every 6 hours (max 3.2 g/day)
Indomethacin	IR: 25–75 mg po every 8–12 hours SR: 75 mg po every 12–24 hours	50 mg po every 6 hours (max 200 mg/day)
Ketoprofen	IR: 50–100 mg po every 6–8 hours SR: 200 mg po/pr every 12–24 hours	75 mg po every 6 hours (max 300 mg/day)
Ketorolac	10 mg po every 6 hours 30–60 mg IV/IM load then 10–30 mg IV/IM every 6 hours	10 mg po every 6 hours (max 40 mg/day) 30 mg IV/IM every 6 hours (max 120 mg/day for $\leq$ 5 days)
Nabumetone	1–2 g po every 12–24 hours	1 g po every 12 hours (max 2 g/day)
Naproxen	250–500 mg po every 8–12 hours	500 mg po every 8 hours (max 1.5 g/day)
Piroxicam	10–20 mg po every 12–24 hours	20 mg every 12 hours (max 40 mg/day)
Sulindac	150 mg po every 12 hours	200 mg po every 12 hours (max 400 mg/day)

Abbreviations: IM, intramuscular; IR, immediate release; IV, intavenous; PO, per os; PR, per rectum; SR, sustained release.

Data from Repchinsky C, editor. Compendium of pharmaceutical specialties. Ottawa (Canada): Canadian Pharmacists Association; 2003.

used with caution in patients who have impaired renal function, liver disease, or congestive heart failure—especially those already receiving angiotension-converting enzyme (ACE) inhibitors, angiotensin II receptors blockers (ARBs) or diuretics. NSAIDS should generally be avoided in patients who have a history of peptic ulcer disease or gastrointestinal bleeding; however, in some cases, potential benefits may outweigh risks. If this is judged to be the case, NSAID use should be limited to the lowest effective dose for the shortest treatment duration, and concurrent gastroprotection should be considered (see below). NSAIDS may cause asthma, urticaria, or severe hypersensitivity in ASA-sensitive patients; thus caution should be exercised in patients at risk. Although a clear causal relationship has not been confirmed, children who have varicella infection or influenza-like illnesses who are treated with salicylates have an increased risk of Reye's syndrome [5].

The administration of NSAIDS late in pregnancy may prolong gestation and interfere with labor. In addition, NSAIDS have been associated with miscarriage and premature closure of the duct arteriosus, and are not recommended in pregnancy (Food and Drug Administration [FDA] category C) [31].

Adverse effects

NSAIDS' most well documented serious adverse effects involve the GI tract, where they cause mucosal injury due to prostaglandin inhibition [11,32]. Rectal or parenteral administration reduces direct mucosal exposure and may mitigate mucosal damage, but NSAID systemic effects remain, and GI injury is possible regardless of the route of administration. Even without direct exposure, systemic COX-1 inhibition compromises gastrointestinal protective mechanisms, including mucosal perfusion, bicarbonate production, and mucus production, thus predisposing to peptic ulcer disease (PUD) and upper gastrointestinal bleeding.

Overall, 10% to 60% of NSAID users develop abdominal pain, dyspepsia, or nausea, and 2% to 4% of patients develop symptomatic ulcers after using NSAIDS for 1 year [32]. The 1-year likelihood of PUD-related hospitalization or death has been estimated at 1% in NSAID users [33,34]. Risk factors associated with NSAID-induced PUD include advanced age and concomitant use of warfarin, corticosteroids, or other NSAIDS (including acetylsalicylic acid) [32,35,36]. Other systemic diseases, such as congestive heart failure, diabetes, and coronary artery disease, also place patients at increased risk [32]. The risk of developing PUD is also correlated with NSAID dose and duration of therapy [35,37,38].

Cytoprotective agents reduce the risk of NSAID-induced PUD. Misoprostol and proton pump inhibitors (PPIs) have the best supporting evidence, whereas the prophylactic benefit of histamine-2 receptor antagonists is less clear [39]. The Misoprostol Ulcer Complications Outcome Safety Assessment (MUCOSA) trial demonstrated that, in patients receiving NSAIDS, prophylactic misoprostol reduced the development of serious upper gastrointestinal complications from 0.95% to 0.56% (absolute risk reduction [ARR] 0.39%; number need to treat [NNT] 256) [40]. Several trials have shown that PPIs reduce the risk of NSAID-induced PUD [41–43]. The Acid Suppression Trial: Ranitidine versus Omeprazole for NSAID-Associated Ulcer Treatment (ASTRONAUT) trial showed that, at 6 months follow-up, 72% of NSAID users treated with omeprazole were ulcer-free, compared with 59% in the ranitidine group (ARR = 13%; NNT = 8) [40]. The Omeprazole versus Misoprostol for NSAID-Induced Ulcer Management (OMNIUM) trial demonstrated that 61% of NSAID recipients treated with omeprazole versus 48% treated with misoprostol remained ulcer-free at 6 months (ARR = 13%; NNT = 8) [42]. Therefore, the best available evidence suggests that high-risk patients receiving NSAIDS should receive prophylaxis with a proton pump inhibitor.

In the kidney, NSAIDS inhibit vasodilatory prostaglandins that maintain renal blood flow and glomerular filtration rate. This may result in renal ischemia and functional damage, especially in volume-depleted patients. NSAID renal effects may cause sodium retention, edema, weight gain, hypertension, hyperkalemia, and acute renal failure [3,16,44]. The risk of NSAID-related nephrotoxicity is dose-dependent, age- and comorbidity-related, and likely to occur during the first month of therapy [16]. Sodium and water retention may aggravate congestive heart failure in patients who have otherwise acceptable symptom control [45]; consequently, caution is warranted when initiating NSAIDS in patients who have congestive heart failure, hypertension, or renal dysfunction.

Other adverse effects may include headache, tinnitus, dizziness, and drowsiness. Severe hepatic reactions, including jaundice, acute hepatitis, hepatocellular necrosis, cholestasis, and fatal fulminant hepatic failure, have been reported rarely in patients receiving NSAIDS. Mild dermatological reactions such as rash or pruritis have been reported, and more serious allergic reactions such as analphylaxis can also occur. Leukopenia, thrombocytopenia, and agranulocytosis are extremely rare [5].

Important drug interactions

Oral anticoagulants

Concurrent use of NSAIDS and oral anticoagulants such as warfarin increases bleeding risk. NSAID antiplatelet effects compound the anticoagulant properties of warfarin, increasing the risk of bleeding complications; therefore concomitant use is not recommended.

Angiotension-converting enzyme inhibitors

Because of effects on glomerular filtration, concurrent use of ACE inhibitors and NSAIDS may result in impaired renal function and loss of antihypertensive effects.

Diuretics

Patients receiving diuretics are at increased risk of developing renal failure if given NSAIDS that reduce renal blood flow. In addition, NSAIDS may interfere with the natriuretic response to diuretics, whose activity depends in part on prostaglandin-mediated alterations in renal blood flow. Thus concomitant use should be avoided.

Glucocorticoids

NSAID therapy may increase the risk of PUD in patients using corticosteroids. The two agents should be combined cautiously if at all.

Lithium

NSAIDS alter the sodium balance at the level of the nephron. As a result, lithium reabsorption is enhanced and lithium levels rise. Some NSAIDS may also directly reduce lithium elimination. If coadministration is necessary, the lithium dosage should be reduced by 50% when a NSAID is added. Physicians should watch carefully for evidence of lithium toxicity involving the central nervous system (drowsiness, confusion, hand tremor, blurred vision, vertigo, and seizures), GI tract (nausea and vomiting) or cardiovascular system (arrhythmias and widening of the QRS complex).

Methotrexate

Concomitant chronic administration of NSAIDS and methotrexate have been associated with severe toxicity associated with prolonged blood concentrations of methotrexate. The exact mechanism of the interaction has not been established, but it has been suggested that NSAIDS may inhibit renal elimination of methotrexate, possibly by decreasing renal perfusion.

Comments and controversies

NSAIDS are effective analgesic and anti-inflammatory agents with low abuse potential. They do not cause sedation or constipation and, at least in short term use, have better side-effect profiles than opioids. Oral NSAIDS are as effective as oral opioids, and parenteral NSAIDS may be as effective as parenteral opioids. There is no good evidence to indicate that any particular NSAID is superior, in terms of analgesic efficacy, to the others, and no good evidence to suggest that parenteral NSAIDS are superior to orally administered NSAIDS. In clinical practice, different patients respond better to different NSAIDS, and experimentation is often necessary to determine the NSAID of choice for a given patient. NSAIDS should be avoided in patients who have gastritis or peptic ulcer disease, and must be used cautiously in the elderly, and in patients who have renal disease or those who have congestive heart failure. Concomitant administration with diuretics and ACE inhibitors may increase risk of adverse renal and cardiovascular effects, and concomitant administration with warfarin and corticosteroids predisposes patients to bleeding complications.

Cyclooxygenase-2 agents

Description

COX enzymes mediate prostaglandin generation in the body. The discovery of distinct COX isoforms—one associated with many important physiological processes and the other associated with pain and inflammation—generated hopes for a new class of analgesics that would control pain and inflammation while causing fewer adverse effects. In reality, COX physiology is much more complex, and the functional distinction between the two isoforms is less clear than initially hoped.

COX-2 inhibitors were designed around the hypothesis that selective inhibition of the COX-2 isoform should reduce pain and inflammation without compromising gastric mucosal integrity. In the ED, these agents are likely to have an increasing role in patients who have acute musculoskeletal pain, headache, and renal or biliary colic. They are somewhat promising, relative to traditional NSAIDS, for patients prone to GI upset and those at higher risk for adverse GI events. Physicians who treat acute pain should be aware of the potential benefits and hazards of COX-2 technology.

Pharmacology

Gastrointestinal

As described in the previous section, traditional NSAIDS that inhibit COX-1 may compromise GI mucosal integrity, predisposing to erosions and ulceration, and may also increase bleeding risk by virtue of antiplatelet effects [14]. Agents that selectively inhibit COX-2 would be expected to cause fewer ulcerations and lower bleeding risk. COX-2 has, however, been identified in normal gastric mucosa, and may have a role in gastroprotection and GI mucosal healing [13].

Cardiovascular

As described in the previous section, anti-inflammatory agents that inhibit primarily COX-1 (eg, NSAIDS) have antiplatelet effects that may be cardioprotective, whereas agents that inhibit prostacyclin more than thromboxane (ie, COX-2 inhibitors) might have prothrombotic effects that increase the risk of cardiovascular events [14,15].

Renal

The beneficial effect of COX-1 on renal perfusion and function was previously described. COX-2 has similar effects on renal prostacyclin production and hence on renal function [44,46,47]. COX-2 inhibitors increase renin activity and reduce sodium excretion by approximately 20%, as do nonspecific NSAIDS [46,48,49]. Although it was hoped that COX-2 agents would have less effect on renal perfusion than traditional NSAIDS, a large amount of existing data suggests that the renal effects associated with COX-2 administration are similar to those reported with prototypical NSAIDS. In addition, cases of acute renal failure (ARF) have occurred in patients who have pre-existing renal disease and who were treated with COX-2 agents [50].

Cyclooxygenase-2 selectivity

In theory, highly selective COX-2 inhibitors should reduce pain, fever, and inflammation while preserving important homeostatic and protective COX-1 functions in the gastrointestinal, cardiovascular, and renal systems. The extent to which an agent inhibits COX-2 activity but not COX-1 activity is referred to as its selectivity. In-vitro selectivity assays suggest that there are large and important differences between agents (Table 2) [51]. Unfortunately, what happens in a test tube may not reflect what happens in a living human. Clinical selectivity—the ability to suppress pain and inflammation without causing COX-1 related adverse events—depends not only on the specificity of the drug for the enzyme, but on how distinct the functions of the two enzyme systems are. Because COX-2 has some physiological roles apart from inflammation, COX-2 inhibitors do in fact have effects on GI mucosa, renal function, and platelets. Clinical selectivity is assessed by clinical trials looking at patient outcomes [51].

Efficacy

COX-2 agents have been studied in several pain models; unfortunately, no studies have been conducted in ED patient populations; thus efficacy must be extrapolated from other settings. The bulk of the efficacy data come from trials comparing celecoxib (Celebrex) or rofecoxib (Vioxx) to various NSAIDS. These trials suggest that there are no clinically relevant efficacy differences between COX-2 agents and traditional NSAIDS for osteoarthritis or rheumatoid arthritis [52–54]. Other studies, more relevant to emergency medicine, showed that COX-2 agents are superior to placebo and as efficacious as naproxen, aspirin, diclofenac, and ibuprofen in acute postoperative dental pain, postoperative orthopedic pain, primary dysmenorrhea, and osteoarthritis [55–61]. It is important to note that COX-2 agents also have antipyretic effects [62]. As yet there are no published studies evaluating COX-2 inhibitors in renal colic, biliary colic, nonspecific abdominal pain, acute gout, headache syndromes, sickle cell crisis, or acute musculoskeletal and soft-tissue injury—conditions of greatest interest in the ED setting.

COX-2 agents have not been adequately studied in the ED setting, but evidence from other therapeutic areas suggests that there are no clinically meaningful efficacy differences between COX-2 inhibitors and traditional NSAIDS for the management of acute pain. Efficacy differences between

Table 2
In-vitro COX-2 selectivity of selected NSAID and COX-2 agents

Agent	COX-1 IC_{50}[a]	COX-2 IC_{50}[a]	COX-1/COX-2 ratio
Indomethacin	0.1	1	0.1
Ibuprofen	38	117	0.14
Diclofenac	.03	.01	3.0
Celecoxib	15	.04	375
Valdecoxib	140	.005	28,000

[a] IC_{50} = drug concentration necessary to reduce enzyme activity by 50%.

Data from FitzGerald GA, Patrono C. Drug therapy: the coxibs, selective inhibitors of cyclooxygenase-2. N Engl J Med 2001;345:433–42.

COX-2 agents may exist, but further research is required to identify and quantify these [12].

Cyclooxygenase-2 interactions with other drugs

Nonsteroidal anti-inflammatory drugs and acetylsalicylic acid (ASA)

Because of pharmacological similarity and the likelihood of additive toxicity, COX-2 agents should rarely be combined with NSAIDS. COX-2 agents can be combined with cardioprotective doses of ASA (in fact it is important not to discontinue cardioprotective ASA when a selective COX-2 inhibitor is prescribed); however, the risk of GI hemorrhage appears to be similar in patients receiving NSAIDS and in patients receiving a COX-2 agent with cardioprotective ASA.

Angiotension-converting enzyme inhibitors and antihypertensives

Because of effects on glomerular filtration, concurrent use of ACE inhibitors and NSAIDS may result in loss of antihypertensive effects and impaired renal function. For the same reason, COX-2 agents may reduce the effects of prescribed loop diuretics.

Anticoagulants

Some NSAIDS are known to displace anticoagulants from plasma protein binding sites, and this effect may occur with COX-2 agents. Celecoxib has been shown not to affect coagulation parameters in healthy subjects, but increased INRs and bleeding episodes have been reported in patients receiving concurrent therapy with warfarin and celecoxib or rofecoxib. If these agents are prescribed for patients on anticoagulants, close INR monitoring is recommended—especially soon after initiation or discontinuation of the COX-2 inhibitor.

Lithium

By reducing glomerular filtration, celecoxib and other COX-2 agents can decrease renal clearance of lithium, which may lead to increased serum lithium concentrations. Patients receiving lithium and a COX-2 agent should be monitored for signs of lithium toxicity, and should have appropriate dosage adjustments when these agents are initiated or discontinued.

Antacids

Magnesium- or aluminum-containing antacids reduce COX-2 plasma concentrations and interfere with clinical effects.

Fluconazole

Fluconazole inhibits cytochrome P450-2C9 isoenzyme activity, and may reduce the metabolism of COX-2 agents. Concurrent use of fluconazole with celecoxib, valdecoxib, or parecoxib may result in increased levels of and side effects from these agents.

Sulfonamide allergy

Celecoxib is structurally similar to the sulfonamides, and hypersensitivity reactions have occurred in patients who have sulfonamide allergy. This effect has not been described with rofecoxib or other COX-2 agents.

Precautions

COX-2 agents should generally be avoided in patients who have a history of ulcer disease or GI bleeding, particularly the elderly and debilitated, who are at higher risk of GI hemorrhage. Because of effects on glomerular filtration, these drugs may exacerbate edema, hypertension, or heart failure, especially in elderly or volume-depleted patients (eg, those who are dehydrated or receiving diuretics), and in those taking ACE inhibitors or ARBs. There are limited data from patients who have severe renal or hepatic impairment, and COX-2 inhibitors are not recommended in such patients.

Agents that modify prostaglandin activity may cause asthma, urticaria, or severe hypersensitivity in aspirin-sensitive patients. Celecoxib and rofecoxib have not been studied in children under 18 years of age or in pregnancy. The administration of prostaglandin inhibitors (including COX-2 agents) late in pregnancy may prolong gestation and interfere with labor. In addition, prostaglandin inhibitors have been associated with miscarriage and premature closure of the duct arteriosus, and are not recommended in pregnancy (FDA category C).

Safety and adverse effects

Tolerability

Adverse reactions to COX-2 agents are usually mild, and most often involve the GI tract, although neurological symptoms including headache, dizziness, and fatigue are reported by 2% to 5% of patients. An analysis of five 3-month trials comparing naprosyn, celecoxib, and placebo found that 12% of naprosyn recipients, 7.8% of celecoxib recipients, and 8.5% of placebo recipients developed moderate to severe abdominal pain, dyspepsia, or nausea (NNT = 25) [63]. Diarrhea, constipation, nausea, heartburn, dyspepsia, or abdominal pain occur in 3% to 10% of COX-2 recipients, but this is statistically similar to rates seen in patients receiving placebo or traditional NSAIDS.

Endoscopic ulcers

The incidence of endoscopic ulcers, defined as mucosal lesions 3 mm or more in diameter, is significantly higher in patients receiving traditional NSAIDS than in patients receiving placebo or COX-2 agents; however, these lesions may be clinically unimportant because they are asymptomatic, not associated with bleeding, and usually detected by endoscopic examinations that are mandated within the study protocol. In an endoscopic study of 742 patients randomly assigned to rofecoxib (25 or 50 mg daily), ibuprofen (800 mg three times a day), or placebo, the incidence of gastroduodenal ulcers 3 mm or larger (at 12 weeks) was 9.9% in the placebo group, 4.1% in the low-dose rofecoxib group, 7.3% in the high-dose rofecoxib group and 27.7% in the ibuprofen group (NNT = 5) [64].

In a 12-week gastroscopy study [65], 537 patients who have osteoarthritis (OA) or rheumatoid arthritis (RA) were randomized to treatment with celecoxib 200 mg twice daily (n = 270) or naproxen 500 mg twice daily (n = 267). Endoscopic ulcer rates were lower with celecoxib at all time intervals: After 12 weeks of treatment, the cumulative incidence of gastroduodenal ulcers was 9% with celecoxib and 41% with naproxen. Efficacy was similar in both treatments, and the incidence of clinical adverse events and withdrawal rates did not differ between treatments.

Significant gastrointestinal events

The manufacturers of rofecoxib pooled 8 trials of 5435 patients [66]. Symptomatic ulcer, perforation, or bleeding occurred in 1.3% of rofecoxib patients compared with 1.8% of NSAID patients per year of exposure (NNT = 200). Fewer rofecoxib patients than NSAID patients (3.5% versus 4.8%) discontinued the study drug due to an adverse GI effect. Most studies show that clinically important upper GI events (perforations, symptomatic ulcers, and bleeding) are less common with COX-2 agents than with prototypical NSAIDS. The best safety data come from the CLASS (Celecoxib Long-term Arthritis Safety Study) and VIGOR (Vioxx GI Outcomes Research) trials, which are discussed below.

Renal effects

In a 6-week trial, 810 patients taking antihypertensives were randomized to celecoxib 200 mg/day or rofecoxib 25 mg/day. The primary endpoints were the development of edema and blood pressure changes. Overall, 9.5% of rofecoxib-treated patients and 4.9% of celecoxib-treated patients reported edema ($P < .05$). At 6 weeks, the change in mean systolic blood pressure was +2.6 mmHg for rofecoxib and -0.5 mmHg for celecoxib. Other trials suggest that the effects of COX-2 inhibitors on renal function are similar to those of nonselective NSAIDS [46,67]. The most common events reported after celecoxib—edema (2.1%), hypertension (0.8%), and exacerbation of preexisting hypertension (0.6%)—were not time- or dose-related.

The cyclooxygenase-2 safety megatrials

It is impossible to discuss COX-2 agents without mention of the COX-2 safety megatrials: CLASS and VIGOR. The CLASS randomized 8059 patients who had osteoarthritis or rheumatoid arthritis to celecoxib 400 mg twice daily (four times the recommended dose), diclofenac 75 mg twice daily, or ibuprofen 800 mg three times daily. The primary outcome was a composite end point incorporating perforation, gastric-outlet obstruction, or upper GI bleeding and referred to as "clinically significant upper GI event" (CSUGIE). Because of controversy around the reporting of the CLASS outcomes in the journal publication [53], we chose to present data from the more comprehensive set submitted to the FDA [68,69].

The CLASS data show that, after a mean treatment duration of 6 months, patients receiving celecoxib had a lower rate of clinically significant upper GI events (0.28%) than those receiving diclofenac or ibuprofen (0.45% and 0.55%, respectively), but the differences were not statistically significant. At 6-month follow-up, celecoxib recipients also had lower rates for the secondary combined outcome measure of CSUGIE or symptomatic gastroduodenal ulcer (0.75%, 1.0%, and 1.5%, respectively; $P = 0.02$ for celecoxib versus pooled NSAIDS). It is important to note, however, that in the 20% of CLASS patients using cardioprotective ASA, there were no significant differences in any of these key outcomes. Although this study was not designed to measure efficacy, these outcomes were also similar between groups: 14.8% of NSAID recipients and 12.6% of celecoxib recipients withdrew due to unsatisfactory treatment effect [69].

Table 3, a summary of GI events seen in the CLASS study (compiled from FDA data), shows that adverse events were relatively common in all three study groups, and that celecoxib recipients suffered fewer events at all time intervals, but that the differences seen were very small. This table also suggests that, for the treatment durations of 7 to 28 days that emergency physicians are likely to prescribe, differences between groups were negligible.

Table 3
Gastrointestinal (GI) adverse events in the CLASS trial

Adverse event	Celecoxib 400 bid	Diclofenac 75 bid	Ibuprofen 800 tid	NNT
Any GI AE	17.5%	22.4%	16.7%	50
GI AE causing withdrawal	7.5%	9.6%	7.5%	100
CSUGIE within 7 days	0%	0.1%	0.1%	1000
CSUGIE within 28 days	0.03%	0.25%	0.20%	500
CSUGIE within 6 mo	0.28%	0.45%	0.55%	450
CSUGIE within 1 yr	0.43%	0.50%	0.55%	1000
Ulcer[a] or CSUGIE within 6 mo	0.75%	1.0%	1.5%	200
Ulcer[a] or CSUGIE within 1 yr	1.1%	1.3%	1.8%	220

Abbreviations: AE, adverse event; bid, twice daily; CSUGIE, clinically significant upper GI event (perforation, obstruction, bleeding); mo, months; tid, three times daily; yr, years.

[a] ulcer symptomatic.

Data from Witter J. NDA-20 998/S-009 Celebrex capsules (Celecoxib) medical officer review. Sept. 20, 2000. Available at: http://www.fda.gov/ohrms/dockets/ac/01/briefing/3677b1_03_med.pdf. Accessed January 29, 2004.

Table 4 shows that there were no clinically relevant differences between the three treatment groups for renal effects, changes in blood chemistry (blood urea nitrogen [BUN], creatinine, electrolytes), or cardiovascular adverse events.

In the VIGOR trial [54], 8076 RA patients were randomized to rofecoxib (50 mg/d) or naproxen (500 mg twice a day) over a treatment period of 9 months. Most were older women, 60% were on long-term steroids, and 8% had prior peptic ulcer disease. Patients who had renal failure, recent coronary artery bypass surgery, or myocardial infarction were excluded, as were those taking ASA. The primary outcome measure was the incidence of confirmed upper GI events.

The VIGOR data suggest that effectiveness was similar for the two drugs, and that the same proportion of patients in each group withdrew from the study because of adverse effects or lack of efficacy [54]. Table 5 shows that rofecoxib caused fewer symptomatic ulcers and GI bleeds, but that it was associated with a higher rate of serious vascular events, including acute myocardial infarction, unstable angina, pulmonary embolism, transient ischemic attack, stroke, and vascular death. It is interesting that the absolute reduction in the rate of complicated ulcers (0.5%) was similar to the absolute increase in the rate of serious vascular events (0.6%).

Cyclooxygenase-2 inhibitors and serious vascular events

NSAIDS and COX-2 agents differ in their antiplatelet effects. Platelet aggregation inhibition is approximately 93% with naproxen, 92% with ASA, 80% with ibuprofen, 40% with diclofenac, and 15% or less with COX-2 agents [15]. COX-2 agents clearly lack a beneficial antiplatelet effect in patients at risk, and may have a prothrombotic effect based on differential inhibition of prostacyclin compared with thromboxane. In the VIGOR trial, 45 (1.1%) of 4047 rofecoxib recipients and 20 (0.5%) of 4046 naproxen recipients suffered serious vascular events, as described above (relative risk [RR] = 2.38; 95% CI, 1.39–4.0), whereas in the CLASS study, no

Table 4
Renal adverse events occurring during entire CLASS study period

Adverse event	Celecoxib	Diclofenac	Ibuprofen	NNT
Hypertension	2.0%	2.0%	3.1%*	200
Generalized edema	0.5%	0.6%	1.0%*	300
Peripheral edema	3.7%	3.5%	5.2%*	150
Cardiac failure	0.3%	0.2%	0.5%	667
Increased BUN	1.1%	1.7%	0.9%	500

* $P < 0.05$ versus celecoxib.

Data from Witter J. NDA-20 998/S-009 Celebrex capsules (Celecoxib) medical officer review. Sept. 20, 2000. Available at: http://www.fda.gov/ohrms/dockets/ac/01/briefing/3677b1_03_med.pdf. Accessed January 29, 2004.

Table 5
Important outcomes in the VIGOR trial

Outcome	Rofecoxib	Naproxen	RR (95% CI)	ARR/ARI	NNT/NNH[a]
Symptomatic ulcer	1.0%	2.1%	0.5 (0.3–0.7)	1.1	91
Complicated ulcer[b]	0.4%	0.9%	0.4 (0.2–0.8)	0.5	200
AE causing withdrawal	16.4%	16.1%	1.02 (0.9–1.1)	0.3	333
Acute MI	0.4%	0.1%	4.0 (1.3–12)	0.3	333
Serious vascular event[c]	1.1%	0.5%	2.38 (1.4–4.0)	0.6	167

Abbreviations: ARI, absolute risk increase; MI, myocardial infarction; NNH, number needed to harm.

[a] For 9 months.

[b] Complicated ulcer = ulcer with perforation or bleeding.

[c] Serious vascular event = acute myocordial infarction, unstable angine, pulmonary embolism, transient ischemic attack, stroke, or vascular death.

cardiovascular hazard was apparent. Mukherjee and associates [15] suggested that acute myocardial infarction (AMI) rates in VIGOR and CLASS were higher than those seen in a large cardiovascular risk meta-analysis, and therefore that COX-2 agents posed a potential cardiovascular hazard; however, no adjustment was made for age or comorbidity, and it is not clear that the patient populations compared are in fact comparable. It is possible that COX-2 agents may increase cardiovascular event rates. If so, the mechanism, the level of increased risk, and the differential toxicity of specific COX-2 agents remain unclear. Physicians should be aware of this potential effect, and assure that patients who have indications for antiplatelet prophylaxis receive an appropriate antiplatelet agent whether or not they are treated with a COX-2 inhibitor.

Specific agents

The best studied COX-2 inhibitors currently available are celecoxib and rofecoxib. Newer, highly selective COX-2 agents include valdecoxib and parecoxib (see Table 2). Trials in dental, gynecologic, and orthopedic pain suggest that these newer highly selective drugs have a similar efficacy to NSAIDS, but fewer GI adverse effects and a prolonged action duration that enables once-daily dosing [69,70]. Like NSAIDS, all of the COX-2 agents have additive effects with morphine and show morphine-sparing effects in acute pain models.

Parecoxib, an intravenous prodrug that is metabolized to valdecoxib, is the first COX-2 agent available in North America that can be given by the IV and intramuscular (IM) routes, providing an opportunity for IV-to-oral progression. In dental, gynecologic, and orthopedic pain, parecoxib (20 mg IV or IM) provided a similar degree and duration of analgesia to intravenous ketorolac (30–60 mg), and more prolonged analgesia than IV morphine (4 mg). Parecoxib (40 mg IV) provided a longer duration of analgesia than morphine or ketorolac [70–73].

Dosing

Celecoxib

Celecoxib is administered orally as a single daily dose or two divided doses. In osteoarthritis trials, daily and twice-daily regimens were equally effective, but this may or may not be true in acute pain. Dosing should be adjusted according to the patient's response, starting at 100 mg twice a day, titrating to effect, and using the lowest effective dose, up to 400 mg twice daily in rare instances.

Rofecoxib

Rofecoxib is available in 12.5 mg, 25 mg, and 50 mg tablets, as well as 12.5 mg/5 mL and 25 mg/5 mL oral suspension. It is administered orally as a single daily dose—most often 25 or 50 mg. Dosage should be adjusted based on individual pain response, using the lowest effective dosage.

Meloxicam

Meloxicam is available as 7.5 and 15 mg tablets. The initial and typical maintenance dosage in adults is 7.5 mg once daily, although doses up to 15 mg/day may provide additional analgesia. As with other agents, the lowest effective dosage for the shortest feasible duration should be used.

Valdecoxib

Valdecoxib is available as 10 and 20 mg tablets. The recommended dosage in adults is 10 to 20 mg once daily. As with other agents, the lowest effective dosage for the shortest feasible duration should be used.

Parecoxib

Parecoxib can be administered as an IM or IV injection in doses of 20 to 40 mg.

Comments and controversies

Unfortunately, COX-2 agents have not been studied in the ED setting. Existing studies from diverse settings use different drugs, different doses, different end points, and different end-point detection methods in diverse patient populations. In addition, they tend to describe adverse events that occur over time periods that are much longer than emergency physicians are likely to prescribe for. Given these limitations, the evidence suggests that COX-2 agents are effective in acute pain, and that they have similar efficacy to NSAID comparators. They are well-tolerated, but cause similar rates of minor GI side effects as traditional NSAIDS. They cause significantly fewer endoscopic ulcers than nonselective NSAIDS, but the clinical importance of these lesions is uncertain. As the selectivity hypothesis predicts, COX-2 agents cause fewer symptomatic ulcers (NNT $\sim$ 100) and slightly fewer bleeding ulcers than nonselective NSAIDS, although the incidence of the latter is very low and the NNT (to prevent one GI bleed) is very high: between 200 to 1000. COX-2 agents are equally likely to cause serious (GI + cardiovascular) adverse events, but these events are uncommon with short treatment durations.

Rofecoxib has been associated with a higher rate of AMI and major vascular events. This may or may not be a class effect; therefore patients eligible for cardiovascular prophylaxis should receive low-dose ASA, recognizing that it reduces thrombotic risk and increases ulcer and bleeding risk.

COX-2 inhibitors have renal effects similar to nonspecific NSAIDS. Both types of drugs should be used with caution in patients who have renal compromise, heart failure, and hypertension. These agents should be considered part of a pain strategy that involves acetaminophen, traditional NSAIDS, COX-2 agents, opioids, and perhaps other analgesics. When used for acute pain, all agents should be prescribed in the lowest effective dose for the shortest time necessary, particularly in elderly and debilitated patients.

Opioid analgesics

Description

Opioids are an essential component of severe pain management and the most important class of analgesics for emergency physicians to be familiar with [74]. Titrated intravenous opioids remain the treatment of choice for most patients who have acute severe pain [75,76], and oral opioids are a mainstay for outpatient management of moderate to severe pain. In recent years, increasing physician awareness of pain management principles has led to increasing use of potent opioids such as fentanyl, oxycodone, hydromorphone, and morphine, yet ED studies continue to suggest that emergency physicians undertreat acute pain [1].

Pharmacology

Opioids bind to receptors in the central nervous system and suppress neuronal pain transmission. In addition, they alter thalamocortical processing of pain signals to modify the subjective experience of pain [2]. The three primary opioid receptors are mu, kappa, and delta receptors. Mu receptors, named for morphine, mediate analgesia, respiratory depression, euphoria, and dependence; kappa receptors mediate analgesia, sedation, and dysphoria; and delta receptors mediate analgesia and mood effects. In addition to their analgesic properties, opioids suppress the medullary cough center (antitussive effects) and decrease the CO2 responsiveness of the medullary respiratory center. This impairs respiratory drive and relieves the sensation of breathlessness (antidyspnea effects). Opioids also activate the chemoreceptor trigger zone and cause nausea and vomiting. In the GI and urinary tract, opioid receptors inhibit bowel motility (antidiarrheal effect) and may cause urinary retention. Opioids produce differing degrees of histamine release, with resultant pruritis, urticaria, and postural hypotension. The ability of opioids to produce euphoria and dependence generates concerns about abuse and addiction. Many patients fear becoming addicted to opioids, and many physicians avoid opioids out of concern about drug abuse. Unfortunately, these legitimate concerns, coupled with limited pharmacological awareness, have led to underprescribing and underdosing, and are a significant roadblock to the appropriate use of opioids for pain management [74].

Opioids provide dose-dependent central analgesia with variable sedation and anxiolysis. Because they lack the "ceiling" effect of other analgesics, opioid titration can relieve any level of pain; hence, the correct opioid dose is not a standard dose or a weight-based dose; it is the dose that relieves the pain. In terms of analgesic efficacy, there is little difference between the different mu receptor agonists. Any of the opioids discussed below can relieve severe pain if they can be tolerated in adequate doses; however, with some agents, notably codeine, limiting side effects appear at relatively low doses. Consequently, when determining the best drug for a specific patient, physicians should consider individual differences, patient experience, and adverse effect profile [77–79].

Mixed opioid agonist-antagonists such as pentazocine, butorphanol, and nalbuphine are not recommended. Their efficacy is limited by a ceiling effect, they have a high rate of adverse effects, and they may cause withdrawal syndromes in patients already using pure agonist opioids [80]. The pure agonist opioids (codeine, hydrocodone, hydromorphone, morphine, and oxycodone) are preferred for acute pain management. These are considered short- or intermediate-acting drugs, and their clinical effects correspond with peak serum levels: Maximal analgesia occurs 60 to 90 minutes after oral dosing, 30 minutes after IM injection, and 6 minutes after IV injection. Significant first-pass metabolism means that oral doses must be substantially higher than parenteral doses to achieve equivalent analgesia (Table 6). In general, the pure opioid agonists are first conjugated in the liver, then the (generally active) metabolites are excreted by the kidneys [80].

Maximum pain control for any given drug and dose is achieved when serum levels reach steady state—at about five half-lives if the drug is dosed regularly. The most effective way to relieve acute continuous pain is therefore to administer short acting opioids on the half-life (ie, every 4-hours rather than merely "as needed") [80]. Using the immediate-release pure opioids listed above, administered on the half-life, steady state can be achieved within 24 hours. As a general rule, shorter-acting strong opioids should be prescribed initially to rapidly control pain and to estimate the daily opioid requirement; then, if ongoing treatment is required, a switch to a longer acting (slow-release) agent is appropriate. When treating acute

Table 6
Analgesic equivalence table

Agent	Dose equivalent to 10 mg morphine (IM)	
	Parenteral	Oral
Morphine sulphate	10 mg	60 mg[a]
Meperidine	100 mg	300 mg
Codeine	120 mg	200–250 mg
Hydrocodone	15 mg	30 mg
Hydromorphone	1.5 mg	8 mg
Oxycodone	15 mg	30 mg
Fentanyl	0.1 mg	NA

[a] For chronic dosing, morphine's oral/IM ratio is approximately 3/1, not 6/1.

Data from Jovey RD. Opioid Analgesics. In: Jovey RD, editor. Managing pain. Toronto (Canada): Healthcare and Financial Publishing, for the Canadian Pain Society; 2002. p. 47–61.

severe pain, it is best to avoid transdermal or delayed release oral formulations, because delayed onset may lead patients to take additional doses before appreciating the effect of the first dose, and prolonged action duration may cause dangerous-dose "stacking" effects [76]. Table 7 lists equivalent doses of opioids for acute pain management.

Specific agents

Morphine

Morphinelike opioids are the foundation of effective pain management [75]. Based on effectiveness, relative lack of toxicity, and longer duration of analgesia—approximately 4 hours compared with meperidine's 2 to 3—morphine is the opioid of first choice for acute severe pain in the ED. Oral morphine preparations are an effective option for moderate and severe outpatient pain, but for acute dosing, it is important to remember that morphine is largely eliminated by first-pass metabolism, with only about 20% of the ingested dose reaching the tissue level. Consequently, oral doses are approximately five times parenteral doses. Table 8 compares standard parenteral doses of morphine to other drugs.

Table 7
Equivalent doses of opioids for acute pain management

Drug	Intramuscular dose	Oral dose
Morphine	10 milligrams	60 milligrams
Meperidine	100 milligrams	300 milligrams
Hydromorphone[a]	2 milligrams	8 milligrams
Codeine	60 milligrams	180 milligrams
Hydrocodone		20 milligrams
Oxycodone		20 milligrams
Fentanyl	0.15 milligrams	

[a] 2 mg hydromorphone po is equivalent to 10 mg morphine solution orally.

Table 8
All drugs compared to standard dose morphine 10 mg IM or 20–30 mg po

	Parenteral			
Drug	PO dose	Dose (IM or SC)	PR dose	Dose frequency
Codeine	200 mg	120 mg		every 4 hours
Oxycodone				
- Percocet (Acet.)	10–15 mg			every 4 hours
- Percodan (ASA)	(2–3 tabs)			
Hydromorphone	4 mg	2 mg	3 mg	every 4 hours
- Dilaudid				
- Sustained Release Capsule		2 × 6 mg	every 12 hours	
Morphine				
- solution (MOS)	20–30 mg			every 4 hours
- MS Contin/MOS-SR	60–90 mg			every 12 hours
- suppository			10, 20 or 30 mg	every 6–8 hours
- injectable		10 mg		every 4 hours
Fentanyl				
Avoid:				
Merperidine	300 mg	75 mg		
- Demerol				

Abbreviations: SC, subcutaneous; Acet, acetaminophen; MOS-SR, morphine sulphate-slow release; PO, per os; PR, per rectum.

Morphine is mainly metabolized by hepatic glucuronidation to several metabolites, including morphine 6-glucuronide (M6G) and morphine 3-glucuronide (M3G), which are eliminated in the urine (Fig. 1). M6G is a more potent analgesic than morphine, and contributes to therapeutic and opioid effects. M3G, known to cause significant central nervous system (CNS) toxicity, including tremors, myoclonic jerks, delirium, and seizures, actually antagonizes morphine's analgesic effects [76]. With repeated administration, particularly in elderly patients and those who have limited renal function, M6G and M3G may accumulate, producing enhanced opioid effects and CNS toxicity.

Like other opioids, morphine causes pruritus, nausea, constipation, and dizziness. Morphine is one of the stronger histamine releasers, and may cause transient urticaria. It is common to see localized urticaria tracking along forearm veins after intravenous morphine administration, but this finding usually resolves quickly without treatment, and by itself should not be construed as an allergic reaction.

Although by itself morphine is a potent and extremely effective analgesic, there is evidence that it can be combined with simple analgesics in an effective multimodal approach to pain. In a double-blind randomized trial, Schug and coworkers [3] compared morphine patient-controlled analgesia (MPCA) with and without acetaminophen in a cohort of postorthopedic surgery patients. Patient satisfaction was significantly higher and mean pain

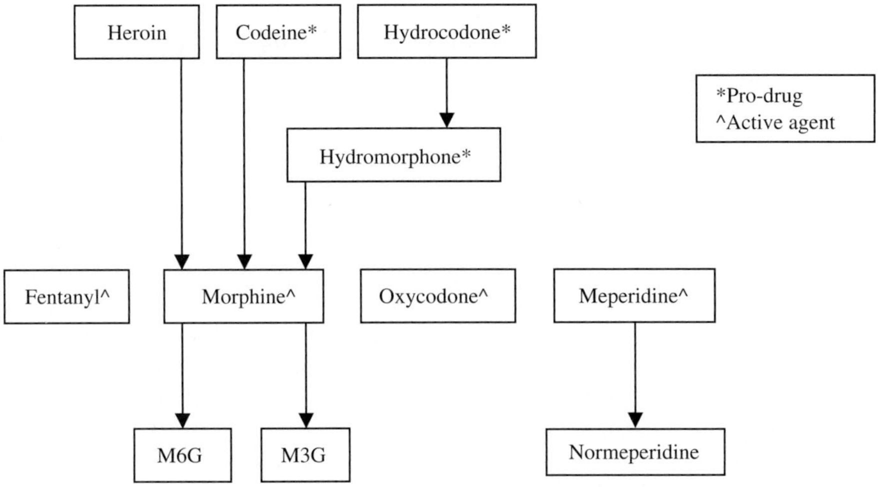

Fig. 1. Pure opioid agonists and key breakdown products.

scores lower when acetaminophen was added to the MPCA regimen. In addition, patients receiving acetaminophen used 16% less self-administered morphine, although the latter difference did not achieve statistical significance.

Some physicians tend to avoid morphine because of historic teaching that it causes more biliary and ureteral spasm than meperidine. Evidence suggests, however, that all opioids cause some smooth-muscle spasm, and that equianalgesic doses of morphine and meperidine have similar effects on renal and biliary smooth muscle. This evidence reduces the "biliary spasm" concept to the level of a medical myth, and mitigates morphine's main perceived disadvantage [81].

Morphine formulations and dosing

There are a large range of morphine preparations available. Those most relevant to acute ED pain management include morphine oral solution, morphine immediate-release tablets (10, 20, and 30 mg) and parenteral morphine for subcutaneous, IM, or IV administration. MS Contin and MOS-SR, or M-ESLON sustained-release preparations are available in strengths of 15, 30, 60, 100, and 200 mg. These are convenient in that they can be given every 12 hours, but they are more appropriate for chronic pain involving prolonged administration. An average oral morphine (immediate release) starting dose in adults is 10 mg orally every 3 to 4 hours as needed, but doses of 20 to 30 mg every 4 hours may be reasonable, depending on patient characteristics and pain severity. An average adult subcutaneous or IM dose is 10 mg (0.15 mg/kg) every 3 or 4 hours. The treatment of choice for acute severe pain in the emergency department is 2.5 to 5 mg IV every 5 to 10 minutes, titrated to effect.

Meperidine (Demerol)

Historically, meperidine is one of the most commonly used agents for the ED treatment of acute pain; however, in recent years, meperidine has fallen from favor and its use has decreased significantly, whereas the use of other opioids has increased [74]. This move away from meperidine may reflect an increasing awareness of its many shortcomings, which include poor bioavailability, a brief duration of analgesia (only 2–3 hours), and toxic side effects [75]. In addition, meperidine is poorly absorbed from the GI tract, and variably absorbed after IM injection, making its effects unpredictable and often inadequate. There is some evidence that meperidine is a less effective analgesic than morphinelike opioids [82]. In addition, oral meperidine is poorly absorbed, and the most commonly prescribed oral dose—50 mg—is no more effective than 650 mg of aspirin or acetaminophen.

When scientists first synthesized meperidine, their intention was to produce an anticholinergic agent; hence meperidine blocks muscarinic receptors and has significant anticholinergic effects, notably visual blurring, constipation, tachycardia, and dry mouth. Central manifestations may include agitation, confusion, delirium, disorientation, and visual hallucinations [83]. In addition, meperidine or its breakdown product normeperidine blocks the reuptake of serotonin and norepinephrine, potentially leading to an overabundance of these neurotransmitters and to clinical consequences related to CNS excitation. As a result, meperidine has been associated with serotonin syndrome [84], and it is contraindicated in patients receiving monoamine oxidase inhibitors, in whom it may precipitate severe hypertensive crises.

In the liver, meperidine is metabolized by the cytochrome P-450 system to normeperidine, a neurotoxic nonopioid metabolite that has weak analgesic effects and potent CNS excitatory effects. These are manifested by anxiety, confusion, dysphoria, hallucinations, hyperreflexia, myoclonus, and occasionally seizures [75,81,85]. Because first-pass metabolism converts much of the active drug to its toxic metabolite, normeperidine blood levels are higher in patients using oral meperidine than in those on parenteral therapy [86]. Although meperidine has a relatively short elimination half-life of 3 to 4 hours, normeperidine has a prolonged half-life of 24 to 48 hours; therefore repeated dosing leads to accumulation and increasing neurotoxicity, particularly in the elderly and in patients with renal dysfunction. The combination of anticholinergic, serotonergic, and adrenergic effects explains why meperidine is the only opioid that causes mydriasis rather than miosis, and why it is perhaps the most neurotoxic opioid—a suboptimal therapeutic choice at the best of times and a particularly bad option in older patients. The major cause for concern with meperidine is the rapid accumulation of the neuroexcitatory metabolite, normeperidine. Although all opioids can cause some degree of CNS excitation, most require prolonged use at high doses. Meperidine can produce subtle changes in a matter of hours and significant toxicity within 1 to 2 days. Because normeperidine is not an opioid, opioid antagonists such as naloxone do not reverse neurotoxic symptoms.

It is a long-held medical myth that meperidine is preferable to morphine in patients who have colicky pain, particularly cholelithiasis [76]. This conclusion is not supported by scientific evidence; in fact, when used in equianalgesic doses, meperidine has as much effect on GI smooth muscle as do other opioids. When the neurotoxic side effects are taken into consideration, it is clear that meperidine has several disadvantages, but no advantages, relative to other opioids; therefore meperidine should rarely if ever be considered the opioid of choice for acute pain.

Meperidine formulations and dosing

Meperidine should generally be avoided, and is rarely the drug of choice for acute pain in the ED. It is available in 50 mg tablets, which should not be prescribed because of the many preferable options, and parenteral formulation for IM and IV administration. An average adult subcutaneous or IM dose is 100 mg (1.5 mg/kg) every 2 to 3 hours as needed. Intravenous doses range from 10 to 50 mg IV every 5 to 10 minutes, titrated to effect.

Codeine

Codeine is the most commonly prescribed opioid, usually given in fixed combination with acetaminophen (eg, Tylenol #3). It is a moderately effective analgesic used for mild and moderate pain, but it causes frequent gastrointestinal adverse effects at doses that have limited euphoric and analgesic effect. These adverse effects reduce both its abuse potential and its therapeutic potential. Codeine's analgesic effects are dose-related, but pushing the dosage above 60 mg produces relatively less pain relief and incrementally more constipation, nausea, and sedation [87]. Codeine is absorbed more completely than morphine (roughly 60% bioavailable); however, it is a prodrug with minimal analgesic effect until it metabolized by hepatic enzymes to morphine and other active metabolites. Unfortunately, 10% of the population are genetically poor metabolizers and experience toxicity, but not pain relief, with codeine. Common side effects include pruritus, nausea, constipation, and dizziness.

Codeine acts additively with acetaminophen, and acetaminophen-codeine combinations are more effective than either drug used alone; however, the evidence is less convincing for codeine-ASA combinations, in which the addition of codeine provides only a small improvement in analgesia relative to ASA alone [87].

In a meta-analysis of 40 trials of moderate to severe dental and postsurgical pain, Moore et al [88] compared the analgesic efficacy of several acetaminophen codeine combinations, presenting their results in terms of the number needed to treat to achieve one additional patient with greater than 50% pain relief. In this analysis, acetaminophen (1000 mg) was more effective than placebo, with an NNT of 4.6, meaning that it is necessary to treat 4.6 patients (with acetaminophen instead of placebo) to have one more patient with at least 50% pain relief. In a similar comparison of acetaminophen-codeine (650 mg/60 mg) versus placebo, the NNT to achieve one additional patient with 50% pain relief was 3.6. These authors concluded that increasing codeine doses up to 60 mg increased pain relief, but that increasing the dose beyond this level led to a disproportionate increase in adverse effects.

Codeine formulations and dosing

Codeine is available as codeine syrup (5 mg/ml), codeine tablets (15, 30, and 60 mg) and codeine phosphate injection (15, 30, and 60 mg/ml). Tylenol 1, 2, and 3 tablets contain 300 mg acetaminophen and 15 mg caffeine, as well as 8, 15, and 30 mg of codeine, respectively. Atasol 15 and 30 tablets contain 300 mg acetaminophen and 30 mg caffeine, as well as 15 and 30 mg of codeine, respectively. Empracet 30 and 60 contain 300 mg acetaminophen with 30 and 60 mg of codeine, but Empracet contains no caffeine, thus may be preferable if insomnia is a concern. Usual codeine dosing is 30 to 60 mg of codeine orally, every 4 to 6 hours as needed. Codeine dosage is limited by GI side effects, and by the acetaminophen content of combination products.

Hydrocodone

Hydrocodone, also a prodrug, is hepatically metabolized to hydromorphone. This drug is often used as an antitussive, but it offers better analgesia with fewer GI adverse effects than codeine. Like codeine, hydrocodone is often combined with simple analgesics such as acetaminophen and ibuprofen, because the combination provides better pain relief than the component analgesics [4,89]. In studies of acute musculoskeletal pain and dental surgery, a hydrocodone-acetaminophen (5 mg/500 mg) combination provided comparable pain relief to a codeine-acetaminophen (30 mg/500 mg) [4,89]. In these studies, hydrocodone caused more drowsiness and dizziness, but fewer GI side effects. In postoperative abdominal surgery studies, hydrocodone-ibuprofen combinations (7.5 mg/200 mg and 15 mg/400 mg) provided better and faster analgesia than corresponding doses of the component drugs used alone [90,91].

Hydrocodone formulations and dosing

Hydrocodone-acetaminophen and hydrocodone-ibuprofen combinations are available as described above. The usual hydrocodone dose range is 5 to 20 mg orally every 4 to 6 hours as needed. Hydrocodone-acetaminophen combinations are limited by adverse effects and acetaminophen content. These compounds are usually prescribed as one or two tablets orally every 4 hours as needed.

Hydromorphone (Dilaudid)

Like codeine, hydromorphone is a prodrug that is metabolized in the liver to morphine. It is effective for moderate and severe pain. Analgesic effects and side effects are dose-related, and its adverse effect profile is similar to other potent mu receptor agonists. Nausea, drowsiness, and pruritus are the most frequent adverse effects, and hydromorphone causes relatively little GI upset [77]. Elderly patients and those who have renal impairment tend to tolerate hydromorphone better than morphine, with less drowsiness and cognitive impairment [92]. Ironically, its euphoric effects and favorable adverse effect profile contribute to a higher abuse potential [77].

With respect to analgesic efficacy and adverse effects, hydromorphone is similar to oxycodone and morphine [77]. A systematic review of 32 acute pain studies comparing hydromorphone and morphine in patients who had postoperative pain, acute trauma pain, burns, biliary colic and ureteral colic concluded that there are no significant differences in terms of efficacy, adverse effects, and patient preference when the two drugs are administered in equianalgesic doses. Conversely, four studies using meperidine as a comparator suggested that hydromorphone provided better analgesia without a increase in adverse effects [77].

Hydromorphone formulations and dosing

Hydromorphone is available in 1, 2, 4, and 8 mg tablets, 3 mg suppositories, and injectable solution. Sustained-release hydromorphone capsules (3 mg and 6 mg) and long-acting Hydromorph Contin are available, but are less appropriate for acute ED pain management. Usual hydromorphone doses are 4 to 8 mg orally every 3 to 4 hours, 1 or 2 mg IM every 3 to 4 hours as needed, or 1 mg IV every 10 minutes titrated to effect.

Oxycodone

Oxycodone is a strong opioid agonist, available in short- or long-acting formulations, and in combination with acetaminophen (Percocet) or ASA (Percodan). Oxycodone preparations are useful for the management of moderate and severe pain. At equianalgesic doses, they cause relatively fewer GI adverse effects than codeine, but it is important to remember that overuse of combination products may result in significant ASA or acetaminophen toxicity. Oxycodone's favorable adverse effect profile, along with its euphoric effects, give it a higher abuse potential.

Analgesic effects are very dose-dependent: A Cochrane meta-analysis [81] showed that, although oxycodone 5 mg is not statistically better than placebo, doses of 10 to 15 mg, with or without acetaminophen, have similar efficacy to IM morphine and NSAIDS. Pooled studies of oxycodone 15 mg versus placebo, in patients who had moderate to severe postoperative pain, show an NNT of 2.4 to achieve one additional patient with 50% pain relief. Oxycodone-acetaminophen (10 mg/650 mg) showed similar superiority over placebo in postabdominal surgery and dental pain patients, with an NNT of 2.2. A dose-response analysis by Edwards and colleagues [78] indicated that oxycodone 15 mg, oxycodone-acetaminophen (5 mg/325 mg), and oxycodone-acetaminophen (10 mg/650 mg) have similar efficacy, which suggests that, in the presence of acetaminophen, oxycodone dosage can be lowered without loss of efficacy. Oxycodone's most common adverse effects are nausea, headache, dizziness, and drowsiness, which are dose-related and rarely severe. At a dose of 5 mg, oxycodone has a similar rate of adverse effects as placebo, but oxycodone 10 mg or 15 mg caused significantly more drowsiness, nausea, and vomiting (RR = 1.8–2.8) [78]. In a recent study of osteoarthritis patients who had NSAID-resistant pain [93], controlled-release oxycodone provided similar analgesia to but less nausea than an immediate-release oxycodone/acetaminophen combination. Both of these active treatments were superior to placebo.

Oxycodone formulations and dosing

Typical oxycodone dosing is 5 to 20 mg every 4 hours as needed. Oxycodone-acetaminophen preparations include Percocet 2.5/325 (5 mg oxycodone/325 mg acetaminophen), Percocet-5/325, Percocet-7.5/500, and Percocet-10/650. Oxycodone-ASA is available as Percodan (5 mg oxycodone/325 mg ASA).

Percocet and Percodan dosing are limited by acetaminophen and ASA content, and they are usually prescribed as one or two tablets every four hours as needed. OxyContin is the sustained release form of oxycodone. It is available in 10 mg, 20 mg, 40 mg, 80 mg, and 160 mg tablet strengths, and is usually administered on a twice-daily basis. Because of problems with dependency, misuse, and diversion, this formulation has generated a great deal of controversy.

Fentanyl

Fentanyl is a synthetic opioid that is highly lipid soluble, giving it a rapid onset within 2 to 3 minutes. Because of rapid redistribution from the CNS into tissues, its clinical duration of action is only 30 minutes, and its elimination half-life is 3 hours, slightly longer than that of morphine. Consequently, after prolonged fentanyl infusions or repeated dosing, when tissue sites are saturated, drug accumulation and toxicity may occur, but this is unlikely after acute dosing in the emergency department. Fentanyl causes less histamine release than morphinelike opioids, and hence produces fewer hemodynamic effects and less hypotension. This makes it a good choice for rapid titration analgesia in ED patients who may be volume-depleted or hemodynamically unstable. The recommended dose is 1 ug/kg given slowly every 3 to 5 minutes, titrated to effect.

Transdermal fentanyl patches (Duragesic) are available for patients who have GI absorption problems or poor compliance with oral regimens. These are a long-acting formulation that takes days to reach steady state after initiating or discontinuing, hence they are rarely appropriate for acute ED pain management [94].

The most appropriate formulation and dosing of fentanyl for acute ED pain management is rapid IV titration, as described above.

Nurse-initiated opioid protocols

Traditionally, ED patients who have acute painful conditions wait for physician assessment before receiving potent analgesics. In settings with experienced ED nurses, nurse-initiated IV morphine protocols for stable adult patients who have acute painful conditions are associated with more rapid and satisfactory pain control, with a low and acceptable rate of complications. Protocols involve IV morphine given as 2.5 mg boluses every 5 minutes until the patient is comfortable, up to 0.1 mg/kg [95].

References

[1] Todd KH, Sloan EP, Chen C, et al. Survey of pain etiology, management practices and patient satisfaction in two urban emergency departments. Can J Emerg Med 2002;4:252–6.
[2] Besson JM. The neurobiology of pain. Lancet 1999;353:1610–5.
[3] Schug SA, Sidebotham DA, McGuinnety M, et al. Acetaminophen as an adjunct to morphine by patient-controlled analgesia in the management of acute postoperative pain. Anesth Analg 1998;87:368–72.
[4] Barkin R. Acetaminophen, aspirin, or ibuprofen in combination analgesic products. Am J Ther 2001;8:433–42.
[5] McEvoy GK. American hospital formulary service. Bethesda (MD): American Society of Health System Pharmacists; 2003.
[6] Bijlsma JW. Analgesia and the patient with osteoarthritis. Am J Ther 2002;9:189–97.
[7] Bradley JD, Brandt KD, Katz BP, et al. Comparison of an antiinflammatory dose of ibuprofen, an analgesic dose of ibuprofen, and acetaminophen in the treatment of patients with osteoarthritis of the knee. N Engl J Med 1991;325:87–91.
[8] Wenzel RG, Sarvis CA, Krause ML. Over-the-counter drugs for acute migraine attacks: literature review and recommendations. Pharmacotherapy 2003;23:494–505.
[9] Williams HJ, Ward JR, Egger MJ, et al. Comparison of naproxen and acetaminophen in a two-year study of treatment of osteoarthritis of the knee. Arthritis Rheum 1993;36: 1196–206.
[10] Hylek EM, Heiman H, Skates SJ, et al. Acetaminophen and other risk factors for excessive warfarin anticoagulation. JAMA 1998;279:657–62.
[11] Schoenfeld P, Kimmey MB, Scheiman J, et al. Review article: nonsteroidal anti-inflammatory drug-associated gastrointestinal complications—guidelines for prevention and treatment. Aliment Pharmacol Ther 1999;13:1273–85.
[12] Loewen PS. Review of the selective COX-2 inhibitors celecoxib and rofecoxib: focus on clinical aspects. Can J Emerg Med 2002;4:268–75.
[13] Feldman M, McMahon AT. Do cyclooxygenase-2 inhibitors provide benefits similar to those of traditional nonsteroidal anti-inflammatory drugs, with less gastrointestinal toxicity? Ann Intern Med 2000;132:134–43.
[14] Lipsky PE, Brooks P, Crofford LJ, et al. Unresolved issues in the role of cyclooxygenase-2 in normal physiologic processes and disease. Arch Intern Med 2000;160:913–20.
[15] Mukherjee D, Nissen SE, Topol E. Risk of cardiovascular events associated with selective COX-2 inhibitors. JAMA 2001;286:954–9.
[16] Gutthann SP. Nonsteroidal anti-inflammatory drugs and the risk of hospitalization for acute renal failure. Arch Intern Med 1996;156:2433–9.
[17] Repchinsky C, editor. Compendium of pharmaceutical specialties. Ottawa (Canada): Canadian Pharmacists Association; 2003.
[18] Catapano MS. The analgesic efficacy of ketorolac for acute pain. J Emerg Med 1996;1: 67–75.

[19] Wood VM, Christenson J, Innes GD, et al. The NARC (nonsteroidal anti-inflammatory in renal colic) trial: single dose intravenous ketorolac vs. titrated intravenous meperidine in acute renal colic. Can J Emerg Med 2000;2:83–9.

[20] Larsen LS, Miller A, Allegra JR. The use of intravenous ketorolac for the treatment of renal colic in the emergency department. Am J Emerg Med 1993;11:197–9.

[21] Koenig KL, Hodgson L, Kozak R, et al. Ketorolac vs meperidine for the management of pain in the emergency department. Acad Emerg Med 1994;1:544–9.

[22] Innes GD, Croskerry P, Worthington J, et al. Ketorolac versus acetaminophen-codeine in the emergency department treatment of back pain. J Emerg Med 1998;16:549–56.

[23] Larkin GL, Peacock WF 4th, Pearl SM, et al. Efficacy of ketorolac tromethamine versus meperidine in the ED treatment of acute renal colic. Am J Emerg Med 1999;17:6–10.

[24] Veenema KR, Leahey N, Schneider S. Ketorolac versus meperidine: ED treatment of severe musculoskeletal low back pain. Am J Emerg Med 2000;18:404–7.

[25] Dula DJ, Anderson R, Wood GC. A prospective study comparing i.m. ketorolac with i.m. meperidine in the treatment of acute biliary colic. J Emerg Med 2001;20:525–34.

[26] Meredith JT, Wait S, Brewer KL. A prospective double-blind study of nasal sumatriptan versus IV ketorolac in migraine. Am J Emerg Med 2003;21:173–5.

[27] Yealy DM. Ketorolac in the treatment of acute pain. Ann Emerg Med 1992;21:985–6.

[28] Wright JM, Price SD, Watson WA. NSAID use and efficacy in the emergency department: single doses of oral ibuprofen versus intramuscular ketorolac. Ann Pharmacother 1994;28: 309–12.

[29] Turturro MA, Paris PM, Seaberg DC. Intramuscular ketorolac versus oral ibuprofen in acute musculoskeletal pain. Ann Emerg Med 1995;26:117–20.

[30] Neighbor ML, Puntillo KA. Intramuscular ketorolac vs oral ibuprofen in emergency department patients with acute pain. Acad Emerg Med 1998;5:118–22.

[31] Li DK, Liu L, Odouli R. Exposure to non-steroidal anti-inflammatory drugs during pregnancy and risk of miscarriage: population based cohort study. BMJ 2003;327:368.

[32] Wolfe M, Lichtenstein DR, Singh G. Gastrointestinal toxicity of nonsteroidal antiinflammatory drugs. N Engl J Med 1999;340:1888–98.

[33] García Rodriguez LA, Walker AM, Gutthann S. Nonsteroidal antiinflammatory drugs and gastrointestinal hospitalizations in Saskatchewan: a cohort study. Epidemiology 1992;3: 337–42.

[34] Langman MJ, Weil J, Wainwright P, et al. Risks of bleeding peptic ulcer associated with individual non-steroidal anti-inflammatory drugs. Lancet 1994;343:1075–8.

[35] Griffin MR, Piper JM, Daugherty JR, et al. Nonsteroidal anti-inflammatory drug use and increased risk for peptic ulcer disease in elderly persons. Ann Intern Med 1991;114:257–63.

[36] Griffin MR. Epidemiology of nonsteroidal anti-inflammatory drug-associated gastrointestinal injury. Am J Med 1998;104(3A):23S–9S.

[37] Garcia Rodriguez LA, Jick H. Risk of gastrointestinal bleeding and perforation associated with individual non-steroidal anti-inflammatory drugs. Lancet 1994;343:769–72.

[38] Henry D, Lim LLY, Garcia Rodriguez LA, et al. Variability in risk of gastrointestinal complications with individual non-steroidal anti-inflammatory drugs: results of a collaborative meta-analysis. Lancet 1996;312:1563–6.

[39] Taha AS, Hudson N, Hawkey CJ, et al. Famotidine for the prevention of gastric and duodenal ulcers caused by nonsteroidal anti-inflammatory drugs. N Engl J Med 1996;344: 1435–9.

[40] Silverstein FE, Graham DY, Senior JR, et al. Misoprostol reduced serious gastrointestinal complications in patients with rheumatoid arthritis receiving nonsteroidal anti-inflammatory drugs. Ann Intern Med 1995;123:241–9.

[41] Agrawal NM, Campbell DR, Safdi MA, et al. Superiority of lansoprazole vs. ranitidine in healing nonsteroidal anti-inflammatory drug-associated gastric ulcers. Arch Intern Med 2000;160:1455–61.

[42] Hawkey CJ, Karrasch JA, Szczepanski L, et al. Omeprazole compared to misoprostol for ulcers associated with nonsteroidal anti-inflammatory drugs. N Engl J Med 1998;338: 727–34.

[43] Yeomans ND, Tulassay Z, Juhasz L, et al. A comparison of omeprazole with ranitidine for ulcers associated with nonsteroidal anti-inflammatory drugs. N Engl J Med 1998;338: 719–26.

[44] Whelton A. Nephrotoxicity of nonsteroidal anti-inflammatory drugs: physiologic foundations and clinical implications. Am J Med 1999;106(5B):13S–24S.

[45] Bleumink GS, Feenstra J, Sturkenboom MC, et al. Nonsteroidal anti-inflammatory drugs and heart failure. Drugs 2003;63:525–34.

[46] Swan SK, Rudy DW, Lasseter KC, et al. Effect of COX-2 inhibition on renal function in elderly persons receiving a low-salt diet. A randomized controlled trial. Ann Intern Med 2000;133:1–9.

[47] Rossat J, Maillard M, Nussberger J, et al. Renal effects of selective COX-2 inhibition in normotensive salt-depleted subjects. Clin Pharmacol Ther 1999;66:76–84.

[48] Brater DC. Effects of nonsteroidal anti-inflammatory drugs on renal function: focus on COX-2-selective inhibition. Am J Med 1999;107:65S–70S.

[49] Whelton A, Schulman G, Wallemark C, et al. Effects of celecoxib and naproxen on renal function in the elderly. Arch Intern Med 2000;160:1465–70.

[50] Perazella MA, Eras J. Are selective COX-2 inhibitors nephrotoxic? Am J Kidney Dis 2000; 35:937–40.

[51] FitzGerald GA, Patrono C. Drug therapy: the coxibs, selective inhibitors of cyclooxygenase-2. N Engl J Med 2001;345:433–42.

[52] Tannenbaum H, Peloso PMJ, Russel AS, et al. An evidence-based approach to prescribing NSAIDS in the treatment of osteoarthritis and rheumatoid arthritis: the Second Canadian Consensus Conference. Can J Clin Pharmacol 2000;7(Suppl A):4A–16A.

[53] Silverstein FE, Faich G, Goldstein JL, et al. Gastrointestinal toxicity with celecoxib vs nonsteroidal anti-inflammatory drugs for osteoarthritis and rheumatoid arthritis: the CLASS study. A randomized controlled trial. Celecoxib Long-term Arthritis Safety Study. JAMA 2000;284(10):1247–55.

[54] Bombardier C, Laine L, Reicin A, et al, for the VIGOR Study Group. Comparison of upper gastrointestinal toxicity of rofecoxib and naproxen in patients with rheumatoid arthritis. N Engl J Med 2000;343:1520–8.

[55] Lane NE. Pain management in osteoarthritis: the role of COX-2 inhibitors. J Rheumatol 1997;24(Suppl 49):20–4.

[56] Mehlisch DR, Mills S, Sandler M. Ex vivo assay of COX-2 inhibition predicts analgesic efficacy in post-surgical dental pain with MK-966. Clin Pharmacol Ther 1998;63:139.

[57] Morrison BW, Daniels SE, Kotey P, et al. Rofecoxib, a specific COX-2 inhibitor, in primary dysmenorrhea: a randomized controlled trial. Obstet Gynecol 1999;94:504–8.

[58] Erhich EW, Dallob A, De Lepeliere I. Characterization of rofecoxib as a COX-2 isoform inhibitor and demonstration of analgesia in the dental pain model. Clin Pharmacol Ther 1999;65:336–47.

[59] Clemett D, Goa KL. Celecoxib: a review of its use in osteoarthritis, rheumatoid arthritis and acute pain. Drugs 2000;59:957–80.

[60] Reuben SS, Connelly NR. Postoperative analgesic effects of celecoxib or rofecoxib after spinal fusion surgery. Anesth Analg 2000;91:1221–5.

[61] Gimbel JS, Brugger A, Zhao W. Efficacy and tolerability of celecoxib versus hydrocodone/acetaminophen in the treatment of pain after ambulatory orthopedic surgery in adults. Clin Therapeut 2001;23:228–41.

[62] Schwartz JI, Chan CC, Mukhopadhyay S, et al. Cyclooxygenase-2 inhibition by rofecoxib reverses naturally occurring fever in humans. Clin Pharmacol Ther 1999;65: 653–60.

[63] Bensen WG, Zhao SZ, Burke TA, et al. Upper gastrointestinal tolerability of celecoxib, a COX-2 specific inhibitor, compared to naproxen and placebo. J Rheumatol 2000;27: 1876–83.
[64] Laine L, Harper S, Simon T, et al, for the Rofecoxib Osteoarthritis Endoscopy Study Group. Randomized trial comparing the effect of rofecoxib, a cyclooxygenase 2-specific inhibitor, with that of ibuprofen on the gastroduodenal mucosa of patients with osteoarthritis. Gastroenterology 1999;117:776–83.
[65] Goldstein JL, Correa P, Zhao LL, et al. Reduced incidence of gastroduodenal ulcers with celecoxib, a novel cyclooxygenase-2 inhibitor, compared to naproxen in patients with arthritis. Am J Gastroenterol 2001;96:1019–27.
[66] Langman MJ, Jensen DM, Watson DJ, et al. Adverse upper gastrointestinal effects of rofecoxib compared with NSAIDS. JAMA 1999;282:1929–33.
[67] Whelton A, Maurath CJ, Verburg KM. Renal safety and tolerability of celecoxib, a novel cyclooxygenase-2 inhibitor. Am J Ther 2000;7:159–75.
[68] Witter J. NDA-20–998/S-009 Celebrex capsules (Celecoxib) medical officer review. Sept. 20, 2000. Available at: http://www.fda.gov/ohrms/dockets/ac/01/briefing/3677b1_03_med.pdf. Accessed January 29, 2004.
[69] Fricke J, Varkalis J, Zwillich S. Valdecoxib is more efficacious than rofecoxib in relieving pain associated with oral surgery. Am J Ther 2002;9:89–97.
[70] Barden J, Edwards JE, McQuay HJ, et al. Oral valdecoxib and injected parecoxib for acute postoperative pain: a quantitative systematic review BMC Anesthesiology 2003, 3:1. Available at: http://www.biomedcentral.com/1471-2253/3/1. Accessed December 4, 2003.
[71] Daniels SE, Grossman EH, Kuss ME, et al. A double-blind, randomized comparison of intramuscularly and intravenously administered parecoxib sodium versus ketorolac and placebo in a post-oral surgery pain model. Clin Ther 2001;23:1018–31.
[72] Rasmussen GL, Steckner K, Hogue C, et al. Intravenous parecoxib sodium for acute pain after orthopedic knee surgery. Am J Orthop 2002;336–43.
[73] Barton SF, Langeland FF, Snabes MC. Efficacy and safety of intravenous parecoxib sodium in relieving postoperative pain following gynecologic laparotomy surgery. Anesthesiology 2002;97:306–14.
[74] Joranson DE, Ryan KM, Gilson AM, et al. Trends in medical use and abuse of opioid analgesics. JAMA 2000;283(13):1710–4.
[75] Acute Pain Management Guideline Panel. Acute pain management: operative or medical procedures and trauma. In: Clinical practice guideline. AHCPR publication 92–0032. Rockville (MD): Agency for Health Care Policy and Research, Public Health Service, US Dept of Health and Human Services; 1992.
[76] McQuay H, Moore A, Justins D. Treating acute pain in hospital. BMJ 1997;314:1531–5.
[77] Quigley C. Hydromorphone for acute and chronic pain. Cochrane Database Syst Rev 2002;(1):CD003447.
[78] Edwards JE, Moore RA, McQuay HJ. Single dose oxycodone and oxycodone plus acetominophen for acute postoperative pain. Cochrane Database Syst Rev 2000;(4): CD002763.
[79] Jovey RD. Opioid Analgesics. In: Jovey RD, editor. Managing pain. Toronto (Canada): Healthcare and Financial Publishing, for the Canadian Pain Society; 2002. p. 47–61.
[80] Ferris FD, von Gunten CF, Emanuel LL. Ensuring competency in end-of-life care: controlling symptoms. BMC Palliative Care 2002;1:5. Availabale at: http://www.biomedcentral.com/1472-684X/1/5. Accessed January 12, 2004.
[81] Latta K, Ginsberg B, Barkin RL. Meperidine: a critical review. Am J Ther 2002;9:53–68.
[82] Jasani NB, O'Connor RE, Bouzoukis JK. Comparison of hydromorphone and meperidine for ureteral colic. Acad Emerg Med 1994;1:539–43.
[83] Barkin RL, Stein ZLG. Drugs with anticholinergic side effects. South Med J 1989;82:547–8.
[84] Weiner AL. Meperidine as a potential cause of serotonin syndrome in the emergency department. Acad Emerg Med 1999;6:156–8.

[85] Kaiko RF, Foley KM, Grabinski PY. Central nervous system excitatory effects of meperidine in cancer patients. Ann Neurol 1983;13:180–5.
[86] Pond SM, Tong T, Benowitz NL. Presystemic metabolism of meperidine to normeperidine in normal and cirrhotic subjects. Clin Pharmacol Ther 1981;30:183–8.
[87] Moore A, Collins S, Carroll D, et al. Paracetamol with and without codeine in acute pain: a quantitative systematic review. Pain 1997;70:193–201.
[88] Moore A, Collins S, Carroll D, et al. Single dose acetaminophen with and without codeine for postoperative pain. Cochrane Database Syst Rev 2000;(2):CD001547.
[89] Turturro MA, Paris PM, Yealy DM, et al. Hydrocodone versus codeine in acute musculoskeletal pain. Ann Emerg Med 1991;20:1100–3.
[90] Sunshine A, Olsen NZ, O'Neill E, et al. Analgesic efficacy of a hydrocodone with ibuprofen combination compared with ibuprofen alone for the treatment of acute postoperative pain. J Clin Pharmacol 1997;37:908–15.
[91] Wideman GL, Keffer M, Morris E, et al. Analgesic efficacy of a combination of hydrocodone with ibuprofen in postoperative pain. Clin Pharmacol Ther 1999;65:66–76.
[92] Hammack JE, Loprinzi CL. Use of orally administered opioids for cancer-related pain. Mayo Clin Proc 1994;69:384–90.
[93] Caldwell JR, Hale ME, Boyd RE, et al. Treatment of osteoarthritis pain with controlled release oxycodone or fixed combination oxycodone plus acetaminophen added to nonsteroidal anti-inflammatory drugs: a double blind, randomized, multicenter, placebo controlled trial. J Rheumatol 1999;26:862–9.
[94] Calis KA, Kohler DR, Corso DM. Drug review. Transdermally administered fentanyl for pain management. Clin Pharm 1992;11:22–36.
[95] Fry M. Nurse-initiated intravenous morphine in the emergency department: efficacy, rate of adverse events and impact on time to analgesia. Emerg Med 2003;14:249.

ELSEVIER
SAUNDERS

EMERGENCY
MEDICINE
CLINICS OF
NORTH AMERICA

Emerg Med Clin N Am 23 (2005) 467–475

The Future of Pain Management in Emergency Medicine

James Ducharme, MDCM, FRCP, DABEM[a,b,*]

[a]Department of Emergency Medicine, Dalhousie University
[b]Department of Emergency Medicine, Atlantic Health Sciences Corporation, 400 University Avenue, Saint John, New Brunswick E2L 4L2, Canada

Other articles in this issue have described the current status of the multiple aspects concerning pain evaluation and management in the emergency setting. This article attempts to chart a path toward future optimal pain care. We cannot attempt to do so without first briefly reiterating the enormity of this symptom in our practices. Cordell et al [1] were able to survey all patients registering during a week's time; they discovered that up to 70% of those patients had pain as part of their presenting complaint. They thus confirmed that pain is indeed the most common symptom in our practice. For more than a decade, we have identified that pain is undertreated in emergency medicine, something we unfortunately share with most other specialties. Wilson and Pendleton [2] coined the term "oligoanalgesia" in 1989 for inadequate use of methods to relieve pain. Studies in the early 1990s by Ducharme, Selbst, and others [3,4] brought further to our attention the degree to which pain was not being treated. Despite a decade of physicians being encouraged to improve this situation, in 2002, Todd and coworkers [5] showed that, unfortunately, things have not improved as much as we had hoped.

Even more disturbing is that we seem unaware of the degree of pain after discharge, and appear to be achieving adequate pain control then even less than during the patient's stay in the emergency department (ED). Sivilotti and colleagues [6] discussed the lack of even basic observational data after discharge for multiple painful conditions. An observational study [7] demonstrated that not one child who had an isolated extremity fracture received an analgesic prescription at discharge. Recommendations for

* Department of Emergency Medicine, Atlantic Health Sciences Corporation, 400 University Avenue, Saint John, New Brunswick E2L 4L2, Canada.
E-mail address: jim_ducharme@bigfoot.com

0733-8627/05/$ - see front matter
doi:10.1016/j.emc.2004.12.011
emed.theclinics.com

acetaminophen were documented in only 20% of charts in that same study. Inadequate pain management after discharge can impact tremendously on functional status: patients who had isolated rib fractures were found to be unable to return to normal work load as a result of pain for a mean of 51 ± 39 days [8]. Although not all studies have been this negative, there are relatively few positive ones. Chan and Verdile [9] were able to attain high levels of pain relief and patient satisfaction after discharge with formal didactic and bedside education of physicians. Inadequate pain management has resulted in the United States in mandated documentation of pain in EDs as a result of a "top-on-down" intervention by the Joint Commission of Accreditation of Health care Organizations (JCAHO), although it is unlikely that this alone will suffice [10].

How then do we improve on our pain management? In the following sections, various aspects of education, evaluation, and therapy that may allow us to optimize pain care in the future are discussed.

Education

Most casual discussions or surveys demonstrate that medical students receive almost no formal training in acute pain assessment or management. Learners therefore infer that pain management is of lesser importance than other aspects of medical care. If we do not include training about pain control from the start of medical school, we risk later being unable to affect attitudes and barriers. Weinstein and associates [11] described attitudes about pain identified in students entering medical school that essentially remain unchanged through their senior year. They showed that the professionalization process of medical training may actually reinforce negative attitudes. Psychologic characteristics associated with reluctance to prescribe opioids and fears of patient addiction and drug regulatory agency sanctions were present from the start of training. Higher scores on reliance on high technology, external locus of control, and intolerance of clinical uncertainty were associated with higher scores on one or more of the three dimensions of opiophobia.

Altering attitudes and eliminating barriers require knowledge. As a result of genomics, knowledge about pain pathways has exploded. The potential number of treatments and medications for pain has increased almost exponentially. To quote R.G. Hill: "To have a frame work in which we can correctly evaluate such a density of information and decide which of the located gene products might be valid drug discovery targets, we must put them in an appropriate context where clinical observation is considered along with that derived from genomics and from carefully conducted preclinical pharmacology" [12]. Wang and coauthors [13], studying rats who had neuropathy, identified 148 genes in the dorsal root ganglion (DRG) that were regulated by greater than a factor of two, suggesting a heretofore-unrecognized complexity of understanding required to successfully control pain. Understanding this new information and increasing the number and type of medications for pain in our daily practice, all the while learning to assess pain and accept patient reporting, requires a commitment of education time that does not presently exist.

This commitment to education must continue into practice. We must learn to recognize that a multidisciplinary approach to pain is optimal. Importantly, critical care and emergency nurses need to not only be aware of research-based pain management practices, but also must lead the way in implementation and continuous evaluation as a measure of decreasing patient pain in the future [14]. Reinforcement and ongoing education are essential: Marquie et al [15] demonstrated that the greater the clinical experience, the greater the risk of "systemic miscalibration." They described how with increasing years of practice, physicians demonstrate increasing discordance in pain scoring when compared with patient self-reporting. Physicians score pain based on their witnessing thousands of patients in pain, not on an individual patient experience. Without ongoing education, senior physicians risk providing less, not more, pain control.

Pain evaluation

Evaluation of pain in emergency medicine has relied primarily on use of unidimensional scales adapted for use in other clinical settings. We may thus be using scales that cannot measure accurately what is happening to the patient. It has been recognized for decades that chronic pain evaluation requires a multidimensional tool; the McGill Pain Questionnaire is the best-known example. Use of this questionnaire may require up to 45 minutes, making it cumbersome for EDs. Although affective disorders such as depression have been identified as major components in chronic pain, we are just learning to what degree emotions impact pain and pain management in the acute setting. In the postoperative setting, Clark and coauthors [16] used a 101-descriptor multidimensional affect and pain survey (MAPS) questionnaire to determine the relative contributions of various dimensions of postoperative pain to a patient's score on a unidimensional numerical pain rating scale (NPRS). They concluded that patient scores on unidimensional pain intensity scales reflect the emotional qualities of pain much more than its sensory intensity or other qualities. Because fear and anxiety in the acute setting played such an important role in patient scoring, they felt that such scales were poor indicators of analgesic requirement.

Optimal recognition of pain is essential. We require better evaluation not only because we wish to decrease suffering, but also because poor pain control worsens patient outcome. Persistent uncontrolled pain suppresses our immune response [17]. It has been shown that there is increased morbidity and mortality in the critical care setting in patients who have inadequate pain control. Even though pain assessment is more difficult in cognitively impaired patients, it is critical to recognize and treat their pain. Elderly people who have hip fractures have been found to have a fivefold greater risk of delirium when their pain is uncontrolled than when adequate analgesia is provided [18].

For many years, if an analgesic study demonstrated a statistical difference in pain relief, we accepted this as proof of superiority of a given agent. Todd and Funk [19] introduced the concept of minimal clinically noticeable changes in pain, suggesting that studies showing less than this minimum change in a pain scale demonstrated no clinical significance. This has still not allowed us to know what measurement is a clinically adequate change. We do not yet know which end point in pain management we should be aiming for in many acute conditions.

We can understand that we need to attempt to eliminate all cardiac-related chest pain, because any persistent pain suggests ongoing ischemia. We seem to recognize that the risk of next-day headache recurrence in migraines is increased if a patient leaves the ED with any degree of headache [20]. Finally, we know that a certain as-of-yet unidentified subset of patients who suffer from acute pain will go on to develop chronic pain, but we do not know if this is from inherent plastification of their pain system or because we fail to initially treat their pain adequately. It appears that a physician-chosen pain-level end point will be unsatisfactory to most patients. Lee and coworkers [21] found a large variance in pain score end points when asking patients when they had obtained adequate pain relief, so a single cutoff may not be acceptable to many. It is possible that our inability to identify a more constant cutoff point may be because we rely on unidimensional scales. We are thus unable to properly assess all aspects of treatment. In patients who had chronic pain, Farrar and associates [22] chose to rely on a simple patient-based question—tell us if you have had enough analgesia—and found very high levels of satisfaction, without high levels of adverse effects. We need to study if this is an acceptable approach in the emergency setting, looking not only at patient satisfaction but also at longer-term outcomes. We should not be relying only on patient satisfaction, because we know that there is little correlation between degree of satisfaction and degree of pain relief [23].

In a busy ED, staff may be unwilling to use complicated scales for measuring pain. Observation of pain-related behavior, although better for acute pain than for chronic, may not compare well with patient reporting [24]. Extent of observer training, relevance of the pain-inducing task, and pain behavior observation measure used did not improve this correlation. Fortunately, a simple verbal numerical rating scale (NRS) does seem to accurately reproduce the findings of written scales [25]. It will have to be in the research setting that we develop and use multidimensional tools to better understand how to control pain in the ED. A "pain-o-meter" that could measure pain as a thermometer measures temperature, as suggested by Cordell [26], still seems to be in the distant future.

Pain management

It is in pain management that we see the future unfolding. Genome research has identified multiple possibilities for novel analgesics as more and more receptors and pathways are identified. It seems almost certain that patients will carry cards or have subcutaneous implants bearing their genomic record, identifying the optimal analgesic medication for their current painful condition with a mere pass through a scanner. Even then, patient and health care worker barriers may still ultimately determine the success of pain control: refusal to take or prescribe medication for fear of addiction, failure to accept patient reporting of pain levels, inability to identify pain in subsets of patients such as infants or the elderly, and so forth. While accepting that we need to strive to overcome these barriers, let us look into the future of pain control.

We have learned that there is considerable variation from one patient to the next, not only in pain expression but in response to analgesics. Cytochrome P450 receptor differences determine our ability to make use of codeine [27]. An individual's response to any particular opioid depends on which of the greater than 15 mu-receptor variants that individual has. Choosing which opioid is optimal for each patient should no longer be guesswork when individual genomic mapping is available. Repetitive prescribing of a few analgesics to all patients will be replaced by tailoring of medication not only to the cause of pain, but to the gene pattern of the individual. Pain will probably have a mechanism-based taxonomy rather than a pathology-related one as at present. Insights into mechanisms will allow understanding of the function of various molecules, permitting targeted medications.

The complexities of pain transmission are becoming ever more apparent; the likelihood of any one pathway or ion channel being exclusively responsive to one medication seems unlikely [12]. The author hopes that both MRI and positron emission tomography (PET) imaging of volunteers receiving painful stimuli will help clarify this issue. At present, many potential neurotransmitters studied in animals have failed due to the degree of complexity involved. What has shown potential?

Cannabinoids

It is now accepted that endogenous opioid and cannabinoid systems interact to produce analgesia [28]. Clinical use of cannabinoids as analgesics has been slowed not only by legal issues, but also by an adverse psychotropic effect profile. It has been difficult to titrate between analgesia and an intoxicated state. Many patients resist the notion of smoking cannabis to achieve analgesia. Cannabinoids act at CB_1 and CB_2 receptors both locally and centrally; they modulate release of neuropeptides from primary afferent receptors, and inhibit the release of calcitonin gene-related peptide (CGRP) from sensory neurons, minimizing local inflammatory response [29,30]. Although there is still a paucity of controlled analgesic trials with cannabinoids, animal studies are suggesting a more important possibility: it appears that endorphins and exogenous opioids also interact with CB_1 receptors, with stimulation of these receptors resulting in almost all drug-seeking or addictive behavior. Animal studies have strongly suggested that a combination of a CB_1 antagonist with an opioid may allow use of opioids for pain control without fear of the development of addiction [31,32]. Clinical trials have just been started in humans to further study this possibility.

Gene therapy

Simply put, the goal of gene therapy is to alter the genome of targeted cells. Nonfunctional cells can be replaced, or overexpressed genes can be downregulated. Within the domain of pain control, the primary goal is to diminish a chronically activated pain system. Yeomans and colleagues [33] have summarized three possible approaches. First, allogenic tissue may be infused into the subarachnoid space, with these cells secreting compounds having analgesic effects. Second, adenoviruses encoded with endogenous beta-endorphins injected intrathecally can "infect" neurons or meningeal cells, causing them to express and secrete this "natural" opioid. Third, recombinant herpes viruses have been used as vectors to alter primary genome nociceptors. At present there seems to be no application under investigation for acute pain scenarios.

Novel approaches to pain control

We know that neuropathic pain responds poorly to standard analgesics. Most effective agents have acted by blockade of sodium channels. Gabapentin, however, was inadvertently found to have neither a gamma-amino-butyric-acid (GABA) effect nor sodium channel action. Rather, it appears to block neurotransmitter release by inhibiting high-threshold calcium currents and to alter amino acid uptake via the NMDA-receptor complex [12]. This suggests further pathways or a combination of pathways that need to be targeted for successful pain control in neuralgia and neuropathic pain. Other new channels exist that, when eliminated in gene-deleted mice, result in profound reductions in response to noxious stimuli. Downstream regulatory element antagonistic modulator (DREAM) is such an example of a calcium-related pain pathway that has been identified [34].

Increased excitability in the dorsal root ganglion (DRG) is now known to occur through a myriad of mechanisms. Several ion channels can be triggered, including acid sensing ion channels (ASICs) as a result of acid production in poorly perfused tissues [35]; tetrodotoxin-resistant sodium channels (neuropathic pain) [36]; and ATP receptor related channels (increases nociceptor recruitment, leading to hyperalgesia) [37]. Cytokines such as tumor necrosis factor and interleukins also increase nociceptor activity [12]. Nociceptor neurons are regulated in activity by neurotrophins such as nerve growth factor [38]. Finally, it has been shown that nerve injury—as with shingles—may result in novel synaptic connections, with adaptation of nerve function to new tasks. The not-insignificant challenge in the next decade will be to identify agents that act via these pathways to provide analgesia for specific conditions while avoiding intolerable adverse effects.

Other initiatives

The author cannot end this look into the future without recognizing the human component of pain management. Fear of punitive action by government agencies, opiophobia, and ignorance of pain management options all restrict physicians from properly controlling pain. There needs to be a collective effort to encourage optimal pain management. Increased prescribing of opioids for pain, as recommended by the World Health Organization, has not led to increased drug abuse. To further improve opioid and analgesic usage while decreasing physician concern of legal action, the American Society of Law, Medicine, and Ethics (ASLME) has undertaken several initiatives to improve the medico-legal atmosphere with respect to the prescription of opioids [39]. The ASLME is initiating a project to identify and modify key educational, administrative, and legal issues in pain management specific to the emergency setting. This combination of system intervention with increasing scientific knowledge augurs well for the next 10 years of pain management.

Summary

How have we as a profession, whose number-one goal is to decrease human suffering, made pain control such a poorly discussed issue in training? From day 1 of medical school, pain and suffering need to be discussed. No clinical area should be taught without discussion of this most common and most important symptom. Although we have shown that up to 70% of our patients have pain as a part of their presenting problem, hospitalized patients also have high rates of pain, often unrecognized [40,41]. Barriers need to be identified and discussed. Alternatives to medications should be as much a part of our armamentarium as caring and compassion. The future of pain control depends on this paradigm shift.

References

[1] Cordell WH, Keene KK, Giles BK, et al. The high prevalence of pain in emergency medical care. Am J Emerg Med 2002;20(3):165–9.
[2] Wilson JE, Pendleton JM. Oligoanalgesia in the emergency department. Am J Emerg Med 1989;7(6):620–3.

[3] Ducharme J, Barber C. A prospective blinded study on emergency pain assessment and therapy. J Emerg Med 1995;13(4):571–5.
[4] Selbst SM, Clark M. Analgesic use in the emergency department. Ann Emerg Med 1990; 19(9):1010–3.
[5] Todd KH, Sloan EP, Chen C, et al. Survey of pain etiology, management practices and patient satisfaction in two urban emergency departments. Canadian Journal of Emergency Medicine 2002;4(4):252–6.
[6] Sivilotti ML, Paris PM, Cantees K, et al. Studying emergency patients outside the emergency department. Ann Emerg Med 1996;27(4):442–7.
[7] Ngai B, Ducharme J. Documented use of analgesics in the emergency department and upon release of patients with extremity fractures. Acad Emerg Med 1997;4(12):1176–8.
[8] Kerr-Valentic MA, Arthur M, Mullins RJ, et al. Rib fracture pain and disability: can we do better? Journal of Trauma-Injury Infection & Critical Care 2003;54(6):1058–63.
[9] Chan L, Verdile VP. Do patients receive adequate pain control after discharge from the ED? Am J Emerg Med 1998;16(7):705–7.
[10] Gallagher RM. Physician variability in pain management: are the JCAHO standards enough? Pain Med 2003;4(1):1–3.
[11] Weinstein SM, Laux LF, Thornby JI, et al. Medical students' attitudes toward pain and the use of opioid analgesics: implications for changing medical school curriculum. South Med J 2000;93(5):472–8.
[12] Hill RG. New targets for analgesic drugs. In: Dostrovsky JO, Carr DB, Koltzenburg M, editors. Proceedings of the 10th World Congress on Pain: progress in pain research and management. Seattle (WA): IASP Press; 2003. p. 419–36.
[13] Wang H, Sun H, Della PK, et al. Chronic neuropathic pain is accompanied by global changes in gene expression and shares pathobiology with neurodegenerative diseases. Neuroscience 2002;114(3):529–46.
[14] Shannon K, Bucknall T. Pain assessment in critical care: what have we learnt from research? Intensive Crit Care Nurs 2003;19(3):154–62.
[15] Marquie L, Raufaste E, Lauque D, et al. Pain rating by patients and physicians: evidence of systematic pain miscalibration. Pain 2003;102(3):289–96.
[16] Clark WC, Yang JC, Tsui SL, et al. Unidimensional pain rating scales: a multidimensional affect and pain survey (MAPS) analysis of what they really measure. Pain 2002;98(3):241–7.
[17] Page GG. The immune-suppressive effects of pain. Adv Exp Med Biol 2003;521:117–25.
[18] Morrison RS, Magaziner J, Gilbert M, et al. Relationship between pain and opioid analgesics on the development of delirium following hip fracture. J Gerontol A Biol Sci Med Sci 2003;58(1):76–81.
[19] Todd KH, Funk JP. The minimum clinically important difference in physician-assigned visual analog pain scores. Acad Emerg Med 1996;3(2):142–6.
[20] Ducharme J, Beveridge RC, Lee JS, et al. Emergency management of migraine: is the headache really over? Acad Emerg Med 1998;5(9):899–905.
[21] Lee JS, Stiell I, Hobden E, et al. Clinically meaningful values of the visual analog scale of pain severity. Acad Emerg Med 2000;7(5):550.
[22] Farrar JT, Portenoy RK, Berlin JA, et al. Defining the clinically important difference in pain outcome measures. Pain 2000;88(3):287–94.
[23] Afilalo M, Tselios C. Pain relief versus patient satisfaction. Ann Emerg Med 1996;27(4): 436–8.
[24] Labus JS, Keefe FJ, Jensen MP. Self-reports of pain intensity and direct observations of pain behavior: when are they correlated? Pain 2003;102(1–2):109–24.
[25] Bijur PE, Latimer CT, Gallagher EJ. Validation of a verbally administered numerical rating scale of acute pain for use in the emergency department. Acad Emerg Med 2003;10(4):390–2.
[26] Cordell WH. Pain-control research opportunities and future directions. Ann Emerg Med 1996;27(4):474–8.

[27] Dresser GK, Bailey DG. A basic conceptual and practical overview of interactions with highly prescribed drugs. Can J Clin Pharmacol 2002;9(4):191–8.
[28] Le Guen S, Mas NM, Canestrelli C, et al. Pain management by a new series of dual inhibitors of enkephalin degrading enzymes: long lasting antinociceptive properties and potentiation by CCK2 antagonist or methadone. Pain 2003;104(1–2):139–48.
[29] De Vries TJ, Homberg JR, Binnekade R, et al. Cannabinoid modulation of the reinforcing and motivational properties of heroin and heroin-associated cues in rats. Psychopharmacology (Berl) 2003;168(1–2):164–9.
[30] Fattore L, Spano MS, Cossu G, et al. Cannabinoid mechanism in reinstatement of heroin-seeking after a long period of abstinence in rats. Eur J Neurosci 2003;17(8):1723–6.
[31] Cossu G, Ledent C, Fattore L, et al. Cannabinoid CB1 receptor knockout mice fail to self-administer morphine but not other drugs of abuse. Behav Brain Res 2001;118(1):61–5.
[32] Solinas M, Panlilio LV, Antoniou K, et al. The cannabinoid CB1 antagonist N-piperidinyl-5-(4-chlorophenyl)-1-(2,4-dichlorophenyl)-4-methylpyrazole-3-carboxamide (SR-141716A) differentially alters the reinforcing effects of heroin under continuous reinforcement, fixed ratio, and progressive ratio schedules of drug self-administration in rats. J Pharmacol Exp Ther 2003;306(1):93–102.
[33] Yeomans DC, Mannes A, Saitoh Y. Gene therapy for pain: different approaches toward a common goal. In: Dostrovsky JO, Carr DB, Koltzenburg M, editors. Proceedings of the 10th World Congress on Pain: progress in pain research and management. Seattle (WA): IASP Press; 2003. p. 521–37.
[34] Cheng HY, Pitcher GM, Laviolette SR, et al. DREAM is a critical transcriptional repressor for pain modulation. Cell 2002;108(1):31–43.
[35] Waldmann R, Bassilana F, de Weille J, et al. Molecular cloning of a non-inactivating proton-gated Na+ channel specific for sensory neurons. J Biol Chem 1997;272(34):20975–8.
[36] Akopian AN, Souslova V, England S, et al. The tetrodotoxin-resistant sodium channel SNS has a specialized function in pain pathways. Nat Neurosci 1999;2(6):541–8.
[37] Jahr CE, Jessell TM. ATP excites a subpopulation of rat dorsal horn neurones. Nature 1983; 304(5928):730–3.
[38] Snider WD, McMahon SB. Tackling pain at the source: new ideas about nociceptors. Neuron 1998;20(4):629–32.
[39] Johnson SH. Providing relief to those in pain: a retrospective on the scholarship and impact of the Mayday Project. J Law Med Ethics 2003;31(1):15–20.
[40] Costantini M, Viterbori P, Flego G. Prevalence of pain in Italian hospitals: results of a regional cross-sectional survey. J Pain Symptom Manage 2002;23(3):221–30.
[41] Salomon L, Tcherny-Lessenot S, Collin E, et al. Pain prevalence in a French teaching hospital. J Pain Symptom Manage 2002;24(6):586–92.

ELSEVIER
SAUNDERS

Emerg Med Clin N Am 23 (2005) 477–502

EMERGENCY
MEDICINE
CLINICS OF
NORTH AMERICA

Local Anesthetics and Peripheral Nerve Blocks in the Emergency Department

Chad S. Crystal, MD, Robert B. Blankenship, MD*

Department of Emergency Medicine, Darnall Army Community Hospital, 36000 Darnall Loop, Fort Hood, TX 76544, USA

Local anesthetics work by blocking the conduction of neural messages. Sodium is mostly an extracellular ion. Closed sodium channels located on the axoplasmic side of the nerve cell prevent its influx into the cell. In this resting state the electrical potential inside a nerve cell is negative in reference to the outside of the cell. This is the resting potential of the nerve cell. After mechanical, chemical, or electrical excitation the sodium channels open and allow sodium ions to move into the cell causing depolarization and propagation of the nerve impulse. In the inactive state, the sodium channels are susceptible to the action of local anesthetic molecules that bind to the channels, causing them to remain inactive and prevent subsequent depolarization [1]. Further conduction by the nerve is blocked until the local anesthetic is displaced from the neural membrane.

Structure of local anesthetics

Local anesthetics are weak bases that require the addition of a hydrochloride salt to be water soluble, facilitating their injection. They usually have an aromatic (hydrophobic) ring structure connected to a tertiary amine (hydrophilic) by an intermediate chain that includes an ester or amide linkage. The chemical composition of local anesthetics determines their potency, duration, and onset of action while the nature of the intermediate chain establishes the two classes of local anesthetics: esters and amides (Table 1).

Lipid solubility determines potency [2]. The more lipophilic a local anesthetic is, the more easily it penetrates the nerve cell membranes, resulting in more effective blockade of the neural signal. The plasma protein binding

* Corresponding author.
E-mail address: robblankenship@gsacep.org (R.B. Blankenship).

doi:10.1016/j.emc.2004.12.012 *emed.theclinics.com*

Table 1
Local anesthetics and their properties

Generic (Trade)	Potency	PKa	Duration	Maximum Dose (mg/kg)
AMIDES				
Bupivacaine (Marcaine)	4	8.1	4	3
Dibucaine (Nupercaine)	4	8.8	4	1
Etidocaine (Duranest)	4	7.7	4	4
Lidocaine (Xylocaine)	2	7.8	2	4.5 (7 with epinephrine)
Mepivacaine (Carbocaine)	2	7.6	2	4.5 (7 with epinephrine)
Prilocaine (Citanest)	2	7.8	2	8
Ropivacaine (Naropin)	4	8.1	4	3
ESTERS				
Chloroprocaine (Nesacaine)	1	9.0	1	12
Cocaine	2	8.7	2	3
Procaine	1	8.9	1	12
Tetracaine (Pontocaine)	4	8.2	3	3

Adapted from Morgan GE, Mikhail MS, Murray MJ, Larson CP. Local anesthetics. In: Morgan GE, Mikhail MS, Murray MJ, Larson CP (editors). Clinical Anesthesiology, 3rd edition. New York: Lange Medical Books; 2002. p. 233–41.

potential determines the duration of action of the local anesthetic molecule [3], presumably because the local anesthetic receptor is also a protein [4]. Those with more protein binding remain associated with the neural membrane for a longer period of time—making it unavailable for metabolism and clearance. For example, procaine is poorly protein bound, and its duration of neural blockade is relatively short. On the other hand, bupivacaine is highly protein bound, and consequently, has a long duration of action [1]. Last, pK_a determines the speed of onset of neural blockade. The pK_a is the pH at which equal percentages of the drug exist in the ionized and nonionized forms. Local anesthetics are weak bases. They therefore tend to become positively charged as the pH of the local milieu declines. Only the nonionized base is able to pass easily through the neural membrane. Local anesthetics with pK_a values closer to the physiologic pH produce higher concentrations of this nonionized base. This equates to a more rapid onset of action. This is why the local anesthetics are less effective in an acidic environment, and why alkalinization speeds onset of action and increases duration. Furthermore, epinephrine is unstable in alkaline environments. Commercially prepared solutions containing it are therefore made more acidic, further increasing the time of onset. Once inside the nerve cell, the nonionized base reaches equilibrium with its ionized form. It is this ionized form (cation) that actually binds to the receptor within the sodium channel and inactivates it.

Toxicity

All local anesthetics have a similar toxic profile predominantly affecting the central nervous and cardiovascular systems. Toxicity is related to the potency of the local anesthetic, total dose delivered, systemic absorption, protein binding, and metabolism and excretion. Of note, most toxic reactions are either dose related or due to inadvertent intraarterial administration.

The rate of systemic absorption of local anesthetics is proportional to the vascularity of the injection site. The absorption rates from highest to lowest are: intercostal > intratracheal > epidural/caudal > brachial plexus > mucosal > distal peripheral nerve > subcutaneous. For this reason, the recommended local anesthetic dose for intercostal blocks is one tenth the maximum for peripheral blocks. Absorption of local anesthetic is slower for those that are highly tissue bound.

The metabolism and excretion of local anesthetics differ between esters and amides. Ester local anesthetics are quickly metabolized by plasma pseudocholinesterase, and the water-soluble metabolites are excreted in the urine. Patients with pseudocholinesterase deficiency (eg, sensitivity to succinylcholine, patients taking cholinesterase inhibitors, and patients with myasthenia gravis) are at an increased risk for systemic toxicity. Of note, cocaine undergoes partial hepatic metabolism and the remainder is excreted into the urine unchanged [4]. Amide local anesthetics are metabolized in the liver. Although the rate of metabolism depends on the agent, the overall time for metabolism is slower than for ester hydrolysis. Consequently, there is a smaller allowance for cumulative dosing over time with amide anesthetics when compared with the esters. Furthermore, decreases in hepatic function or liver blood flow will reduce the metabolic rate and predispose to systemic toxicity. Metabolites of prilocaine (*o*-toluidine derivatives), a component of EMLA cream, may accumulate after high doses of the drug, and can convert hemoglobin to methemoglobin. Benzocaine may also cause methemoglobinemia.

Central nervous system toxicity

The central nervous sytsem (CNS) toxic effects of local anesthetics are directly related to lipid solubility [1]. As the lipid solubility of a local anesthetic increases, the gap between the wanted clinical effect and systemic toxicity narrows. This is why bupivacaine has more risk for systemic toxicity than lidocaine. Furthermore, local anesthetics that exhibit strong protein binding cross the blood–brain barrier more effectively as they remain in the nonionic state more often.

Symptoms of CNS toxicity range from lightheadedness, tongue numbness, metallic taste, and restlessness at low levels, to perioral paresthesias, slurred speech, and excitability or drowsiness at higher levels. Seizures and coma are manifestations of severe toxicity. The CNS effects are believed to be due to the depression of inhibitory neurons, leaving the excitatory pathways unopposed [5]. Treatment of local anesthetic-induced seizures is with benzodiazepines, which raise the seizure threshold. One caveat to this treatment is benzodiazepines, which, like certain local anesthetics, are highly protein bound in the plasma. Intravenous administration of benzodiazepine can compound toxicity by displacing the anesthetic from plasma proteins, contributing to the free, active form [6]. An alternate anticonvulsant is thiopental 0.5 to 2 mg/kg. However, the duration of action is shorter with thiopental, and it may require repeat dosing should the seizures reoccur. Careful attention should be given to oxygenation and ventilation as hypoxia, hypercarbia, and acidosis worsen the toxicity of local anesthetics.

Cardiac toxicity

Cardiac toxicity occurs secondary to blockade of the sodium channels in the cardiac conduction system [1]. The resultant increased activity in reentrant pathways and reduction of the refractory period predisposes the heart to ventricular dysrhythmias. At higher plasma concentrations, myocardial contractility is depressed. Smooth muscle dilation may cause hypotension. Symptoms of cardiac toxicity include palpitations, cardiac dysrhythmias, hyper- or hypotension and cardiovascular collapse [7]. It usually occurs after the stimulant phase of CNS toxicity. Cardiac toxicity may result from any of the local anesthetics; however, it is more likely in the more lipophilic agents such as etidocaine and bupivacaine. Cardiac toxicity is worsened by the use of epinephrine [3], hypoxia, hypercarbia, and acidosis.

Bupivacaine is notorious for cardiac toxicity, often associated with accidental intravascular injection. A range of effects including hypotension, atrioventricular block, and dysrhythmias has occurred. The proposed reason for its increased cardiotoxicity when compared with other agents includes its higher degree of depolarization changes and high degree of protein binding.

Management of cardiovascular collapse from local anesthetic toxicity should follow advanced cardiac life support (ACLS) guidelines, with a few notable exceptions. First, as lidocaine is a local anesthetic, its use should be avoided. Animal models suggest increased benefit with high-dose epinephrine to treat bupivacaine-induced cardiac toxicity, although this is controversial. Bretylium, 5 mg/kg repeated up to 30 mg/kg, can occasionally convert ventricular tachyarrhythmias to normal sinus rhythm, or at least facilitate electrical cardioversion. Unfortunately, the effects of Bretylium may take 30 minutes to occur, so prolonged resuscitation is needed [8].

Allergic reactions

True allergy to local anesthetics is rare. A careful history is paramount to discriminate the true allergic reactions. Many times what the patient reports as an allergy was actually an uncomfortable drug effect, vagal reaction, or intraarterial injection of the local anesthetic or epinephrine. True allergic reactions will usually produce some form of skin or upper airway involvement. When an allergic reaction does occur it is usually due to the metabolite *para*-aminobenzoic acid (PABA) in ester anesthetics and the preservative methylparaben (MPB) in amide anesthetics. If a true allergy is suspected, based on history or documentation, a preservative-free agent from the other class should be used. Most true allergic reactions are due to the esters. Therefore, if in doubt as to the class of local anesthetic that caused the previous allergic reaction, it is safest to administer a preservative-free amide local anesthetic (eg, cardiac lidocaine). The risk of a hypersensitivity reaction to this agent is extremely low.

Alternatively, agents such as saline with benzyl alcohol, benzyl alcohol with epinephrine or 0.5% to 1% diphenhydramine may be used. Benzyl alcohol is the preferred agent, as initial studies suggest it is the most effective alternative [9]. Diphenhydramine has been shown to cause severe pain on injection, prolonged analgesia, and prolonged rebound hyperesthesia [10]. Furthermore, diphenhydramine carries the additional risk of local irritation and necrosis of the skin when used in the fingertips or areas supplied by the end arteries [11].

Topical anesthetics

Overview

Topical anesthetics began to be used in the latter half of the 19th century with the advent of cocaine. It took almost another century for more effective and safer topical anesthetic agents to become available. A laceration repair no longer requires a painful injection for anesthetic delivery. An injection may be avoided altogether, or performed painlessly through an area treated with a topical anesthetic. Additionally, topical anesthesia avoids the wound edge distortion that subcutaneous infiltration may produce. Topical anesthesia can be divided into three main categories of use: mucosal membranes, nonintact skin, and intact skin.

Topical anesthetics for mucosal membranes

Cocaine and lidocaine are two agents that may used to numb the mucosa of the nose, mouth, and pharynx. Cocaine is a unique anesthetic in that it has intrinsic vasoconstrictor properties, making it useful both intranasally and during surgery to reduce blood loss. Cocaine in a 4% solution provides rapid and effective anesthesia for approximately 45 minutes. The maximum dose given should be less than 3 mg/kg. Unfortunately, cocaine has some disadvantages. Due to its potential for coronary artery vasoconstriction, hypertension, and tachycardia it should not be used in patients with known or suspected coronary artery disease. In addition to concerns of systemic toxicity, cocaine's expense and federal regulatory issues make it a somewhat unattractive agent.

Lidocaine provides adequate anesthesia in this region when used in the 1% to 4% concentration. Although it does not have any intrinsic vasoconstrictor properties, epinephrine or phenylephrine can be added for this effect. Topical application of lidocaine results in a high level of absorption, so caution must be used to avoid exceeding the maximum weight-based dose. To minimize error, it is best to calculate the maximum dose based (5 mg/kg of lidocaine without epinephrine or phenylephrine, 7 mg/kg of lidocaine with epinephrine or phenylephrine) before administering the anesthetic. To determine the amount of anesthetic in a given volume, simply multiply the concentration of the anesthetic by 10 to determine the milligrams of anesthetic in 1 mL of solution. For example, 2 mL of 4% viscous lidocaine contains 80 mg of lidocaine. More dilute solutions may be used in situations requiring high volumes.

Several alternatives are available for applying local anesthetic to mucous membranes. An atomizer can be used to create a fine mist. Lidocaine jelly can be rubbed between the cheek and gums. Cotton swabs or pledgets can be soaked in the solution and introduced into the nose to either numb the entire mucosal surface or a selective area. A vaporizer, such as one might use for albuterol, is effective in anesthetizing the entire oropharynx, often including the vocal cords [12]. The measured amount of lidocaine is placed into the vaporizer and the patient then inhales the mist produced.

Topical anesthetics for intact skin

There are three choices available for topical anesthesia to intact skin: Eutectic mixture of local anesthetics (EMLA), ELA-Max, and iontophoretic preparations. EMLA contains a mixture of 2.5% lidocaine and 2.5% prilocaine in a 1:1 ratio by weight. Each gram of cream contains 25 mg of lidocaine and 25 mg of prilocaine, purified water, carboxypolymethylene (a thickening agent), and sodium hydroxide (to adjust the pH to 9.4). The suggested dose is 2.5 g on 20 to 25 cm^2 of skin, with a maximum dosage of 2 g on 10 cm^2 of skin. The Federal Drug Administration (FDA) approved EMLA cream in 1992 for use on intact skin; however, more recent studies suggest EMLA might be effective and safe for use in lacerations [13]. Further studies are needed before EMLA can be recommended for nonintact skin, due to its high cost (approximately $5.00 per application) and prolonged onset of action.

EMLA has a slow onset of action, and takes at least 45 to 60 minutes to achieve anesthesia. EMLA should be applied to intact skin for at least 1 hour but not longer than 2 hours before the planned procedure. Once it has been applied, it should be covered with an occlusive dressing. Studies have shown anesthetic depth of 3 mm after a 60-minute application and 5 mm after a 120-minute application [14]. Anesthesia lasts for 1 to 2 hours. Advantages of EMLA are its ease and comfort of use and benign safety profile. Complications of EMLA include blanching of skin, redness at the application site, and contact dermatitis. In infants less than 3 months of age there is a theoretical risk of methemoglobinemia due to inadequate levels of methemoglobin reductase. For this reason EMLA should not be used in patients less than 3 months old. However, at least one metanalysis has demonstrated no increased risk of methemoglobinemia when EMLA cream was used in neonates. Although toxicity from lidocaine and prilocaine is possible, it should not occur if EMLA is used as directed. It can be used in the emergency department for venipuncture, arterial puncture, lumbar puncture, and arthrocentesis, yet its slow onset of action makes it impractical for the large majority of emergency medicine patients.

ELA-Max is a recent addition to the topical anesthetics. It contains 4% lidocaine cream in a liposomal matrix and is FDA approved for the temporary relief of pain resulting from minor cuts and abrasions. Liposomes enhance the action of the lidocaine by facilitating the rate and extent of its absorption. Consequently, ELA-Max achieves adequate anesthesia in only 30 minutes, as opposed to EMLA's 60-minute onset of action [15,16]. An occlusive dressing does not need to be applied over ELA-Max, but it may be beneficial in preventing active children from displacing the ELA-Max. In limited trials it appears to be a safe topical anesthetic. ELA-Max does not contain prilocaine or its metabolites that have recently been implicated in EMLA-induced methemoglobinemia in older children. Thus, ELA-Max theoretically should not increase the risk of methemoglobinemia—even in young infants.

Another method for dermal anesthesia of intact skin is lidocaine iontophoresis. Iontophoresis allows the introduction of soluble, positively charged lidocaine hydrochloride into the skin by the use of a small external electrical current. In recent studies, this technique appears to be safe and efficacious [17], with an insignificant systemic absorption of lidocaine [18–20]. Lidocaine iontophoresis achieves anesthesia in 10 to 20 minutes, making it a more rapid alternative to EMLA cream. Undesirable effects of this delivery method include the sensation of electrical current flowing through the skin, and temporary erythema, blanching, itching, and urticaria at the application site. Another disadvantage of this technique is only one site can be anesthetized at one time. Last, an iontophoresis device costs approximately $400, and the one-time use disposable electrodes are $6 to $7.50 each, making this slightly more expensive than EMLA. However, the time saved by using iontophoresis may outweigh the slightly higher costs of its use.

Topical anesthetics for nonintact skin

Two primary choices exist to painlessly provide anesthesia over nonintact skin: TAC and LET. TAC was introduced in 1980, and is composed of tetracaine 0.5%, adrenaline 0.05%, and cocaine 11.8%. Five to 10 mL of TAC is applied to an open wound and covered with gauze. The gauze should be held in place for 10 to 20 minutes with either tape or a gloved hand to prevent inadvertent absorption of the medication by a well-intentioned parent. TAC works best on the scalp and face, but it can be used on extremities. However, due to its adrenaline content, it should not be used in areas with end arteries. Use of TAC on or near mucous membranes should be avoided to prevent toxicity from the systemic absorption of tetracaine and cocaine. There are significant concerns over the use of TAC due to reported cases of respiratory arrest, seizures, and death in children due to its improper application leading to increased systemic absorption [21]. Other drawbacks to TAC include its high cost, potential for abuse and the regulatory issues involved with dispensing and administering a cocaine-containing medication. These problems have led most emergency departments to abandon its use.

LET (lidocaine 4%, epinephrine 0.1%, and tetracaine 0.5%) is an excellent alternative agent to TAC. LET is as effective as TAC [22–24], possesses a superior safety record, is more cost effective, and does not contain a controlled substance. LET comes in both a solution and gel form. They are equally efficacious [25], although the gel may be easier to apply with less run off. One to 3 mL of LET should be applied directly to the wound and then covered for 15 to 30 minutes. Like TAC, LET should not be applied directly to or near mucous membranes, the pinna of the ear, the nose, penis, fingers, or toes.

Local anesthetics used for subcutaneous infiltration

General

Local anesthetics are classified into two groups: amides and esters (Table 1). Certain key differences exist between the two broad classes, especially with regard to metabolism and allergic potential. Esters are hydrolyzed in the plasma by pseudocholinesterase, a much more rapid process than the hepatic metabolism of the amides. The slower metabolism of the amides increases the possibility of toxicity, especially in a patient with liver dysfunction. The breakdown of the ester compounds by pseudocholinesterase produces *para*-aminobenzoic acid, a potentially allergenic substance. Because metabolism of the amide compounds does not result in this byproduct, most allergic reactions to the local anesthetics are due to the esters.

Lidocaine

Lidocaine (Xylocaine) is the most commonly used local anesthetic for intradermal infiltration. This is most likely due to its excellent clinical efficacy and good safety record. It is prepared commercially as a 1.0 to 2.0% solution with a pH of 6.5 in solution and a pK_a of 7.9. Onset of action usually begins 4 to 7 minutes after injection. The maximum dose is 3 to 5 mg/kg, up to 300 mg in a single dose. The addition of epinephrine prolongs its duration of action and decreases its systemic absorption, allowing a maximal dose of 7 mg/kg. A 1% solution without epinephrine has an average duration of action of approximately 1.5 hours. The duration is extended to approximately 3.5 hours with epinephrine. Traditionally, it was taught that epinephrine should *never* be used in the hands or feet due to the risk of ischemia from significant constriction of end arterioles. However, a few citations in the recent literature suggest that, with careful screening, epinephrine may be used in the hands and feet on a *limited* basis [26,27]. Given the preponderance of data that states otherwise, it would be prudent to avoid using epinephrine in the digits, and to use it in the hands and feet only very selectively until more data is available [28]. To reverse digital artery vasospasm due to intentional or inadvertent local injection of epinephrine locally inject 2 mg of phentolamine.

Bupivacaine

Bupivacaine (Marcaine) is a very potent local anesthetic with anesthesia equivalent to lidocaine. Due to its high pK_a and protein binding, its onset of action may take up to 20 minutes, with duration of action of 3 to 6 hours. It is clinically available as either a 0.25% or 0.5% solution. Maximal doses of bupivacaine are 2 to 2.5 mg/kg without epinephrine and 3 to 3.5 mg/kg with epinephrine. A dose of bupivacaine may be repeated every 3 hours, but the total dose in a 24-hour period should not exceed 400 mg. Although bupivacaine is well suited for longer procedures, it should be noted that the risk of systemic toxicity with bupivacaine is much higher than most other local anesthetics due to its high potency and protein binding. The toxic potential of bupivacaine has led to the development of newer agents such as ropivacaine and levobupivacaine.

Ropivacaine (Naropin)

Ropivacaine is a new amide local anesthetic approved by the FDA in 1996. It is very similar to bupivacaine in terms of potency, onset time, and duration of action, but it is 70% less likely to cause the cardiotoxic effects associated with bupivacaine. It does have some intrinsic vasoconstrictive properties, so it probably should not be used on end arterial areas. It costs eight times more than bupivacaine [29].

Levobupivacaine

Levobupivacaine is the S-isomer of bupivacaine. This pure S-enantiomer has fewer cardiovascular and CNS side effects when compared with its racemic cousin bupivacaine. The potency of the two drugs is similar. It costs five times more than bupivacaine [30].

Mepivacaine

Mepivacaine (Carbocaine) is structurally similar to lidocaine. Its onset of action is similar to lidocaine, but its duration of action is much longer

(3 hours). Epinephrine increases the duration of action by 20% to 30%. It is prepared for local infiltration as a 0.5% or 1.0% solution. Despite its quick onset and longer duration of action, mepivacaine's reputation for being more toxic than lidocaine has limited its clinical use.

Reducing the pain of injection of local anesthetics

Many techniques may be employed to lessen the degree of pain from the injection of a local anesthetic. The use of a small needle (27–30 gauge) and slow administration of the anesthetic (30 seconds per mL) [31] in a proximal to distal direction tend to lessen the pain of injection. Infiltration of local anesthetics inside the cut wound edge is less painful than injection through intact skin [32].

Many studies have shown that buffering of lidocaine reduces the pain of infiltration [33–37]. To make a buffered lidocaine solution, add sodium bicarbonate (44 mEq/50 mL) to lidocaine in a 1:10 ration (1 mL of bicarbonate is added to 10 mL of lidocaine). Buffering of lidocaine decreases its shelf life to 7 days because buffered lidocaine undergoes biodegradation at room temperature. The limiting factor in the addition of sodium bicarbonate to local anesthetic solutions is the tendency for the more lipid-soluble agents to precipitate. For example, mixing sodium bicarbonate and bupivacaine in a 1:10 ratio causes precipitation. Therefore, bupivacaine is buffered in a 1:50 ratio (0.1 mL of bicarbonate is added to 5 mL of bupivacaine).

The literature is equivocal on whether warming an anesthetic will reduce the pain of administration. What is reasonable is to ensure the anesthetic is at least room temperature. Lidocaine can be warmed in either dry heat, such as a blanket warmer, or in temperature-regulated water baths at 37°C. If the lidocaine has not been buffered, it will not suffer degradation in shelf life with heating.

Addition of vasoconstrictors to local anesthetics

The addition of a vasoconstrictor, such as epinephrine, offers several advantages to most local anesthetics. First, a vasoconstrictor will decrease local blood flow, allowing for better hemostasis in the surgical field. This is beneficial, as local anesthetics, with the exceptions of cocaine and ropivacaine, are vasodilators by a direct action on smooth muscle vessel walls causing relaxation. Vasoconstriction also decreases the rate of systemic absorption of the local anesthetic. This allows an increased maximum dose of local anesthetic to be administered while reducing the risk of systemic toxicity. Last, by decreasing local blood flow metabolism and redistribution of the local anesthetic, the duration of action is prolonged.

Commercially prepared solutions of lidocaine or bupivacaine with epinephrine in concentrations of 1:100,000 (10 μg/mL epinephrine) to

1:200,000 (5 μg/mL epinephrine) are available and widely used for subcutaneous infiltration. These preparations are acidified to a pH of 3 to 4.5 to stabilize the epinephrine component. Therefore, these solutions will have a slower onset of action and be associated with more pain on injection.

Regional anesthesia

General indications and contraindications

The general indication for regional anesthesia is pain, in an area amenable to a blockade of a specific peripheral nerve (or group of nerves) in a clinical situation that nerve block provides an advantage over other techniques. In reality, the route of anesthesia chosen is a decision made between the physician and the patient. It often involves a variety of factors including patient preference, physician comfort with the techniques involved, and the time constraints of a busy emergency department. As always, the risks and benefits of the proposed procedure(s) should be explained to the patient, who may then make a decision based on informed consent. Indications for the individual nerve blocks are contained within their respective sections below.

Contraindications to the specific regional anesthetic techniques are discussed in their sections below. In general, nerve blocks are contraindicated in uncooperative patients and patients who are unable to communicate severe pain on injection (eg, those patients suffering from dementia or psychosis and children). Severe pain is often an indicator of intraneural injection, which may produce ischemic nerve injury. Infection directly overlying the injection site, distortion of the anatomical landmarks, and allergy to the local anesthetic being used are also contraindications [38].

Advantages

In the emergency department a variety of methods exist to reduce the discomfort of painful conditions procedures. Peripheral nerve blocks are just one of these techniques. Considered as a group, they have multiple benefits over local infiltration anesthesia. Often less local anesthetic may be used leading to a lower risk of systemic toxicity. They are often less painful to perform than subcutaneous injection and result in less anxiety for the patient. In regions with great cosmetic significance (such as the lip and face), a peripheral nerve block avoids the tissue distortion produced by directly injecting a local anesthetic into the wound margins.

Disadvantages

Regional anesthesia requires a high degree of patient cooperation, especially in areas where success is guided by a patient's ability to detect subtle paresthesias. There is a risk of systemic toxicity (approximately 7.5 per

10,000), especially due to inadvertent intravascular injection, and a small risk of peripheral nerve damage (1.9 per 10,000) [39]. Peripheral nerve blockade is a "blind" technique, as it is most often performed in the emergency department without the benefit of a nerve stimulator. This results in a risk of failure that is probably closely related to the clinical experience of the practitioner performing the block. For this reason, the patient should be informed before the procedure of a possible need for additional anesthesia.

General techniques

Due to the risk of systemic toxicity, the majority of peripheral nerve blocks should be performed in an area with adequate monitoring and resuscitation equipment. Immediate toxicity is often due to accidental intravascular injection of the local anesthetic. Careful aspiration of the syringe before injection and the use of the "immobile needle" technique (intravenous tubing between the needle and syringe allows the operator to use both hands for needle stabilization and anatomic palpation while an assistant aspirates and injects the syringe) may reduce this risk. Delayed toxicity occurs when an excessive amount of local anesthetic is absorbed into the systemic circulation. The timing of this event depends on the anesthetic agent used and the area being injected. A high index of suspicion is required to diagnose the first signs of both immediate and delayed toxicity.

The patient may be premedicated with a systemic benzodiazepine or opiod to reduce the anxiety and pain of injection. However, the sedation must be light to facilitate patient cooperation.

The skin should be prepared in an antiseptic fashion before needle insertion. Povidone-iodine (Betadine) is one acceptable agent. Preparation of the oral mucosa before an intraoral procedure is discussed below.

The majority of the procedures described herein are "blind" techniques, and knowledge of the local anatomy must be combined with patient cooperation to facilitate a successful block. When a needle comes into contact with a peripheral nerve, it produces a paresthesia in that nerve's sensory distribution. For a successful block to occur, the local anesthetic must be injected in proximity to the nerve (perineural) but not directly within it (intraneural), as intraneural injection may produce ischemic nerve injury secondary to the high pressures it produces. The intensity of the pain and its duration serve as clues to the injection site of the anesthetic agent. Perineural injection causes a brief increase in the paresthesia, whereas intraneural injection produces an intense and prolonged pain. If intraneural positioning is suspected, the injection should be terminated immediately and the needle repositioned [38].

Wrist blocks

For many injuries to the hand, local infiltration or a digital block may be more effective than a wrist block. Wrist blocks have a variable and possibly slow time to onset and can be time-consuming to perform if all three nerves must be blocked. Examples of situations that are amenable to a wrist block include: "road rash," thermal burns requiring debridement, hydrofluoric acid burns, injury to more than one finger, and lacerations to the palm.

Radial nerve

To begin, identify the radial artery and radial styloid. At the level of the styloid inject 3 mL of local anesthetic just lateral to the radial artery. From this point proceed dorsally and subcutaneously inject local anesthetic along the dorsum of the wrist until the dorsal midline is reached. Approximately 5 mL of local anesthetic is required [40].

Ulnar nerve

The ulnar nerve lies deep to the flexor carpi ulnaris tendon at the level of the proximal palmar crease. It runs into the wrist alongside the ulnar artery. The flexor carpi ulnaris tendon is found just proximal to the pisiform bone when the wrist is flexed against resistance. At the proximal palmar crease the artery and nerve both run on the radial side of the tendon, but the nerve lies deep to the artery. This makes the volar approach difficult. The lateral approach is therefore recommended [41]. A 25-gauge needle is inserted at the proximal palmar crease on the ulnar side of the wrist. It is advanced 1.0 to 1.5 cm in a horizontal plane under the flexor carpi ulnaris. Three to 5 mL of local anesthetic is injected. Cutaneous nerves branch off the ulnar nerve, wrap around the wrist, and supply the dorsum of the hand. These may be blocked by injecting 5 to 6 mL of local anesthetic subcutaneously from the lateral border of the flexor carpi ulnaris tendon to the dorsal midline. The same injection site may be used, which may minimize the pain of injection [41].

Median nerve

The median nerve is located between the flexor carpi radialis tendon and palmaris longus tendon at the level of the proximal volar crease. In 20% of the population no palmaris longus tendon is present. In these patients the median nerve is found 1 cm ulnar to the flexor carpi radialis tendon. Insert a 25-gauge needle vertically through the skin and penetrate the deep fascia of the flexor retinaculum at a depth of approximately 1 cm. A slight "pop" should be appreciated and a paresthesia elicited. Inject 5 to 7 mL of local anesthetic just radial to the palmaris longus tendon. If the deep fascia has been penetrated a cutaneous wheal should not develop. It is better to begin injecting the local anesthetic too deep and continue injecting as the needle is withdrawn than to inject too superficially, as the retinaculum acts as a barrier to superficially injected anesthetic [41].

Hand

Digital nerve

Four digital nerves course into each digit. The two dorsal nerves run alongside the phalanx at the 2 and 10 o'clock positions, while the two palmar nerves occupy the 4 and 8 o'clock positions. The palmar nerves supply sensation to the volar aspects of the fingers, while the dorsal digital nerves supply the dorsal aspect of the digits. The palmar nerves of the middle three fingers also supply sensation to the dorsum of the fingertips, including the nailbed. Therefore, in the middle three fingers only the palmar digital nerves must be blocked to provide anesthesia to the area distal to the DIP joint. In the thumb and fifth finger all four nerves must be blocked to obtain adequate anesthesia of the fingertip and nailbed [41].

A variety of approaches may be used to perform a digital block. A few of them will be described here. When an option exists, the dorsal approach may be preferred to the volar approach as the dorsal skin is thinner and less painful to inject.

A 3.75-cm 25-gauge or 27-gauge needle is inserted at the web space, lateral to the bone and just distal to the knuckle. A subcutaneous wheal of 0.5 mL to 1.0 mL of local anesthetic is injected at this point. This will anesthetize the dorsal digital nerve and injection site. The needle is advanced lateral to the bone until the palmar skin begins to tent. At this point the needle is withdrawn 1 mm and 0.5 mL to 1.5 mL of local anesthetic is injected. This is repeated on the opposite side of the digit so that all four nerves are blocked [42].

A variation of this technique may cause less pain to the patient. One side of the digit is injected as described above, but rather than withdrawing the needle, the clinician redirects it across the dorsum of the digit to anesthetize the opposite side. The needle is then withdrawn, and may be reinserted into the area that was previously anesthetized. The block then proceeds as usual.

As noted above, the palmar approach may be more painful than dorsal needle insertion. However, in the middle three fingers, where only the volar nerves must be blocked for most common fingertip injuries, it is a useful technique. The needle is inserted over the center of the metacarpal head and local anesthetic is injected while the needle is advanced to the bone. The needle is then withdrawn 3 to 4 mm and angled to the left and right to block both volar nerves. Four to 5 mL of local anesthetic should be injected in total. A variation of this technique can be used in children to provide anesthesia for the most common fingertip injuries. The finger is pinched just distal to the proximal finger crease such that the skin overlying the finger crease is tented. A needle is inserted here and 0.5 to 1.0 mL of local anesthetic is injected subcutaneously. This single injection will anesthetize both volar digital nerves [41].

As discussed above, some clinicians perform digital blocks with epinephrine-containing solutions. At this time, most emergency medicine authorities advise against this practice. If epinephrine is accidentally injected into a digit, phentolamine may be used to reverse the alpha-agonism.

Metacarpal and intrathecal blocks

At least one study has suggested that a digital block provides more rapid and consistent anesthesia than a metacarpal block [43]. The transthecal technique is probably equivalent to the traditional digital block [44]. These techniques are therefore not discussed here.

Bier block (intravenous regional anesthesia)

Intravenous regional anesthesia (known as a Bier block) has been shown in numerous studies to be a safe and effective form of regional anesthesia for procedures involving the upper or lower extremities [45–48]. It is a reliable method to achieve consistent anesthesia, a bloodless field, and muscle relaxation. No deaths have ever been directly linked with its use. The procedure may be used in any patient who is able to cooperate. Contraindications include an allergy to the local anesthetic being used, uncontrolled hypertension, severe peripheral vascular disease, and soft tissue damage in the proximal extremity.

The procedure should be explained to the patient and an intravenous line placed in the unaffected extremity as a "backup" for resuscitation; 0.5% lidocaine without epinephrine is used. This can either be purchased as such or made by diluting 1% lidocaine in equal parts sterile saline. The usual dose is 3 mg/kg (recall there are 10 mg of lidocaine in 1 mL of 1% lidocaine), but a dose of 1.5 mg/kg is nearly as efficacious, and should be used as the starting point in the emergency department [49]. More lidocaine may always be given if needed. The lidocaine solution should be premixed in a 50-mL syringe.

Other anesthetic agents have no advantage over lidocaine, and should not be used. Bupivacaine should never be used due to the risk for severe cardiovascular and neurologic sequelae.

A pneumatic tourniquet is applied over cotton padding proximal to the pathology. A double-cuff pneumatic system is ideal. A standard blood pressure cuff should not be used, as it is prone to failure under prolonged high pressures.

The tourniquet is inflated and a 20-gauge catheter is inserted in a superficial vein, at least 10 cm distal to the tourniquet. Some studies show a higher success rate with more distal catheter placement. The tourniquet is now deflated and the extremity exsanguinated by either elevating it or wrapping it with an elastic bandage. Elevation is less painful to the patient, but must be done for at least 3 minutes and may be somewhat less effective than wrapping. As some authorities do not believe exsanguination is essential, one should be careful to avoid causing the patient unnecessary pain with the wrapping. The wrapping is done in a distal-to-proximal direction with the extremity elevated, being careful not to dislodge the previously placed catheter. With the arm still elevated, the pneumatic cuff is inflated to 250 mmHg (or 50 mmHg above the systolic pressure in a child). The extremity is lowered and the wrap, if used, is removed.

The lidocaine solution is slowly injected into the catheter at the predetermined dose. The patient will begin to note paresthesias or warmth in 3 to 5 minutes. It begins at the fingertips and progresses to the elbow to complete the anesthesia in 10 to 20 minutes. Muscle relaxation follows. If adequate anesthesia is not achieved in 15 minutes, more lidocaine may be infused, but the 3 mg/kg limit should never be exceeded. Another option is to inject 10 to 20 mL of saline solution. Once adequate anesthesia is achieved, the catheter is removed, the site is tightly taped to prevent leakage of the local anesthetic, and the procedure is performed [45].

A double-cuff tourniquet system may be used to alleviate tourniquet discomfort, which many patients experience after 20 to 30 minutes. In this system there is both a proximal and distal cuff. The proximal cuff is inflated at the beginning of the procedure and the anesthetic solution infused. Anesthesia will be obtained under the distal cuff. When the patient complains of pain under the proximal cuff, the distal cuff may be inflated. Be careful to not deflate the proximal tourniquet until the distal cuff is adequately inflated. Most patients are only able to endure approximately 1 hour of tourniquet time, limiting this block to procedures that can be performed in less than this amount of time [50].

At the completion of the procedure, a careful sequence must be followed to avoid potential lidocaine toxicity. If the procedure was completed in less than 30 minutes, the lidocaine may not have achieved adequate tissue fixation, and deflation of the cuff may produce a high peak plasma level of lidocaine. Therefore, the clinician should wait a full 30 minutes before attempting to deflate the tourniquet. At this point, the tourniquet is deflated for 5 seconds and reinflated for 1 to 2 minutes. This cycle is repeated three to four times and the patient observed for 20 minutes before being discharged [45].

Severe complications are rare, and include seizures and cardiovascular problems. High blood levels of lidocaine may be avoided by cautiously preventing a large intravascular bolus from reaching the systemic circulation. This may be accomplished by not deflating the cuff until at least 30 minutes have elapsed, not using blood pressure cuffs as tourniquets, never exceeding the 3 mg/kg dosage recommendation, and avoiding the placement of the catheter proximal to the tourniquet.

Femoral nerve block

The femoral nerve block has been used in the treatment of femoral shaft fractures for over 50 years. It has been shown to be effective for hip fractures as well [51]. Some studies suggest that patients with femoral neck fractures prefer this block to opiod analgesia [52]. Complications are rare, but careful aspiration of the syringe must be performed before injection of the local anesthetic, given the proximity of the femoral vein and artery [53]. A careful neurovascular exam must be performed both before and after the procedure.

To perform this block, the patient is placed in a supine position. The skin overlying the femoral triangle is prepared in the usual fashion. The femoral artery is palpated 1 to 2 cm distal to the inguinal ligament, and a subcutaneous wheal of local anesthetic is injected 1 to 2 cm lateral to this point. The nondominant hand is kept on the femoral artery throughout the remainder of the procedure. A 1.25-cm 22-gauge needle is attached to an extension tube setup and a 20-mL syringe. It is inserted just lateral to the artery at a 90° angle, and is advanced until a paresthesia is produced or the needle pulsates laterally. If a paresthesia is elicited, the needle is assumed to be in close proximity to the nerve and 10 to 20 mL of local anesthetic is injected. If no paresthesia is elicited, 10 to 20 mL of local anesthetic is injected in a fan-like distribution lateral to the artery in an attempt to anesthetize the nerve [41].

3 in 1 block (inguinal perivascular block)

The 3-in-1 block may be used to block the femoral, obturator, and lateral femoral cutaneous nerves with a single injection. The femoral nerve runs down the thigh in a fascial sheath that is continuous with a nerve sheath that contains all three nerves more proximally. If a large amount of local anesthetic is injected into this sheath it will track proximally and block all three nerves. This block demands injection of the local anesthetic into the nerve sheath. Although 20 to 30 mL of local anesthetic is being injected, the nondominant hand must be used to apply firm pressure distal to the injection site both during and for 5 minutes after the injection. It may take up to 30 minutes for this block to reach its peak efficacy [41].

Ankle blocks

Five peripheral nerve branches supply sensation to the foot. The superficial peroneal, deep peroneal, and saphenous nerves are anterior and supply sensation to the dorsum of the foot. At the level of the ankle, the superficial peroneal nerve consists of several branches, all of which lie superficially between the lateral malleolus and extensor hallucis longus tendon. These branches provide sensory supply to a large part of the dorsum of the foot. At the ankle, the deep peroneal nerve runs under the extensor hallucis longus tendon. It supplies the sensation for the web space between the first and second toes. The saphenous nerve parallels the saphenous vein between the medial malleolus and tibialis anterior tendon. It supplies sensation to the medial foot, around the arch. The posterior tibial and sural nerves are posterior and supply sensation to the volar aspect of the foot. The sural nerve lies superficially between the lateral malleolus and Achilles tendon. It supplies the lateral aspect of the foot, both volar and dorsal. The posterior tibial nerve lies deep and posterior to the posterior tibial artery between the medial malleolus and Achilles tendon. It provides sensation to most of the volar surface of the foot and toes [41].

Posterior tibial nerve

With the patient prone, and the foot off the end of the bed in slight dorsiflexion, the posterior tibial artery is located just posterior to the medial malleolus [54]. A point is selected 0.5 to 1.0 cm superior to this. A 3.75-cm 25-gauge needle is inserted here, just posterior to the artery, and directed at a 45° angle to the mediolateral plane. When 0.5 to 1.0 cm deep, the needle is moved side to side in an attempt to produce a paresthesia. If one is produced, 3 to 5 mL of local anesthetic is injected after aspiration. If a paresthesia is not produced, the needle is advanced further until it contacts the posterior border of the tibia. It is withdrawn 1 mm, and 5 to 7 mL of local anesthetic are injected while the needle is withdrawn another 1 cm [41].

Sural nerve

The sural nerve lies superficially, and is easily blocked by subcutaneously injecting 3 to 5 mL of local anesthetic between the Achilles tendon and lateral malleolus at a level 1 cm above the lateral malleolus. The patient should be positioned as for the posterior tibial nerve block [54].

Superficial peroneal nerves

The patient should be placed in a supine position. These nerves are superficial and are blocked by depositing 4 to 10 mL of local anesthetic subcutaneously between the extensor hallucis longus tendon and the lateral malleolus [41]. Alternatively, a wheal of 0.5 to 1.0 mL of local anesthetic may be deposited midway between the anterior tibial edge and the lateral malleolus [54].

Deep peroneal nerve

The deep peroneal nerve is blocked 1 cm above the base of the medial malleolus with the patient supine. The anterior tibial tendon is palpated while the patient dorsiflexes the foot. The extensor hallucis longus tendon is palpated by having the patient dorsiflex the great toe. The needle is placed between these two tendons and a SQ wheal of local anesthetic is deposited. The needle is then advanced under the extensor hallucis longus tendon (about 30° laterally) until it contacts the tibia. This occurs at a depth of less than 1 cm. At this point the needle is withdrawn 1 mm and 1 mL of local anesthetic is injected [41,54].

Saphenous nerve

The saphenous nerve is superficial, and is blocked by subcutaneously injecting 3 to 5 mL of local anesthetic between the medial malleolus and anterior tibial tendon.

Digital toe blocks

Digital nerve blocks in the foot are more efficacious and comfortable for the patient than local infiltration of local anesthetic into the toes. Due to the fibrous septa and limited subcutaneous space, local infiltration here may be painful, ineffective, and causative of local tissue ischemia.

Two volar and two dorsal digital nerves supply each toe. The dorsal digital nerves are branches of the deep and superficial peroneal nerves, while the volar digital nerves branch from the posterior tibial and sural nerves. In the toes, the nerves lie close to the bone at the 2, 4, 8, and 10 o'clock positions. More proximally, they parallel the tendons and are further from the bone [41].

Multiple sites for injection may be considered. The metatarsal approach is performed by inserting the needle dorsally between the metatarsal bones and injecting 1 mL of local anesthetic in a subcutaneous wheal. The needle is advanced until it tents the volar skin, and 2 mL of local anesthetic are deposited as the needle is withdrawn. The needle is then redirected laterally and this procedure repeated. Due to sensory overlap, this procedure must be performed in two or three adjacent spaces for one toe to be blocked. It is difficult to achieve consistent block of the digital nerves using this approach as the nerves do not lie in a predictable location at this level of the foot.

The recommended approach to achieve a digital block of the toe is the web space block. A 27-gauge 3.75-cm needle is inserted at the lateral edge of the bone just proximal to the base of the toe. A subcutaneous wheal is made by injecting 0.5 to 1.0 mL of local anesthetic, and then the needle is advanced until it is seen to almost exit the volar skin; 0.5 to 1.0 mL of local anesthetic is injected and the needle is withdrawn while simultaneously injecting another 0.5 mL of local anesthetic. This is repeated on the opposite side of the toe. Variations such as those used in the finger may be used to minimize patient discomfort and repetitive needle sticks. If the block is performed more distally, in the toe itself, the technique is the same but less local anesthetic is used due to the risk of vascular compromise in such a small subcutaneous space [41].

Intercostal block

An intercostal nerve block provides pain relief over the cutaneous area supplied by the nerve blocked. It is commonly employed in the emergency department for patients with broken or contused ribs. Although theoretically advantageous in that it may decrease hypoventilation, atelectasis, and pneumonia, there are no good studies that show it to be more effective than oral analgesics in the outpatient setting [41]. It is contraindicated in patients with flail chest or an overlying skin infection.

Pneumothorax occurs in up to 1.4% of individual intercostal nerves blocked, with an increased incidence in patients with underlying lung disease. When this fact is combined with a less than desirable success rate and duration of relief far less than what is required, it is important to thoroughly counsel the patient beforehand. A trial of oral analgesics may be indicated first [55].

An understanding of the anatomy involved is essential to obtaining a successful block. Each thoracic nerve exits the spinal column at the intervertebral foramen. The posterior cutaneous branch immediately branches off and supplies the paraspinal area. The intercostal nerve runs along the subcostal groove with the vein and artery. At the midaxillary line it gives off the lateral cutaneous branches. These nerves provide the sensory supply to the anterior and posterior lateral chest wall, and must be anesthetized to obtain adequate pain relief.

It should be noted that posteriorly only a thin layer of fascia separates the nerve from the pleura. However, at the posterior axillary line, the internal intercostal muscle lies between the nerve and the pleura. Because most rib fractures occur in the anterior or lateral portion of the ribs, the clinician can take advantage of this anatomical advantage by performing most blocks at the posterior axillary line [41].

The injured rib is palpated and followed posteriorly with the patient sitting upright and leaning forward on a Mayo stand [56]. The overlying area is prepared in a sterile manner. The index finger of the nondominant hand retracts the skin at the inferior border of the rib superiorly and over the rib. A 25-gauge needle, 3.75 cm long, on a 10-mL syringe is then directed by the dominant hand to puncture the skin at the tip of this finger. The needle should be directed at an 80° angle pointing cephalad. It is advanced until it contacts the rib. Skin retraction is now released, which will move the needle perpendicular to the chest wall and to the inferior edge of the rib. The syringe is switched to the nondominant hand. The palm is rested against the chest wall and the middle finger walks the needle off the inferior edge of the rib. The needle is slowly advanced 3 mm and aspirated. Two to 5 mL of local anesthetic is deposited while the needle is slowly moved in and out 1 mm. This maneuver ensures the compartment between the internal and external intercostal muscles (which contains the nerve) is penetrated. Due to innervation from overlapping nerves, this technique is then repeated on the two ribs above and below.

The patient should be observed for up to 30 minutes after the procedure. If no symptoms suspicious of a pneumothorax develop, he or she may be discharged home with return precautions. Symptomatic patients should have a chest radiograph taken, and those with pneumothoraces treated in the usual fashion [41].

Facial and oral blocks

General recommendations

Bupivacaine is probably the best local anesthetic for ED procedures in this area due to its prolonged duration of action when compared with lidocaine. Epinephrine should be added (when not contraindicated) when dental blocks are performed due to the high vascularity of the oral cavity. One exception is the maxillary supraperiosteal injection. Lidocaine with epinephrine provides the most prolonged anesthesia for this procedure [57].

A 27-gauge or larger needle should be used to facilitate aspiration and prevent intravascular injection of the local anesthetic. Aspirating syringes, which contain thumb rings or finger grips, are recommended, as they facilitate aspiration. Topical anesthetics should be used in the oral cavity before needle insertion. The area should be completely dried with gauze and then painted with anesthetic applied to a cotton-tipped applicator. Low concentrations of anesthetic (eg, 2% viscous lidocaine) are ineffective. Agents such as 20% benzocaine or 5% to 10% lidocaine must be used. Benzocaine has the advantages of rapid onset (30 seconds), brief duration (5 to 15 minutes), and low systemic absorption. In addition to the modalities described above, distraction techniques such as shaking the lip may decrease the pain of injection [58].

Supraperiosteal

A supraperiosteal block is useful for providing anesthesia to a single tooth. The area to be injected should be prepared as previously described. The mucous membrane is then pulled to expose the mucobuccal fold. For maxillary teeth the mucosa is pulled downward and out, while for the mandibular teeth it is pulled upward and out. The needle should enter the mucobuccal fold with the bevel facing the bone. One to 2 mL of local anesthetic is deposited at the apex of the tooth, close to the periosteum. Complete anesthesia may take 5 to 10 minutes. Because the nerve to be anesthetized lies inside the cortex of bone, this technique may fail if the local anesthetic is placed too far from the periosteum or the root [58].

Anterior superior alveolar nerve

This block provides anesthesia to the maxillary canine, the central and lateral incisors, and one half of the upper lip. The area should be prepared as previously discussed. The needle is inserted with the bevel facing bone superior to the apex of the canine and directed into the canine fossa. Two milliliters of local anesthetic are injected [59].

Middle superior alveolar nerve

Blocking this nerve will provide anesthesia to the maxillary premolars and part of the first molar. The needle is inserted with the bevel facing bone superior to the apex of the second premolar tooth. Two milliliters of local anesthetic are injected [57].

Posterior superior alveolar nerve

This block will provide anesthesia to the maxillary molars. The first maxillary molar sometimes must be separately anesthetized with a middle superior alveolar nerve block to gain complete anesthesia.

The area should be prepared as previously discussed. The patient's mouth should be half-open. The physician should retract the cheek laterally and insert the needle in the mucosal reflection just distal to the distal buccal root of the upper second molar. The needle is advanced along the curvature of the maxillary tuberosity to a depth of 2 to 2.5 cm. Two to 3 mL of local anesthetic is then injected after aspiration, being careful to avoid injection into the pterygoid plexus [57].

Infraorbital nerve

When local anesthetic is injected adjacent to the infraorbital foramen, it anesthetizes the middle and superior alveolar nerves and the infraorbital nerve. Therefore, this block will provide anesthesia to the intraoral areas previously discussed as well as the skin of the lower eyelid, nose, and upper lip. The infraorbital foramen is located on the inferior border of the infraorbital ridge on a vertical line with the pupil. The intraoral approach is preferred to the extraoral variation, as one study showed it provided a longer duration of anesthesia [60].

The intraoral approach is as follows. While holding one finger over the inferior border of the infraorbital rim a needle is inserted in the labial mucosa opposite the apex of the first premolar tooth approximately 0.5 cm from the buccal surface. The needle is advanced in a plane parallel to the axis of the tooth until it is palpated near the foramen at a depth of approximately 1.5 cm. Two to 3 mL of local anesthetic is deposited near, but not within, the foramen [58,61].

Inferior alveolar nerve block

This block will provide anesthesia to the ipsilateral mandibular teeth and the lower lip and chin via the mental nerve. The area should be prepared in the usual fashion, and the physician should stand on the side opposite to the one being injected. The syringe should be help parallel to the occlusal surfaces of the teeth and angled such that it overlies the first and second premolars on the opposite side of the mandible. A 25-gauge needle may be bent 30° to facilitate this angle. The coronoid process of the mandible is palpated with the non-dominant hand and the cheek retracted laterally. A triangle is visualized in the mucosa posterior to the molars. The needle is inserted in this triangle 1 cm above the occlusal surface of the molars. It is advanced until it contacts the mandibular bone, which is the posterior surface of the mandibular sulcus. The needle is withdrawn slightly and 1 to 2 mL of local anesthetic is injected after aspiration (3 to 4 mL if the needle is placed suboptimally). The bone must be contacted. If it is not it may indicate an approach that was too posterior and directed toward the parotid gland. If the local anesthetic is deposited too far posterior into the parotid gland the facial nerve may be anesthetized. This may produce a temporary Bell's palsy that will resolve when the local anesthetic wears off. If more local anesthetic is deposited while the needle is withdrawn, the lingual nerve may be anesthetized. The long buccal nerve may be blocked as well to provide anesthesia of the mucosa opposite the second and third molars. After the needle is withdrawn, it is reinserted into the buccal mucosa opposite the second molar; 0.5 mL of local anesthetic is injected [58,62].

Mental nerve block

The mental nerve is a continuation of the inferior alveolar nerve. It emerges from the mental foramen inferior to the second premolar tooth (in children the foramen lies between the first and second primary molars), and innervates the skin and mucosa of the ipsilateral lip with some midline crossover. For this reason, both mental nerves must be blocked for midline lip anesthesia.

If topical anesthesia is used, the intraoral approach is generally less painful than the extraoral approach [63]. The mental foramen is located approximately 1 cm inferior and anterior to the second premolar (just medial to the pupil along a vertical line). It should be palpated before this block is attempted. The area is prepared in the usual fashion, and the needle is inserted in the lower mucobuccal fold at a 45° angle. One to 3 mL of local anesthetic is injected into the area around the mental foramen [58,64].

Ophthalmic nerve block

This technique will provide anesthesia of the forehead and scalp as far posteriorly as the lambdoid suture. The lateral and medial branches of the supraorbital, supratrochlear, and infratrochlear nerves all emerge from the superior aspect of the orbit. The supraorbital notch is along the supraorbital rim directly above the pupil. The supraorbital nerves emerge from it. The supratrochlear nerve emerges 0.5 to 1.0 cm medial to this, and the infratrochlear nerve can be found on the most medial portion of the supraorbital rim.

To perform the block 1 to 3 mL of local anesthetic are deposited adjacent to the supraorbital notch. If this does not produce an adequate block, local anesthetic may be infiltrated subcutaneously along the entire supraorbital rim by injecting 5 mL of local anesthetic superior to the entire length of the eyebrow. A finger should be placed just below the supraorbital rim to reduce the risk of eyelid swelling [58,65].

Summary

The emergency physician has a variety of options for providing effective pain relief. A solid understanding of the local anesthetic agents and regional anesthetic techniques is an essential component of every emergency physician's analgesia armamentarium.

References

[1] Tetzlaff JE. The pharmacology of local anesthetics. Anesthesiol Clin North Am 2000;18(2): 217–33.

[2] Piccinini F, Chiarra A, Villani F. The active form of local anesthetic drugs. Experientia 1972; 28:140–1.
[3] Covino BG. Pharmacology of local anesthetic agents. Br J Anaesth 1986;58:701–16.
[4] Morgan GE, Mikhail MS, Murray MJ, et al. Local anesthetics. In: Morgan GE, Mikhail MS, Murray MJ, Larson CP, editors. Clinical anesthesiology. 3rd edition. New York: Lange Medical Books; 2002. p. 233–41.
[5] Stoelting RK, Miller RD, editors. Basics of anesthesia. 3rd edition. New York: Churchill Livingstone; 1994.
[6] Ahlstrom KK, Frodel JL. Local anesthetics for facial plastic procedures. Otolaryngol Clin North Am 2002;35(1):29–53.
[7] Rodriguez E, Jordan R. Contemporary trends in pediatric sedation and analgesia. Emerg Med Clin North Am 2002;20(1):199–222.
[8] Markakis DA. Regional anesthesia in pediatrics. Anesthesiol Clin North Am 2000;18(2): 355–81.
[9] Bartfield JM, Jandreau SW, Raccio-Robak N. Randomized trial of diphenhydramine versus benzyl alcohol with epinephrine as an alternative to lidocaine local anesthesia. Ann Emerg Med 1998;32(6):650–4.
[10] Xia Y, Chen E, Tibbits DL, et al. Comparison of effects of lidocaine hydrochloride, buffered lidocaine, diphenhydramine, and normal saline after intradermal injection. J Clin Anesth 2002;14(5):339–43.
[11] Dire DJ, Hogan DE. Double-blinded comparison of diphenhydramine versus lidocaine as a local anesthetic. Ann Emerg Med 1993;22(9):1419–22.
[12] Wilder RT. Local anesthetics for the pediatric patient. Pediatr Clin North Am 2000;47(3): 545–58.
[13] Zempsky WT, Karasic RB. EMLA versus TAC for topical anesthesia of extremity wounds in children. Ann Emerg Med 1997;30:163–6.
[14] Bjerring P, Arendt-Nielson L. Depth and duration of skin analgesia to needle insertion after topical application of EMLA cream. Br J Anaesth 1990;64:173–7.
[15] Eichenfield LF, Funk A, Fallon-Friedlander S, et al. A clinical study to evaluate the efficacy of ELA-Max (4% liposomal lidocaine) as compared with eutectic mixture of local anesthetics cream for pain reduction of venipuncture in children. Pediatrics 2002;109(6): 1093–9.
[16] Bucalo BD, Mirikitani EJ, Moy RL. Comparison of skin anesthetic effect of liposomal lidocaine, EMLA nonliposomal lidocaine, and EMLA using 30-minute application time. Dermatol Surg 1998;24:537–41.
[17] Wallace MS, Ridgeway B, Jun E, et al. Topical delivery of lidocaine in healthy volunteers by electroporation, electroincorporation, or iontophoresis: an evaluation of skin anesthesia. Reg Anesth Pain Med 2001;26:229–38.
[18] Kim MK, Kini NM, Troshynski TJ, et al. A randomized clinical trial of dermal anesthesia by iontophoresis for peripheral intravenous catheter placement in children. Ann Emerg Med 1999;33(4):395–9.
[19] Schultz AA, Strout TD, Jordan P, Worthing B. Safety, tolerability, and efficacy of iontophoresis with lidocaine for dermal anesthesia in ED pediatric patients. J Emerg Nurs 2002;28(4):289–96.
[20] Dailey RH. Fatality secondary to misuse of TAC solution. Ann Emerg Med 1988;17: 159–60.
[21] Jacobsen S. Errors in emergency practice. Emerg Med 1987;19:109.
[22] Blackburn PA, Butler KH, Hughes MJ, et al. Comparison of tetracaine-adrenaline-cocaine (TAC) with topical lidocaine-epinephrine (TLE): efficacy and cost. Am J Emerg Med 1995; 13(3):315–7.
[23] Ernst AA, Marvez-Valls E, Nick TG, et al. LAT (Lidocaine-adrenaline-tetracaine) versus TAC (tetracaine-adrenaline-cocaine) for topical anesthesia in face and scalp lacerations. Am J Emerg Med 1995;13(2):151–4.

[24] Schilling CG, Bank DE, Borchert BA, et al. Tetracaine, epinephrine (adrenaline), and cocaine (TAC) versus lidocaine, epinephrine, and tetracaine (LET) for anesthesia of lacerations in children. Ann Emerg Med 1995;25(2):203–8.
[25] Resch K, Schilling C, Borchert BD, et al. Topical anesthesia for pediatric lacerations: a randomized trial of lidocaine-epinephrine-tetracaine solution versus gel. Ann Emerg Med 1998;32:693–7.
[26] Wilhelmi BJ, Blackwell SJ, Miller J, et al. Epinephrine in digital blocks: revisited. Ann Plast Surg 1998;41(4):410–4.
[27] Green D, Walter J, Heden R, et al. The effects of local anesthetics containing epinephrine on the digital blood perfusion. J Am Podiatr Med Assoc 1992;82(2):98–110.
[28] Wagner MJ. Anesthesia. In: Hart RG, Vehara DT, Wagner MJ, editors. Emergency and primary care of the hand. ACEP, Dallas, TX; 2001.
[29] Panni M, Segal S. New local anesthetics: are they worth the cost? Anesthesiol Clin North Am 2003;21(1):19–35.
[30] Santos AC, DeArmas PI. Systemic toxicity of levobupivacaine, bupivacaine, and ropivacaine during continuous intravenous infusion to nonpregnant and pregnant ewes. Anesthesiology 2001;95(5):1256–64.
[31] Scarfone RJ, Jasani M, Gracely EJ. Pain of local anesthetics: rate of administration and buffering. Ann Emerg Med 1998;31:36–40.
[32] Bartfield JM, Sokaris SJ, Raccio-Robak N. Local anesthesia for lacerations: pain of infiltration inside vs outside the wound. Acad Emerg Med 1998;5(2):100–5.
[33] McKay W, Morris R, Mushlin P. Sodium bicarbonate attenuates pain on skin infiltration with lidocaine, with or without epinephrine. Anesth Analg 1987;66:572–4.
[34] Christoph RA, Buchanan L, Begalla K, et al. Pain reduction in local anesthetic administration through pH buffering. Ann Emerg Med 1988;17:117–20.
[35] Bartfield JM, Gennis P, Barbera J, et al. Buffered versus plain lidocaine as a local anesthetic for simple laceration repair. Ann Emerg Med 1990;19(12):1387–9.
[36] Matsumoto AH, Reifsnyder AC, Hartwell GD, et al. Reducing the discomfort of lidocaine administration through pH buffering. J Vasc Interv Radiol 1994;5:171–5.
[37] Colaric KB, Overton DT, Moore K. Pain reduction in lidocaine administration through buffering and warming. Am J Emerg Med 1998;16:353–6.
[38] Morgan GE, Mikhail MS, Murray MJ, et al. Peripheral nerve blocks. In: Morgan GE, Mikhail MS, Murray MJ, Larson CP, editors. Clinical anesthesiology. 3rd edition. New York: Lange Medical Books; 2002. p. 283–308.
[39] Faccenda KA, Finucane BT. Complications of regional anaesthesia: incidence and prevention. Drug Saf 2001;24(6):413–42.
[40] Ducharme J. Wrist blocks. In: Rosen P, Chan TC, Vilke GM, Sternbach G, editors. Atlas of emergency procedures. St. Louis: Mosby; 2001. p. 170–3.
[41] Kelly JJ, Spektor M. Nerve blocks of the thorax and extremities. In: Roberts JR, Hedges JR, editors. Clinical procedures in emergency medicine. 4th edition. Philadelphia: WB Saunders; 2004. p. 567–90.
[42] Taleghani NN, Sternbach G. Digital nerve block. In: Rosen P, Chan TC, Vilke GM, Sternbach G, editors. Atlas of emergency procedures. St. Louis: Mosby; 2001. p. 174–5.
[43] Knoop K, Trott A, Syverud S. Comparison of digital versus metacarpal blocks for repair of finger injuries. Ann Emerg Med 1994;23(6):1296–300.
[44] Hill RG Jr, Patterson JW, Parker JC, et al. Comparison of transthecal digital block and traditional digital block for anesthesia of the finger. Ann Emerg Med 1995;25(5):604–7.
[45] Roberts JR. Intravenous regional anesthesia. In: Roberts JR, Hedges JR, editors. Clinical procedures in emergency medicine. 4th edition. Philadelphia: WB Saunders; 2004. p. 591–5.
[46] Colbern EC. Intravenous regional anesthesia: the perfusion block. Anesth Analg 1966;45(1): 69–72.

[47] Dunbar RW, Mazze RI. Intravenous regional anesthesia: experience with 779 cases. Anesth Analg 1967;46(6):806–13.
[48] Roberts JR. Intravenous regional anesthesia—"Bier Block". Am Fam Physician 1978;17(2): 123–6.
[49] Farrell RG, Swanson SL, Walter JR. Safe and effective IV regional anesthesia for use in the emergency department. Ann Emerg Med 1985;14(4):288–92.
[50] Gerancher JC. Regional anesthesia: upper extremity nerve blocks. Anesthesiol Clin North Am 2000;18(2):297–317.
[51] Ducharme J. Acute pain and pain control: state of the art. Ann Emerg Med 2000;35(6): 592–603.
[52] McGlone R, Sadhra K, Hamer DW, et al. Femoral nerve block in the initial management of femoral shaft fractures. Arch Emerg Med 1987;4(3):163–8.
[53] Dilger JA. Regional anesthesia: lower extremity nerve blocks. Anesthesiol Clin North Am 2000;18(2):319–40.
[54] Taleghani NN, Sternbach G. Foot blocks. In: Rosen P, Chan TC, Vilke GM, Sternbach G, editors. Atlas of emergency procedures. St. Louis: Mosby; 2001. p. 176–7.
[55] Shanti CM, Carlin AM, Tyburski JG. Incidence of pneumothorax from intercostal nerve block for analgesia in rib fractures. J Trauma 2001;51(3):536–9.
[56] Barton ED. Intercostal nerve block. In: Rosen P, Chan TC, Vilke GM, Sternbach G, editors. Atlas of emergency procedures. St. Louis: Mosby; 2001. p. 34–5.
[57] Yagiela JA. Oral-facial emergencies: anesthesia and pain management. Emerg Med Clin North Am 2000;18(3):449–70.
[58] Amsterdam JT, Kilgore KP. Regional anesthesia of the head and neck. In: Roberts JR, Hedges JR, editors. Clinical procedures in emergency medicine. 4th edition. Philadelphia: WB Saunders; 2004. p. 552–66.
[59] Amsterdam JT. Internal maxillary-superior alveolar nerve block. In: Rosen P, Chan TC, Vilke GM, Sternbach G, editors. Atlas of emergency procedures. St. Louis: Mosby; 2001. p. 162–3.
[60] Lynch MT, Syverud SA, Schwab RA, et al. Comparison of intraoral and percutaneous approaches for infraorbital nerve block. Acad Emerg Med 1994;1(6):514–9.
[61] Taleghani NN, Sternbach G. Facial and oral blocks: infraorbital nerve block. In: Rosen P, Chan TC, Vilke GM, Sternbach G, editors. Atlas of emergency procedures. St. Louis: Mosby; 2001. p. 160–1.
[62] Amsterdam JT. Mandibular and inferior alveolar nerve block. In: Rosen P, Chan TC, Vilke GM, Sternbach G, editors. Atlas of emergency procedures. St. Louis: Mosby; 2001. p. 164–5.
[63] Syverud SA, Jenkins JM, Schwab RA, et al. A comparative study of the percutaneous versus intraoral technique for mental nerve block. Acad Emerg Med 1994;1(6):509–13.
[64] Amsterdam JT. Mental nerve block. In: Rosen P, Chan TC, Vilke GM, Sternbach G, editors. Atlas of emergency procedures. St. Louis: Mosby; 2001. p. 166–7.
[65] Taleghani NN, Sternbach G. Facial and oral blocks: supraorbital nerve block. In: Rosen P, Chan TC, Vilke GM, Sternbach G, editors. Atlas of emergency procedures. St. Louis: Mosby; 2001. p. 158–9.

ELSEVIER
SAUNDERS

Emerg Med Clin N Am 23 (2005) 503–517

EMERGENCY
MEDICINE
CLINICS OF
NORTH AMERICA

Procedural Sedation and Analgesia: A Review and New Concepts

Elizabeth L. Bahn, MD*, Kurtis R. Holt, MD, FACEP

Department of Emergency Medicine, Madigan Army Medical Center, Fort Lewis, WA 984431, USA

Providing sedation and analgesia (PSA) to patients to accomplish painful procedures or difficult diagnostic imaging is becoming a standard practice in every emergency department (ED). Emergency physicians (EPs) are called upon daily to provide this service. Despite the emergence as a common procedure, PSA is as yet an evolving area of emergency medicine marked with tradition, unchallenged dogma, and unanswered questions.

Heretofore we used the term "conscious sedation" to define the act of giving sedatives and analgesics to patients. This term has since been abandoned for a more precise and meaningful title. Conscious sedation implies an alert patient yet sedated. It is an oxymoron. In addition, it is an imprecise description of the patient. During this procedure patients experience a spectrum of sedation, most of which is not in the "conscious" zone. The term conscious sedation is not recognized by the Joint Commission on Accreditation of Health Care Organizations (JCAHO) as a measurable level of sedation, and has since been abandoned for a more inclusive yet flexible title, "procedural sedation and analgesia" [1].

In 2001, JCAHO created sedation guidelines in an attempt to define the spectrum of procedural sedation and analgesia and provide a qualitative measurement for EPs [2]. The spectrum ranges from minimal sedation to general anesthesia, with defined criteria at each level. Minimal sedation is equivalent to anxiolysis. It is a drug-induced state during which patients respond normally to verbal commands. Respiratory and cardiovascular functions are not affected [2]. Next in the spectrum is moderate sedation/analgesia. This describes a depression of consciousness during which patients respond purposefully to verbal commands, either alone or accompanied by light tactile stimulation. Spontaneous ventilation is adequate, and cardiovascular function is usually maintained [2].

* Corresponding author.
E-mail address: elizabeth_bahn@hotmail.com (E.L. Bahn).

doi:10.1016/j.emc.2004.12.013 **emed.theclinics.com**

The deeper levels of the spectrum range from "deep sedation" to "general anesthesia." Deep sedation/analgesia describes a depression of consciousness during which patients cannot be easily aroused but respond purposefully following repeated or painful stimuli. Patients may require assistance in maintaining a patent airway and spontaneous ventilation. Cardiovascular function is usually maintained [2]. General anesthesia is the point at which consciousness is lost and the patient is not rousable to stimuli. The patient requires respiratory assistance and cardiovascular function is often impaired [2].

Another level of sedation, which may be placed along with moderate sedation, is dissociative sedation. This is a relatively new description since the introduction of ketamine as a sedative agent. It is characterized as a trance-like cataleptic state induced by a dissociative agent that provides profound analgesia and amnesia. Protective airway reflexes and spontaneous respirations are maintained along with cardiovascular stability [2].

The JCAHO sedation guidelines provide qualitative goals for the EP when he/she is conducting PSA. The ideal is to fulfill all the goals of PSA, which are to alleviate anxiety, minimize physical pain and discomfort, and maximize amnesia. In addition, PSA should assist in controlling behavior to expedite the procedure while minimizing negative psychologic responses to treatment. Last, the EP strives to maintain safety by minimizing risks and ensuring safe discharge.

PSA continues to evolve within emergency medicine. This field of practice is becoming more defined. Clinical dogma is being challenged, resulting in new concepts and application to emergency medicine. Last, EPs are building experience with multiple drugs, which adds to our armamentarium. By understanding the current and new concepts of PSA, becoming familiar with the pharmacologic agents, and appreciating the spectrum of sedation, the EP can reach his clinical goals.

Review of medications

Midazolam

Otherwise known as Versed, midazolam is a benzodiazepine with both amnestic and anxiolytic properties. With no analgesic effects, it is commonly combined with fentanyl as probably the most well-known "cocktail" used for "conscious sedation." It has many properties that make it the preferred benzodiazepine for procedural sedation. When comparing it to diazepam (Valium) it has a much more rapid onset of action and rarely causes phlebitis. When compared with lorazepam (Ativan), the relatively rapid onset of action makes it more useful in the ED setting. Midazolam appears to have superior amnestic properties when compared with diazepam and lorazepam [3].

Midazolam can be given intravenously (IV), intramuscularly, or orally. When using it for procedural sedation in the ED, IV is the much-preferred route secondarily to the delayed onset of action and erratic absorption by the intramuscular or oral routes. Additionally, the onset of action is delayed at least 15 minutes with the intramuscular route. The IV dose is 0.03 mg to 0.1 mg/kg. Onset of sedation is typically 2 to 5 minutes, and duration of action is 30 to 60 minutes. When using in the elderly population or with concomitantly administered analgesics, the above-mentioned dosing should be decreased accordingly. Additionally, in the elderly population the duration of action can be markedly increased secondary to decreased metabolic clearance. A common dosing regimen, when used in conjunction with fentanyl, is 0.5 μg/kg of fentanyl with 0.05 mg/kg of midazolam to a total dose of 1 to 2 μg/kg of fentanyl and a maximum dose of 4 mg of midazolam.

In a recent study by Burton et al [4], in the Annals of Emergency Medicine midazolam was compared with etomidate for procedural sedation. A dose of 0.033 mg/kg was used for midazolam. The median time for PSA was 23 minutes for midazolam with an average of 2.1 doses of midazolam used, compared with an etomidate dose of 0.1 mg/kg, with 10 minutes to PSA and average of 1.6 doses needed [4].

Side effects of midazolam are dose dependent, and include hypoventilation and hypoxemia. These side effects are more prominent when midazolam is combined with other central nervous system depressants such as narcotics. Hypotension also occurs with high doses.

Fentanyl

A synthetic opioid and 1000 times as potent as meperidine, Fentanyl is the narcotic of choice for analgesia in PSA. Extremely rapid onset of action and short duration of action make it a relatively easily titrated narcotic. Fentanyl has the added benefits of a not causing a histamine release and minimal cardiovascular effects. Fentanyl has minimal amnestic effects, and should not be used as a sole agent for PSA. It is commonly combined with amnestics and anxiolytics such as midazolam, etomidate, and others, for PSA.

Fentanyl is best given IV at a dose of 0.5 to 1 μg/kg every 1 to 2 minutes. As with most medications used in PSA, lower doses should be used when given to the elderly. Intramuscular and oral preparations are available, but should not be used in the adult population for PSA secondary to erratic absorption and delayed onset of action.

Fentanyl is not without side effects, and most are potentiated by the addition anxiolytics and amnestics. These side effects include hypoxemia, apnea, vomiting, and pruritus. An advantage over other narcotics is that fentanyl seems to have minimal cardiovascular; therefore, it is less likely to cause hypotension.

Methohexital

Of all the barbiturates used for PSA, methohexital (Brevital) is the most popular among ED physicians. Pentobarbital, used more frequently in children, appears to have a longer half-life in adults. Thiopental is used more often as an induction agent for intubation, but has minimal evidence that it can be used safely for PSA. Methohexital has an onset of action of less than 1 minute and a duration of action of less than 10 minutes. These properties make it an excellent choice for short procedures such as reduction of fractures or cardioversions. Although methohexital induces a state of unconsciousness, airway protective measures are preserved. It is purely an amnestic agent and has no analgesic properties; consequently, small doses of opioids are commonly given for that reason. The one caveat is that the opioids appear to potentiate the respiratory depression that is an uncommon but potential side effect. Methohexital does have a direct myocardial depressant effect that can lead to a drop in blood pressure with a concomitant elevation in heart rate. Therefore, its use in the hemodynamically unstable patient should be questioned [5].

As with most agents used for PSA, the IV route is much preferred. Methohexital is dosed at 0.75 to 1 mg/kg, and can be redosed at 2-minute intervals of 0.5 mg/kg. In a study by Miner et al [6], methohexital was compared with propofol for PSA in patients undergoing fracture and dislocations reductions. Both were given as 1 mg/kg doses and then redosed at 0.5 mg/kg at 2-minute intervals if needed. The authors were unable to detect a significant difference in the level of subclinical respiratory depression or level of sedation. Out of 109 patients, six required bag–valve–mask-assisted ventilations all for less than 1 minute and not requiring hospitalization.

The benefit of having an ultrashort acting agent is that the effects are transient and brief. Overall, methohexital is an appealing option for short procedures requiring PSA. Its safety has been proven, and should be in every emergency medicine physician's armamentarium for PSA.

Ketamine

Well known as an agent used for the pediatric population for PSA, ketamine is emerging as a popular agent for adult PSA as well. A member of the street drug phencyclidine, it is unusual in the fact that it is a "dissociative" agent; meaning that it causes a dissociation between the thalamoneocortical and limbic systems, preventing the higher centers from perceiving visual, auditory, or painful stimuli. Muscle tone is maintained; therefore, airway protective measures are preserved. With its almost immediate onset of action and ultrashort acting properties, it seems to be the perfect agent for PSA. The disadvantages of ketamine, which have kept it largely out of the adult population, are the presence of the "emergence phenomena" and the hypertension and tachycardia that has been associated with its use. It has been suggested that vomiting associated with emergence has the potential to cause aspiration pneumonia. That has been recounted secondary to the fact that almost all cases of vomiting that occurred with ketamine use were once the patient was alert and oriented with protective airway reflexes in effect. The "emergence phenomena," manifested by hallucinations and nightmares, is seen in up to 50% of the adult population. A study by Chudnofsky et al [7] indicated that the addition of a small dose of midazolam to ketamine reduced the incidence of the "emergency phenomena" to five patients out of 70 experiencing a mild emergence reaction. The dosing of the medications used was 0.07 mg/kg of IV midazolam and 2 mg/kg of IV ketamine.

In the adult population the IV route is again the preferred method of delivering the medication: 1 to 2 mg/kg over 1 to 2 minutes, followed by doses of 0.25 to 0.5 mg/kg every 5 to 10 minutes, as needed. Anticholinergic agents, such as glycopyrrolate and atropine at doses of 0.2 mg and 0.02 mg/kg, respectively, are given to blunt the hypersalivation that occurs in some patients. Contraindications to the use of ketamine include history of airway instability, high predisposition to laryngospasm, severe cardiovascular disease, cerebral spinal fluid obstructive states, intraocular pressure pathology, and hypersensitivity [8].

Nitrous oxide

An ultrashort-acting agent with immediate onset of action, combined with the fact that it has little effect on other organ systems other than the central nervous system; nitrous oxide would appear to be an ideal agent for PSA. It also has analgesic properties that are overshadowed by its sedative and anxiolytic effects. The difficulty with nitrous oxide is that it requires a well-ventilated room with a scavenger system to prevent inhalation by the ED staff. It also has extremely high potential for misuse among the ED staff as well.

The dosing for PSA ranges from 30% to 50%, and must be administered with 30% oxygen to avoid hypoxia. This requirement may result in deep sedation with loss of protective airway reflexes.

New concepts in PSA

Monitoring

Objective measurements quantifying the depth of sedation have not yet been fully established. Currently, several qualitative tools are used to measure sedation depth. These are clinical scoring systems that have previously been validated in the intensive care unit (ICU) setting. The most commonly used scores are the Observer's Assessment of Alertness/Sedation Scale [9] and the Ramsay Sedation Scale (OAA/S) [10]. Recently, the

Ramsey Sedation Scale was modified to be consistent with the JCAHO definitions of sedation depth [11]. These are used both in research as comparative tools and in the ED for documentation of sedation depth, but neither can be objectively used to predict deep sedation with subsequent respiratory depression, which is clearly an endpoint that should be avoided.

In accordance with JCAHO and institutional guidelines, patients are to be monitored continuously both with objective physiologic monitors and with qualitative clinical assessments. Although noninvasive monitoring of blood pressure, cardiac activity, and pulse oximetry are routinely performed, it is unknown how these measurements add to the assessment of sedation depth or to the prediction of respiratory depression. Recently, there have been several investigations evaluating the utility of the end tidal carbon dioxide ($ETCO_2$) monitor and the Bispectral Index (BIS) monitor in the assessment of sedation depth and the detection of respiratory depression.

End tidal CO_2 monitoring is routinely used during general anesthesia. It is the measurement of carbon dioxide emitted throughout expiration. A predictable waveform is recorded. The normal range for $ETCO_2$ is between 40 to 48 mmHg. Changes in $ETCO_2$ occur before changes in the SaO_2 in the face of respiratory depression, as patients can maintain normal oxygen saturation for several minutes even during ventilatory failure or airway obstruction. During airway obstruction the $ETCO_2$ waveform flattens, while during ventilatory failure the $ETCO_2$ will rise above 50 mmHg. These two findings precede oxygen desaturation. Many studies have suggested that $ETCO_2$ is an accurate predictor of respiratory depression, and can be used as a tool for monitoring during PSA [12].

Minor et al [12] sought to determine the utility of $ETCO_2$ to detect respiratory depression in patients undergoing PSA. They also sought to determine whether the depth of sedation, as perceived by clinical assessment, could be predicted by the amount of respiratory depression detected by the $ETCO_2$. This was a prospective, observational study of patients undergoing PSA in the ED. They compared $ETCO_2$ measurements with the OAA/S and the development of respiratory depression. They found no correlation between the $ETCO_2$ and the OAA/S. Although an absent waveform, an absolute change in $ETCO_2$ $>$10 mmHg, or an $ETCO_2$ $>$50 mmHg predicted all cases of clinically significant respiratory depresson [12]. $ETCO_2$ monitoring may not predict the depth of sedation, but it can be used for early detection of respiratory depression.

Recently, bispectral encephalographic analysis has been studied in the PSA population to determine its utility as a measure of sedation depth. Bispectral analysis is a processed EEG parameter that measures a patient's level of sedation [11]. The BIS has formerly been used by anesthesiologists during general anesthesia to monitor a patient's level of alertness. The BIS is based on a 100-point scale, with 1 being without brain activity and 100 being fully awake and alert [13]. A BIS score below 60 is associated with a low probability of a response to verbal stimuli [13].

Bispectral monitoring has already been validated as a tool in the OR setting [13]. It has yet to be validated as a tool for sedation monitoring in the PSA population. However, recently Gill et al [11] used the BIS monitor in comparison to a modified Ramsey Sedation Scale to determine a correlation between the scores. This study was a prospective observational study of 270 patients undergoing PSA in the ED setting. They ultimately determined that the correlation between the BIS and the modified Ramsey Sedation Scale was only moderate and displayed wide variability. However, a score of greater than 83 excluded deep sedation, and a score of less than or equal to 70 reliably identified general anesthesia [11].

Miner et al [14] conducted a prospective observational study on patients undergoing PSA to determine a correlation between the BIS score and rates of respiratory depression, and the patient's perception of pain and recall. Respiratory depression was defined by $ETCO_2$ and oxygen saturation. An absent $ETCO_2$ waveform, a change from baseline >10 mmHg, or an SaO_2 <90% delineated respiratory depression. Patients also completed a visual analog scale concerning their perception of pain and recall. There was statistical significance in the rates of respiratory depression between patients with a BIS score of 70 to 85 and those with a score of 60 to 69 and those with a score <60 ($P = 0.0003$ and $P = 0.006$), respectively. There was no statistically significant difference in respiratory depression between patients with a BIS score >85 and those with a score of 70 to 85. In addition, among patients with a BIS score <85 there was no difference in the visual analog scores for pain and recall. However, the visual analog scores for pain and recall were significantly different between those with a BIS score >85 and those with scores <85. The results of this study indicate that achieving a BIS score between 70 and 85 results in an optimal depth of sedation without increasing the risk of respiratory depression [14].

Depth of sedation monitoring is essential to maintaining patient safety, minimizing complications such as respiratory depression and aspiration, and providing adequate analgesia, amnesia, and anxiolysis. JCAHO provides goals for sedation depth and standards to maintain, but as of yet, there is no one quantitative tool to adequately measure sedation depth. $ETCO_2$ monitoring can be used as an adjunctive device to help the EP predict and detect respiratory depression regardless of sedation depth. Currently, the American Society of Anesthesiologists (ASA) mandates that capnography be used for all cases of general anesthesia care both in and out of the operating room setting [15]. The BIS monitor is evolving into a tool that can assist with sedation management by providing a range of values that may predict an optimal sedation depth. However, we are yet to determine how to achieve those goal values with our pharmacologic agents and doses. This remains as an area of future investigation.

Preprocedural fasting

The risk of pulmonary aspiration of gastric contents is a concern inherent to any practitioner who is sedating a patient. The preprocedural fasting time and the depth of sedation are two variables that have historically and universally been thought to contribute to the risk of aspiration. In most institutional guidelines and those set forth by JCAHO, assessing the fasting time and limiting the depth of sedation are standards that have to be met. In some instances strict requirements must be met that may not be practical nor feasible when applying them to the emergency patient. For example, few patients presenting to the ED have met the standard fasting time requirement. In addition, the level of sedation necessary to perform a particular procedure may be deeper than the goal of "moderate sedation." Due to the unique nature of the emergency patient it is obvious that these two standards have been challenged in an attempt to incorporate them more feasibly into the practice of emergency medicine.

Most of the research done to evaluate and describe pulmonary aspiration and the risk factors leading to this complication has come from the general anesthesia literature. Based upon early animal models, it was determined that the extent of pulmonary injury was directly related to the acidity and volume of gastric contents that were aspirated. In the primate model it was shown that a minimum of 0.8 mL/kg was needed to produce changes in the lung consistent with aspiration pneumonitis [16]. From this and other studies on animal models the concept of preprocedural fasting was born.

More recent studies, however, have challenged this original thinking. First, it has been determined that silent aspiration occurs both in normal sleep and during general anesthesia both with and without cuffed endotracheal tubes [17]. Second, fasting more than 2 hours produces no significant difference in gastric volume and pH compared with a 2-hour fast [17]. Because of the many studies supporting these findings the ASA changed their consensus statements [18]. For clear liquids, "evidence is silent on the relationship between fasting times, gastric volume, or gastric acidity and the risk of emesis/reflux or pulmonary aspiration in humans." For solid foods, "there is insufficient published evidence to address the safety of any preoperative fasting period" [18]. The recommendation, therefore, is 2 hours for clear liquids and 6 hours for solids [18].

The application of the general anesthesia literature to the emergency medicine arena has been questioned [17]. A recent analysis pooled the existing studies on clinically apparent aspiration during general anesthesia. The combined data showed the overall incidence of aspiration to be 1:3420, with aspiration mortality in 1:125,109 [17]. These results indicate that in modern anesthesia the risk of clinically significant aspiration is low. So far there are no reported cases of aspiration during ED PSA in the medical literature.

The argument has been made that the relative risk of aspiration during ED PSA is significantly lower than that of general anesthesia [17]. Several points are to be considered in this argument. (1) Aspiration occurs mostly during manipulations of the airway. During PSA endotracheal intubation and extubation should ideally not occur. (2) The depth of sedation in PSA is targeted to a point where the individual maintains their protective reflexes. (3) The practice of PSA does not employ inhalational agents, which are emetogenic. Last, the majority of PSA is performed on young, healthy adults and children, and in general, those with an ASA clinical classification I or II. The elderly and ASA class III, IV, and V, who represent the majority of the general anesthesia population, are at higher risk of aspiration [17] and complications of sedation in general.

The question of the incidence of clinically significant aspiration during PSA still remains. However, in a recent prospective analysis of children undergoing PSA in the ED it was noted that 56% of the study group did not meet fasting guideline criteria [19]. Adverse events occurred in 68 of the 1014 patients studied (6.7%). These included, O_2 desaturation $<90\%$, transient apnea, emesis, hypotension, emergence reaction, and laryngospasm. All events were successfully treated. Interestingly, there was no difference in adverse events between patients who met fasting criteria and those who did not [19]. Of significant note, there were no episodes of aspiration in this study population [19].

The guidelines that apply to general anesthesia may not be applicable to PSA in the ED setting. The emergency practitioner should, however, be aware of the potential risks of aspiration and control those variables that he/she can. As there is no basis in the literature for specific fasting times, and the guidelines currently in effect were generated by consensus opinion [17,20], the EP must use prudence when selecting patients for PSA. An emergent fracture/dislocation reduction with a full stomach may be appropriate, while an incision and drainage of an abscess with a full stomach would not. EPs should also be prepared to manage the complications of PSA, which could include aspiration. Proper equipment preparation, choice of sedative drug, and depth of sedation are all under the control of the EP to minimize risk. Until there is more literature on aspiration during PSA the incidence and risk factors will remain largely speculative. The EP must use the current guidelines as a reference point, but good clinical judgment and preparation should determine the course.

New concepts in the pharmacology of PSA

Etomidate use In PSA

Etomidate is a sedative hypnotic agent that has gained wide acceptance and use as an effective drug for rapid sequence induction. Many EPs prefer this drug because of its rapid onset, short duration of action, and minimal effect on respiratory and cardiovascular function. The features that make it a desirable induction agent also make it useful for PSA. Increasingly, EPs are using etomidate in the ED for sedation for a variety of procedures. There is limited but promising research on the safety and efficacy of etomidate use for PSA.

In 2001, Ruth et al [21] published their results of a two-part feasibility study of etomidate use in the ED for PSA. The pilot phase was a retrospective chart review of patients who had received etomidate for PSA. Nine patient charts were evaluated. Etomidate was used for dislocation/reductions, abscess drainage, cardioversion, and foreign body removal. All procedures were successful. All patients received an IV bolus dose of 0.1 mg/kg, with each achieving adequate sedation and no complications, particularly oxygen desaturation and/or apnea [21]. During the feasibility phase of this study the use of etomidate was prospectively studied. Adequate sedation was achieved in 98% based on physician assessment. Although there were five cases of oxygen desaturation below 90%, no patient needed assisted ventilation or endotracheal intubation [21]. Retrospective data on patients who have received etomidate for PSA is promising in regard to safety. Keim et al [22] report that one patient (2%) in their study experienced transient apnea and one patient (2%) had oxygen desaturation. Both had been given opioids in conjunction with the etomidate, and neither required intubation. Vinson et al [23] also retrospectively studied ED patients receiving etomidate for PSA and noted few adverse events. Of 134 patients, five (3.3%) experienced oxygen desaturation below 94% [23]. These patients were all >55 years of age and had received higher doses (0.23 mg/kg). In addition, none required endotracheal intubation. Of note, the mean dose of etomidate used in this study was 0.20 mg/kg. Moderate sedation was achieved in 32% and deep sedation with verbal unresponsiveness was noted in 68% [23].

Another attractive feature of etomidate is its quick onset and its short duration of action. This profile makes it an efficient drug to use in a busy ED. Ruth et al [21] report a return to a baseline-modified Aldrete postanesthetic recovery score in an average of 12.6 minutes. Vinson et al [23] showed that 95% of patients in their study attained full recovery to the preprocedural level of alertness within 30 minutes. Furthermore, a recent prospective, double-blinded, randomized controlled trial comparing etomidate and midazolam showed a significant difference in total PSA times between the groups [24]. The median PSA time was 10 minutes in the etomidate group and 23 minutes in the midazolam group ($P > 0.001$) [24].

The side effect profile of etomidate also makes it attractive for ED use in PSA. The most common side effects reported are nausea, vomiting, and myoclonus [21–24]. One case of hyperemesis resistant to antiemetic therapy, which required a 3-hour stay in the ED, was reported [21]. Otherwise, the incidence of postprocedural nausea and vomiting was low [21–24]. Etomidate has been associated with myoclonus in 0% to 80% of patients, and is considered dose related [22]. Burton et al [24] reported mild myoclonus in three patients and severe myoclonus in one patient. Ruth et al [21] reported myoclonus in four cases. Three episodes were described as brief tremors while one was described as "total body stiffness" lasting 1 minute. None of these events required intervention. Another side effect of etomidate reported in the literature is adrenal suppression [22]. Etomidate inhibits 11-*b*-Hydroxylase, an enzyme that promotes conversion of 11-deoxycortisol to cortisol and can temporarily suppress the adrenal axis [22]. Reports on adrenal suppression have involved patients who received continuous infusion of etomidate for sedation. However, a decline in plasma cortisol levels after one induction dose has been reported [22].

Etomidate use, a sedative agent during PSA, is gaining wider acceptance as more research is being done. Etomidate offers many advantages, including its rapid onset, short duration of action, and its stable hemodynamic profile. In addition, etomidate has a relatively low adverse effect profile and has been shown to be safe for use in PSA [21–24]. The biggest concern for its use is that it can quickly and easily induce deep sedation and/or general anesthesia. With proper monitoring and dosing, etomidate is a safe and effective choice in the ED for adult PSA.

Propofol use for PSA

Few topics in emergency medicine have generated as much debate and controversy as the use of propofol for PSA. Propofol is classified as a nonopioid, nonbarbiturate, sedative-hypnotic agent. It has gained wide acceptance as an agent to induce general anesthesia, but has met much resistance for use as an agent for PSA. The properties that make it so desirable for PSA are its rapid onset, short duration of action, and predictable efficacy for inducing deep sedation. However, these characteristics are also what drive the debate as to whether propofol is appropriate for use in the ED. The primary criticism is that it potently and rapidly induces a deep level of sedation, which can easily tend toward general anesthesia.

Most studies involving propofol have been conducted in the pediatric population for brief, painful procedures both in the ED and in the ICU setting. Propofol has been found to be as effective as midazolam for achieving adequate sedation without significant adverse effects [25]. However, the mean recovery time for the propofol was significantly shorter then the midazolam, 15 minutes versus 76 minutes, respectively [25]. Propofol has also been shown to be as effective as ketamine in optimizing comfort without increasing the rate of adverse effects during procedures in the pediatric ICU [26]. Again, recovery time was minimized significantly with propofol use compared with ketamine [26]. Other small prospective studies have showed similar utility in the use of propofol without an increase in morbidity and mortality [27].

Recently, two trials have evaluated the safety and efficacy of propofol for both emergent and elective painful procedures in the ED and short-stay units. Basset et al [28] used propofol in 393 emergent pediatric sedations. They used an initial IV bolus dose of 1 mg/kg then titrated by 0.5 mg/kg to the desired sedation level. They additionally used fentanyl or morphine before the procedure as an adjunct for analgesia. Ninety-five percent of patients maintained an SaO_2 >90%. Three patients experienced apnea, requiring bag–valve–mask for less then 1 minute, and none needed endotracheal intubation. Ninety-two percent sustained a brief duration of hypotension with an SBP <82 mmHg, and 6% experienced a transient bradycardia <60 bpm. The median duration of sedation was 30 minutes and the median time from procedure completion to ED discharge was 18 minutes [28]. Guenther et al [29] experienced similar findings using the same propofol protocol for elective pediatric procedures in a short-stay unit. They used 1 mg/kg IV bolus dose then 0.5 mg/kg titration. The median total dose used was 3.5 mg/kg. They noted similar recovery times and an adverse event profile as reported by Basset et al [28]. Of note, this study was conducted on a pediatric population that was predominantly ASA class III. Patients of a higher ASA classification are generally considered at higher risk for complications during procedural sedation [30].

Propofol has yet to be fully introduced into the adult PSA realm. However, Coll-Vinent et al [31] recently used propofol in a randomized, controlled trial comparing it to etomidate and midazolam for sedation during cardioversion. The dose of propofol was 1.5 mg/kg IV bolus, followed by 0.5 mg/kg, as needed. All drugs were uniformly effective for completing the procedure, and there was no significant difference in adverse events among the agents. Propofol was well tolerated, received high patient satisfaction, and demonstrated the quickest recovery time (median, 10 minutes, $P = 0.002$) [31]. Although a small study, it shows promise for using propofol for PSA in the adult ED.

Propofol appears to be a desirable agent for use as a sedative for brief, painful procedures like fracture reduction or cardioversion. It has an immediate clinical effect after administration, a predictable potency that reliably produces sedation, and a short duration of action that minimizes recovery time. However, such characteristics make it easy for the EP to overshoot the level of sedation desired and induce a general anesthesia. Care must be taken with this agent. Begin with low doses and titrate to the desired level of sedation and prepare to manage any complications associated with deep sedation or general anesthesia. Basset el al [28] and Guenther et al [29] used a 1 mg/kg IV bolus dose with a 0.5 mg/kg titration dose in pediatric patients. They also used fentanyl or morphine as adjuncts. The adverse event rate was not substantially higher than that seen with midazolam and fentanyl [28–30].

Propofol use still meets resistance in some institutions. JCAHO does not prohibit its use by EPs [30]; rather, they allow for individual hospitals to set their own policies. In light of recent studies supporting the safety and efficacy of propofol use for procedural sedation in the pediatric population, many EDs may be adding this to their list of available agents for PSA. However, more research needs to be conducted for its use in adult PSA.

Summary

Procedural sedation and analgesia has become a commonplace procedure in the ED, certainly falling under the domain of the EP. Every EP should approach PSA as a complex procedure requiring high-level skills and knowledge. Initially, understand that PSA represents a spectrum of goals, from anxiolysis and pain relief to deep sedation. Assess the needs of the patient and the concomitant procedure and set goals accordingly. There is a pharmacopia of drugs that provide sedation and analgesia. Become familiar with their pharmacology, advantages and disadvantages, and indications. This will allow for appropriate usage and achievement of sedation goals. Several drugs that are commonly used for general anesthesia are proving themselves to be safe and efficacious for PSA. Both etomidate and propofol have emerged as useful drugs for PSA. Continued research and practice with these agents will add to our understanding and help define their use for PSA.

Performing PSA as a procedure itself requires preparedness, diligent monitoring, and risk awareness. Knowing the patient's comorbid state and choosing agents that will not exacerbate their baseline status minimize risk. Following fasting guidelines is appropriate in certain clinical situations, and is prudent when time permits. However, these guidelines are a benchmark for minimizing risk and are not supported by evidence-based medicine. It is important to be cognizant of the guidelines but also to identify the emergency scenario where action must be taken despite the fasting guidelines. Controlling sedation depth also minimizes the risk of aspiration and other complications. The $ETCO_2$ monitor and Bispectral Index may prove to be useful adjuncts for monitoring sedation depth. However, there is nothing yet that measures sedation depth quantitatively that can replace the qualitative assessment of the EP.

More and more PSA is falling under the domain of the EP. It is important for the EP to be involved in hospital policy and guidelines associated with this procedure, and to remain aware of new research in this field. EPs can thereby contribute to quality assurance throughout the medical community by setting a standard in the practice of PSA, as they are not the only practitioners using this procedure. With continued practice and research, expertise in this field will grow measurably.

References

[1] Green SM, Krauss B. Procedural sedation terminology: moving beyond "conscious sedation." Ann Emerg Med 2002;39:433–5.

[2] Joint Commission on Accreditation of Healthcare Organization. 2001 sedation and anesthesia care standards. Oakbrook Terrace (IL): JCAHO (Web page: www.jcaho.org/standard/aneshap).
[3] Muse DA. Conscious and deep sedation. In: Harwood-Nuss A, Wolfson AB, editors. The clinical practice of emergency medicine. 3rd edition. Philadelphia: Lippincott/Williams and Wilkins; 2001. p. 1761.
[4] Burton J, Bock A, Strout T, et al. Etomidate and midazolam for reduction of anterior shoulder dislocation: a randomized, controlled trial. Ann Emerg Med 2002;40(5): 496–504.
[5] Chudnofsky CR, Lozon MM. Sedation and analgesia for procedures. In: Marx JA, Hockberger RS, Walls RM, editors. Rosen's emergency medicine, concepts and clinical practice. 5th edition. St. Louis: Mosby; 2002. p. 2581.
[6] Miner J, Biros M, Krieg S, et al. Randomized clinical trial of propofol versus methohexital for procedural sedation during fracture and dislocation reduction in the emergency department. Acad Emerg Med 2003;10(9):931–7.
[7] Chudnofsky C, Weber J, Stoyanoff P, et al. A combination of Midazolam and Ketamine for procedural sedation and analgesia in adult emergency department patients. Acad Emerg Med 2000;7(3):228–35.
[8] Cromhout A. Ketamine: its use in the emergency department. Emerg Med 2003;15:155–9.
[9] Chernik DA, Gillings D, Laine H, et al. Validity and reliability of the Observer's Assessment of Alertness/Sedaton Scale: study with intravenous midazolam. J Clin Psychopharmacol 1990;10:244.
[10] Frenzel D, Greim C, Sommer C, et al. Is the bispectral index appropriate for monitoring the sedation level of mechanically ventilated surgical ICU patients? Intens Care Med 2002;28: 178–83.
[11] Gill M, Green SM, Krauss B. A study of the bispectral index monitor during procedural sedation and analgesia in the emergency department. Ann Emerg Med 2003;41:234–41.
[12] Miner JR, Heegaard W, Plummer D. End-tidal carbon dioxide monitoring during procedural sedation. Acad Emerg Med 2002;9:275–80.
[13] Rowow C, Manberg P. Bispectral index monitoring. Anesthesiol Clin North Am 1998;2: 89–107.
[14] Miner JR, Biros MH, Heegaard W, et al. Bispectral electroencephalographic analysis of patients undergoing procedural sedation in the emergency department. Acad Emerg Med 2003;10:638–43.
[15] American Society of Anesthiologists. Standards for basic anesthetic monitoring. Available at: http://www.asahq.org/publicationsAndServices/standards/02.html.
[16] Raidoo DM, Rocke DA, Brock-Utne JG, et al. Critical volume for pulmonary acid aspiration: reappraisal in a primate model. Br J Anaesth 1990;65:248–50.
[17] Green SM, Krauss B. Pulmonary aspiration risk during emergency department procedural sedation—an examination of the role of fasting and sedation depth. Acad Emerg Med 2002; 9(1):35–41.
[18] American Society of Anesthesiologists. Practice guidelines for preoperative fasting and the use of pharmacologic agents to reduce the risk of pulmonary aspiration: application to healthy patients undergoing elective procedures. Anesthesiology 1999;90:896–905.
[19] Agrawal D, Manzi SF, Gupta R, et al. Preprocedural fasting state and adverse events in children undergoing procedural sedation and analgesia in a pediatric emergency department. Ann Emerg Med 2003;42(5):636–45.
[20] Green SM. Fasting is a consideration—not a necessity—for emergency department procedural sedation and analgesia. Ann Emerg Med 2003;42(5):647–50.
[21] Ruth WJ, Burton JH, Bock AJ. Intravenous etomidate for procedural sedation in emergency department patients. Acad Emerg Med 2001;8(1):13–8.
[22] Keim SM, Erstad BL, Sakles JC, et al. Etomidate for procedural sedation in the emergency department. Pharmacotherapy 2002;22(5):586–91.

[23] Vinson DR, Bradbury DR. Etomidate for procedural sedation in emergency medicine. Ann Emerg Med 2002;39(6):592–8.
[24] Burton JH, Bock AJ, Strout TD, et al. Etomidate and midazolam for reduction of anterior shoulder dislocation: a randomized, controlled trial. Ann Emerg Med 2002;40(5):496–504.
[25] Havel CJ, Strait RT, Hennes H. A clinical trial of propofol vs. midazolam for procedural sedation in a pediatric emergency department. Acad Emerg Med 1999;6(10):989–97.
[26] Vardi A, Salem Y, Padeh S, et al. Is propofol safe for procedural sedation in children? A prospective evaluation of propofol versus ketamine in pediatric critical care. Crit Care Med 2002;30(6):1231–5.
[27] Guenther-Skokan EG, Pribble C, Bassett KE, et al. Use of propofol sedation in a pediatric emergency department: a prospective study. Clin Pediatr 2001;40:663–71.
[28] Bassett KE, Anderson JL, Pribble CG, et al. Propofol for procedural sedation in children in the emergency department. Ann Emerg Med 2003;42(6):773–82.
[29] Guenther E, Pribble CG, Junkins EP, et al. Propofol sedation by emergency physicians for elective pediatric outpatient procedures. Ann Emerg Med 2003;42(6):783–91.
[30] Green SM, Krauss B. Propofol in emergency medicine: pushing the sedation frontier. Ann Emerg Med 2003;42(6):792–7.
[31] Coll-Vinent B, Sala Z, Fernandez C, et al. Sedation for cardioversion in the emergency department: analysis of effectiveness in four protocols. Ann Emerg Med 2003;42(6):767–72.

ELSEVIER
SAUNDERS

EMERGENCY
MEDICINE
CLINICS OF
NORTH AMERICA

Emerg Med Clin N Am 23 (2005) 519–527

Establishing an Emergency Department Pain Management System

Christopher F. Richards, MD

Center for Policy and Research in Emergency Medicine, Oregon Health and Science University, 3181 S.W. Sam Jackson Park Road, Mail Code, CDW-EM, Portland, OR 97239-2984, USA

Other articles in this edition will describe multiple aspects of pain management in the emergency department (ED). Many of those authors have cited multiple works that describe our current failure to achieve optimal pain control for our patients. Providing optimal pain control with the pitfalls and caveats described in other articles is a challenge. Education of individuals is not sufficient to effect process change, particularly one of the magnitude required to repair some current systems. Education may change the way an individual acts, but only changing the culture and infrastructure will result in a change in the care provided by the system.

Forces both within and outside medicine have made pain management a priority. The Joint Commission on Accreditation of Health Care Organizations pain standards is well known, but cases of failure to treat pain being considered malpractice are also on the rise [1–6]. Fortunately, designing and establishing a system can improve pain management outcomes [7].

This article will attempt to outline some strategies to systematically improve departmental pain management. Many departments have already established protocols and guidelines addressing effective and adequate pain assessment and management. Although some of these approaches and modifications to existing systems may not be effective or appropriate for all systems, and may seem excessive to some, the goal of these strategies described above is to provide an effective systems approach for effective pain management in the ED setting.

E-mail address: richarch@ohsu.edu (C.F. Richards).

doi:10.1016/j.emc.2004.12.014 **emed.theclinics.com**

Implications of the current state

The emergency medicine literature on pain control and pain management reveals a rift between patient expectations and provider behavior. Up to 70% of patients presenting to the ED have pain as part of their presenting complaint [8]. This makes pain the most prevalent symptom in the ED. Patient expectations with regard to control of pain are quite high; some might say unreasonably so. Fosnocht [9] found that ED patients felt that 23 minutes from arrival to pain relief was a reasonable interval, while the actual interval to receiving pain medication was 78 minutes. This directly translated into patient satisfaction scores. Perhaps of greater importance, multiple studies have demonstrated that when patient satisfaction is compromised, malpractice risk rises [10,11].

The idea that we undertreat pain in the ED is not new, and unfortunately, it is not uniform across race and other boundries [12–15]. Disparities in the administration of analgesia in the ED among various ethnic groups have been studied, showing that Black and Hispanic patients are often less likely to receive appropriate analgesia than are Whites [16–18]. Further research is necessary to further delineate the scope of the disparities in the ED and to study potential solutions [19]. Improvements in the overall treatment of pain should help to reduce such disparities.

If our treatment of pain is less than ideal, our documentation of that treatment is worse. In a recent study of ED patients, 15% of nurses and 10% of physicians used a pain scale to document pain initially, with even lower rates for reassessments [20]. Such levels are in profound contrast to the Joint Commission on Accreditation of Health Care Organizations standard that all ED patients have their pain assessed.

Setting up the program

Any ED guideline for the management of pain in the ED should consider the following: assessment of pain, acute versus chronic pain, potential medication tolerance, concurrent anxiety and psychiatric issues, communication with other members of the health care team, assessment tools, program monitoring, and a continuous quality assurance program.

Assessment of pain

The first step in developing a pain management program is assessment. A uniform method of assessment must be available and used in your department. Staff may initially be resistant to the idea of such a scale; however, many are available. Staff were initially resistant to the idea of pulseoximetry, but now it is obtained on every patient in our ED. As such, assessment and screening for pain with an objective scale should be required for all patients. Documentation of that assessment and any reassessment necessary due to treatment or other intervention should also be recorded. Policies and procedures need to reflect these expectations, and staff training and form revisions provide tools for maintaining changed behavior patterns. If pain is really to be the sixth vital sign, a sixth column should be added to the ED chart.

Once assessment and appropriate reassessments of pain is universal in your department, the next step is appropriate management of pain. Many practice guidelines exist to aid clinicians in the management of specific types of pain or conditions. Some examples are listed in Table 1. Unfortunately, most of these guidelines deal with chronic pain, osteoarthritis for example, or acute exacerbations of chronic pain, such as low back pain. Although these conditions are certainly staples of emergency practice, they are in no way inclusive. Protocols and guidelines are useful, but rather than focusing on what medications and what route, the focus should be on the assessment and reassessment of pain after appropriate interventions. Some very specific conditions, such as sickle cell crisis and fracture, are amenable to a critical pain pathway where very frequent assessment and titration of medications can be ordered.

There are a number of pain assessment tools available. Many of these tools are impractical for daily ED use, but serve a useful research function. The multidimensional McGill Pain Questionnaire is one example; it, unfortunately, takes 30 to 45 minutes to administer [21]. Although multidimensional tools are used for research purposes and as initial assessment tools in pain clinics, they are impractical for ED use. Even the short form of the McGill Pain Questionnaire tool is too cumbersome for ED use [22]. One-dimensional tools can be practical for ED use, and fall into three categories: numeric rating scales, visual analog scales, and categoric scales. Most EDs use a verbal numeric rating scale such as the classic 1 to 10 scale. The visual analog scale, used extensively in emergency medicine research, can be used as a day-to-day tool [23]. Unfortunately, it requires the clinician to measure the line with a ruler to assess and record the pain accurately. Categoric

Table 1
Pain management guidelines for specific types of pain or conditions

AHCPR	Clinical Practice Guideline: Management of Cancer Pain [41]
AHCPR	Acute Low Back Pain Problems in Adults [42]
AAOS	Clinical Guidelines:
	Hip Pain [43]
	Knee Pain
	Wrist Pain
AAFP and AAN	Guidelines on Migraines [44–48]
AAFP	Management of Pain in Sickle Cells Crises [49]

Abbreviations: AAFP, American Academy of Family Physicians; AAN, American Academy of Neurology; AAOS, American Academy of Orthopaedic Surgeons; AHCPR, The Agency for Health Care Policy and Research (Currently called the Agency for Healthcare Research and Quality).

scales work by asking the patient to rate the pain intensity using visual or verbal descriptors. The most familiar are scales using faces to describe the pain [24–27]. One-dimensional scales work well for acute pain but has limited value for complex multidimensional pain often referred to as chronic pain [24]. A multidimensional pain assessment tool that may be of use in some ED settings is the Brief Pain Inventory, although it will likely be more useful for research [28].

Aspects of a pain guideline

The guideline should recognize the differences in pathophysiology and human response to acute versus chronic pain. Acute pain is not classified in terms of duration, but rather as a "complex unpleasant experience with emotional, cognitive, and sensory features occurring in response to tissue trauma" [29]. On the other hand, chronic pain is pain that extends beyond the period of healing, with levels of identified pathology that are often insufficient to explain the presence or extent of the pain [21,30]. Acute pain, while usually concordant with the extent of tissue damage, results in neurohumoral responses that can have adverse effects. Although the emotional effects are obvious, the effects on neuronal remodeling and subsequent chronic pain are less obvious but equally important [21]. Chronic pain, unlike its cousin acute pain, does not have an adaptive function. It may be caused by remote injury, malignancy, arthritis, or a host of other nonlife-threatening conditions. To a much greater extent than acute pain, affective disorder and social and other environmental stressors influence the perception of chronic pain and ED presentation. Although acute pain should be managed aggressively to promote tissue healing and facilitate evaluation and treatment of injuries, chronic pain must be evaluated and treated in the larger context. Complementary therapies such as antidepressants and antianxiety medications can be useful here, and should be incorporated into a guideline.

The potential for medication tolerance and side effects should be considered in the guideline. Many analgesics such as acetaminophen have a single dose range, but others such as the opiates should be titrated to effect. Opiate tolerance is an issue; medication interactions and side effects can also be a problem. Medication selection can be tailored to the specific environment. For example, our ED, and many others around the country, are completely Meperidine free.

It goes without saying that the ED is not equivalent to an outpatient clinic environment. Current access to care issues aside, the patient population perceives their problem as more acute than those presenting to an outpatient clinic environment. This patient anxiety must be considered and treated where appropriate. In addition, many of our patients present to us because they have concurrent psychiatric and social issues. No ED pain guideline is complete without consideration of these issues. In our ED, we rely heavily upon our ED social workers for assistance in this regard.

Communication with other members of the health care team is a central part of emergency practice. Unfortunately, a number of factors prevent us, the health care team, from communicating effectively. There are provider availability issues related to time or distance, system issues, and patient issues. Documenting attempts to locate the appropriate provider is essential, and should be included in the guideline and the accompanying documentation forms. This is especially important for the chronic pain patient or the patient with potential drug-seeking behavior, as these patients often concurrently obtain care from multiple health care settings [31]. System issues such as consultants who do not have 24/7 coverage can create communication issues. In addition, patient factors such as travel distant from home and dishonesty regarding having a primary care physician or narcotic contract can create impediments to communications and patient care. We have recently developed a protocol for dealing with "patients who have forgotten their identity" to prevent some of these issues, as well as minimize fraudulent usage of health care resources.

Treatment of pain in the ED

Although the assessment of pain can be protocolized and mandated in the ED, I will not be so bold as to suggest a protocol for doing so here. However, when establishing a pain management system, one must make the necessary tool available to the ED staff and provide some guidance in their use. The tools available to emergency physicians in the ED for the treatment of pain fall into three broad categories: opiate analgesics, nonopiod analgesics, and adjuvants. In addition, use of nonpharmacologic adjuvants should be encouraged.

The opiate analgesics include the mu opiate agonists like morphine, the mu opiate agonist-antagonists like butorphanol, and opiate analgesic combinations or various varieties like acetaminophen with an opiate. These agents are available for parenteral, oral, and transdermal use. Tramadol is a mixed mu agonist and norepinephrine and serotonin reuptake blocker. A variety of these agents should be available for use in the ED. As stated above, rapid titration or ideally patient controlled analgesia should be used for defined conditions.

The nonopiate analgesics consist of acetaminophen, aspirin, and nonsteroidal anti-inflammatory drugs (NSAIDs), including the newer cyclooxygenase-2 selective NSAIDs. Again, physicians should be familiar with these, and a variety of these agents should be available for use in the ED.

Adjuvant therapy with tricyclic antidepressants, antiepileptic drugs, corticosteroids, beta-blockers, calcium channel blockers, and local anesthetics (transdermally or via injection therapy) can be very helpful, and should be considered when appropriate.

Nonpharmacologic approaches to pain management should supplement but usually do not replace medications. Psychologic interventions such as behavioral therapy, biofeedback, or psychotherapy, and physical rehabilitative methods such as massage, strengthening exercises, or nonallopathic (alternative) approaches are available.

Managing the ED pain control program

Program monitoring should be a continuous process. Adding assessment of your local pain protocol to you list of continuous quality assurance indicators is important. Increasing use of electronic health records and electronic charting enhances such tracking and promises to improve adherence to such protocols. Intermittent chart audits can also be used. Results of monitoring should be shared with staff on a routine basis. We post results and graphicl trends of these types of audits in our staff bathrooms for easy accessibility. The results should be reviewed by the departments Continuous Quality Improvement (CQI) committee at regular intervals to assure compliance and adequacy and to address any changes necessary.

Special features for consideration in the emergency department

Drug-seeking behavior

All emergency physicians are familiar with drug-seeking behavior. The behavior of these patients and emergency physician interactions with them likely color many of our perceptions of pain in the ED. Zechnich and Hedges [31] describe a cohort of 30 patients described as at risk for drug-seeking behavior. These patients visited an average of 4.1 different EDs on 12.6 separate occasions during the 1-year study period. Even after being told that they would receive no further "narcotics" in the ED, 71% of them received controlled substances in that ED and 93% received controlled substances in another ED. Two of 30 overdosed and died of a drug overdose. But drug-seeking behavior is like pornography; you know it when you see it, but are not quite sure what to do with it. "Drug seekers" are a subset of serial patients. Repeat patients represent 62% of visits and 30% of patients, but serial patients (those with four or more visits a year) represent 5% of patients and 21% of visits [32]. Some centers including our own have used case management interventions with some success with serial patients, including those with drug-seeking features. Pope [33] described a cohort of 24 patients in whom the annual number of ED visits decreased from a median of 26.5 to 6.5 visits in the years preceding and after implantation of an aggressive multidisciplinary approach to repeat visits.

Some EDs track these patients with either official or unofficial lists [31]. The term "habitual patient files" has been proposed as a replacement for "repeated file," "problem patient file," "frequent flyer file," "special needs list," and other more pejorative names for such lists [34]. Such lists have ethical, legal, confidentiality, and other issues to consider. An alternative is an electronic ED tracking system that displays the number of pervious visits in a given interval. EMSTAT (A4 Healthsystems) list the number of visits for a given patient in the last year next to the patient's time in the ED for this visit. The number turns red if a there is a visit within the last 72 hours. Such a system alerts providers of previous encounters for all patients and avoids any pejorative labels. Other systems use flags on charts to alert providers of important clinical or nonclinical issues. It is important that such flags be appropriate and current, as they suffer from many of the issues associated with habitual patient lists. Whatever system that is used to identify habitual user of the ED or patients who may potentially be using the ED as a method for obtaining medications for secondary gain, a multidisciplinary approach to include case management, social work, primary care, and drug-addiction treatment programs is necessary to effectively treat these patients. Such systems are further discussed in the chapter by Hansen elsewhere in this issue.

Special populations

Some populations of ED patients are particularly susceptible oligoanalgesia. Ethnic minorities are a well-known example [16–18]. Other populations at risk include pediatrics, the mentally retarded, the elderly, and patients with psychiatric illnesses [35–40]. In some cases, guidelines specific for these populations or for specific disease states may be appropriate.

Summary

Any ED system for the management of pain in the ED should consider the following: assessment of pain including mandatory use of some assessment tool, a guideline for treatment of pain, communication with other members of the health care team, assessment tools, program monitoring, and a continuous quality assurance program. The treatment guideline should consider acute versus chronic pain, potential medication tolerance, concurrent anxiety and psychiatric issues, special populations, and disease-specific conditions.

References

[1] Acello B. Meeting JCAHO standards for pain control. Nursing 2000;30:52–4.
[2] Dahl JL, Saeger L, Stein W, et al. The new JCAHO pain assessment standards: implications for the medical director. J Am Med Dir Assoc 2000;1:S24–31.

[3] Furrow BR. Pain management and liability issues. Hematol Oncol Clin North Am 2002; 16:1483–94.
[4] Shapiro RS. Health care providers' liability exposure for inappropriate pain management. J Law Med Ethics 1996;24:360–4.
[5] Shapiro RS. Legal bases for the control of analgesic drugs. J Pain Symptom Manage 1994; 9:153–9.
[6] Shapiro RS. Liability issues in the management of pain. J Pain Symptom Manage 1994;9: 146–52.
[7] Somers LJ, Beckett MW, Sedgwick PM, et al. Improving the delivery of analgesia to children in pain. Emerg Med J 2001;18:159–61.
[8] Cordell WH, Keene KK, Giles BK, et al. The high prevalence of pain in emergency medical care. Am J Emerg Med 2002;20:165–9.
[9] Fosnocht DE, Swanson ER, Bossart P. Patient expectations for pain medication delivery. Am J Emerg Med 2001;19:399–402.
[10] Hickson GB, Federspiel CF, Pichert JW, et al. Patient complaints and malpractice risk. JAMA 2002;287:2951–7.
[11] Usha Kiran TS, Jayawickrama NS. Complaints and claims in the UK National Health Service. J Eval Clin Pract 2002;8:85–6.
[12] Ducharme J. Emergency pain management: a Canadian Association of Emergency Physicians (CAEP) consensus document. J Emerg Med 1994;12:855–66.
[13] Selbst SM. Managing pain in the pediatric emergency department. Pediatr Emerg Care 1989; 5:56–63.
[14] Selbst SM, Henretig FM. The treatment of pain in the emergency department. Pediatr Clin North Am 1989;36:965–78.
[15] Wilson JE, Pendleton JM. Oligoanalgesia in the emergency department. Am J Emerg Med 1989;7:620–3.
[16] Todd KH, Deaton C, D'Adamo AP, et al. Ethnicity and analgesic practice. Ann Emerg Med 2000;35:11–6.
[17] Todd KH, Lee T, Hoffman JR. The effect of ethnicity on physician estimates of pain severity in patients with isolated extremity trauma. JAMA 1994;271:925–8.
[18] Todd KH, Samaroo N, Hoffman JR. Ethnicity as a risk factor for inadequate emergency department analgesia. JAMA 1993;269:1537–9.
[19] Richards CF, Lowe RA. Researching racial and ethnic disparities in emergency medicine. Acad Emerg Med 2003;10:1169–75.
[20] Eder SC, Sloan EP, Todd K. Documentation of ED patient pain by nurses and physicians. Am J Emerg Med 2003;21:253–7.
[21] Turk DC. Understanding pain sufferers: the role of cognitive processes. Spine J 2004;4:1–7.
[22] Melzack R. The short-form McGill Pain Questionnaire. Pain 1987;30:191–7.
[23] Bijur PE, Silver W, Gallagher EJ. Reliability of the visual analog scale for measurement of acute pain. Acad Emerg Med 2001;8:1153–7.
[24] Bieri D, Reeve RA, Champion GD, et al. The Faces Pain Scale for the self-assessment of the severity of pain experienced by children: development, initial validation, and preliminary investigation for ratio scale properties. Pain 1990;41:139–50.
[25] Wong DL, Baker CM. Pain in children: comparison of assessment scales. Okla Nurse 1988; 33:8.
[26] Wong DL, Baker CM. Pain in children: comparison of assessment scales. Pediatr Nurs 1988; 14:9–17.
[27] Wong DL, Baker CM. Smiling faces as anchor for pain intensity scales. Pain 2001;89:295.
[28] Cleeland CS, Ryan KM. Pain assessment: global use of the Brief Pain Inventory. Ann Acad Med Singapore 1994;23:129–38.
[29] Chapman CR, Nakamura Y. A passion of the soul: an introduction to pain for consciousness researchers. Conscious Cogn 1999;8:391–422.

[30] Turk DC, Okifuji A. Psychological factors in chronic pain: evolution and revolution. J Consult Clin Psychol 2002;70:678–90.
[31] Zechnich AD, Hedges JR. Community-wide emergency department visits by patients suspected of drug-seeking behavior. Acad Emerg Med 1996;3:312–7.
[32] Cook LJ, Knight S, Junkins EP Jr, et al. Repeat patients to the emergency department in a statewide database. Acad Emerg Med 2004;11:256–63.
[33] Pope D, Fernandes CM, Bouthillette F, et al. Frequent users of the emergency department: a program to improve care and reduce visits. CMAJ 2000;162:1017–20.
[34] Geiderman JM. Keeping lists and naming names: habitual patient files for suspected nontherapeutic drug-seeking patients. Ann Emerg Med 2003;41:873–81.
[35] AGS Panel on Chronic Pain in Older Persons, American Geriatrics Society. The management of chronic pain in older persons. Geriatrics 1998;53(Suppl 3):S8–24.
[36] Chan L, Russell TJ, Robak N. Parental perception of the adequacy of pain control in their child after discharge from the emergency department. Pediatr Emerg Care 1998;14:251–3.
[37] Friedland LR, Pancioli AM, Duncan KM. Pediatric emergency department analgesic practice. Pediatr Emerg Care 1997;13:103–6.
[38] Gloth FM 3rd. Pain management in older adults: prevention and treatment. J Am Geriatr Soc 2001;49:188–99.
[39] Grossman SA, Richards CF, Anglin D, et al. Caring for the patient with mental retardation in the emergency department. Ann Emerg Med 2000;35:69–76.
[40] O'Brien JG. Acute pain in the elderly. Postgrad Med Spec 199;49–55.
[41] Jacox A, Carr DB, Payne R. New clinical-practice guidelines for the management of pain in patients with cancer. N Engl J Med 1994;330:651–5.
[42] Bigos SJ. United States Agency for Health Care Policy and Research: acute low back problems in adults. Rockville, MD: US Dept. of Health and Human Services, Public Health Service, Agency for Health Care Policy and Research; 1994.
[43] Clinical Guideline on Hip Pain. In: American Academy of Orthopedics. www.aos.org: Accessed December 13, 2003.
[44] Morey SS. Guidelines on migraine: part 2. General principles of drug therapy. Am Fam Physician 2000;62:1915–7.
[45] Morey SS. Guidelines on migraine: part 3. Recommendations for individual drugs. Am Fam Physician 2000;62:2145–8.
[46] Morey SS. Guidelines on migraine: part 4. General principles of preventive therapy. Am Fam Physician 2000;62:2359–60.
[47] Morey SS. Guidelines on migraine: part 5. Recommendations for specific prophylactic drugs. Am Fam Physician 2000;62:2535–9.
[48] Silberstein SD. Practice parameter: evidence-based guidelines for migraine headache (an evidence-based review): report of the Quality Standards Subcommittee of the American Academy of Neurology. Neurology 2000;55:754–62.
[49] Preboth M. Management of pain in sickle cell disease. Am Fam Physician 2000;61:1544–50.

EMERGENCY
MEDICINE
CLINICS OF
NORTH AMERICA

ELSEVIER
SAUNDERS

Emerg Med Clin N Am 23 (2005) 529–549

Complementary and Alternative Pain Therapy in the Emergency Department

James N. Dillard, MD, DC, CAc, FAAPM&R[a,b], Sharon Knapp, MS, FNP, NP-C[c,*]

[a]*Columbia University College of Physicians and Surgeons, 630 West 168th Street, New York, NY 10032, USA*

[b]*Rosenthal Center for Complementary and Alternative Medicine, 630 West 168th Street, New York, NY 10032, USA*

[c]*Oregon Health and Sciences University, 3181 S.W. Sam Jackson Park Road, Mail Code CDW-EM, Portland, OR 97239-2984, USA*

Comprehensive care of patients with pain and the complexities in treating it requires understanding the physiologic dynamics of pain, pharmacologic methods for treatment, as well as other measures available for treatment outside of the emergency department that may be part of the patients self-care and belief system. A brief review of the pathophysiology of pain pathways, a review of pain management principles, and a review of complementary and alternative medicine (CAM) therapies used will be discussed. Using CAM strategies with conventional treatments is becoming increasingly popular among patients. Understanding all treatment modalities will allow the practitioners to better meet the needs of their patients and be aware of potential interactions, which may complicate their medical management in the emergency department.

Management of pain in the emergency department is a seemingly simple task, but one that reportedly has been done poorly [1–3]. Very few medical schools have acute pain control as part of a core curriculum. With little formal training it may be assumed that pain control is not a priority. Extensive teaching is not necessarily the answer, but some focused teaching and increased awareness may be what is needed to improve pain management [4]. Pain has a predictable presence in patients, but the management of pain is often a single modality of therapy. Traditionally, a one-shot [sic] approach to pain is the approach in the emergency

* Corresponding author.
E-mail address: knappsh@ohsu.edu (S. Knapp).

0733-8627/05/$ - see front matter
doi:10.1016/j.emc.2004.12.015

department. This amounts to intravenous, intramuscular, or oral narcotics as the method of choice for most pain and injection of anesthetic agents for local or regional pain as prevention.

The Joint Commission on Accreditation of Hospitals Organizations mandates evaluation, treatment, and assessment of effectiveness of pain treatment. As of 2001, pain assessment has become the fifth vital sign (http://www.jcaho.org/, accessed 1/25/03). With this mandate, treating pain has become a priority of health care providers. It is estimated that as many as 75 million Americans live with chronic pain, and 22% of patients in primary care report poorly controlled pain [5,6]. Pain is a costly national problem in lost workdays, hospitalization, physical therapy, disability, and pharmaceutical cost, as well as litigation costs surrounding pain. Chronic pain accounts for 21% of all emergency room visits, and causes 25% of days lost in the workplace [6]. It is the third most common health care problem, behind heart disease and cancer, but disables more individuals than heart disease and cancer put together.

Studies indicate that, on average, only 57% of a patient's pain is relieved with the best prescribing practices (Steven Passik, PhD, presentation at APS meeting, March 2002, Baltimore). This remaining 43% then is open to improvement in prescribing or in the absence of a clear surgical or other invasive option, and presents an opportunity for the application of nonpharmacologic and complementary therapies to provide additional relief.

There are a number of key factors to be mindful of in pain management. Pain intensity and quality are important to understanding underlying pathophysiology. Pain syndromes are associated with distinct etiologies, and have prognostic and therapeutic implications. Our understanding of pain has recently moved forward with our increased knowledge of pain neuromodulators and the discovery of neurobiologic processes of pain.

Pathophysiology of pain

Two major types of pain exist: nociceptive and neuropathic. Nociceptors are free afferent nerve fibers that distinguish noxious from innocuous stimuli. These are located in the skin, subcutaneous tissue, and visceral and somatic structures.

Somatic nociceptive pain arises from bone, joint, muscle, skin, or connective tissue. Direct trauma to tissues is the typical cause of this type of pain. Visceral pain arises form visceral organs like the gastrointestinal tract or pancreas. Visceral nociceptive pain may arise from the organ or capsule or from obstruction of a hollow viscus causing intermittent, poorly localized pain. Somatic nociceptive pain is described as sharp, aching, throbbing, pressure, or vise like. Visceral nociceptive pain is often described as gnawing or cramping, or if due to obstruction of a hollow viscus, may be described as aching, sharp, or throbbing. This is the pain often associated with appendicitis, cholecystitis, or pleurisy.

There are a number of important neuromodulator substances that act on peripheral and central receptors. Peripheral receptor activation begins with injury and the release of inflammatory substances such as mast cells, macrophages and lymphocytes, bradykinin, and histamine. There is also neurogenic activation that occurs with the inflammatory response. These substances sensitize the nociceptor, during early tissue injury. This response to injury results in the release of pro-inflammatory mediators producing vasodilation and extravasation of plasma proteins in the arachidonic acid metabolic pathway, prostaglandin, leukotriene, and other inflammatory substances such as potassium, serotonin, and substance P. These either serve to sensitize or excite primary afferent nerves or trigger vasodilatation in response to the injury. Such tissue damage also results in peripheral site release of local endogenous opioids [7].

Moving from tissue injury toward the central nervous system additional neuromodulators exist that play a role in pain. Those acting on receptors in the dorsal horn include opioid (mu, kappa, and delta), alpha adrenergic, gamma-aminobutryic acid (GABA), serotonin, and adenosine, neurokinin, N-methyl-D-aspartate (NMDA), and non-NMDA receptors such as alpha-amino-3-hydroxy-5-methyl-4-isoxazolepropioic acid (AMPA). The periaquaductal gray of the midbrain is involved in central mediation of pain. This area contains both opiate or endorphin receptors and significant levels of endorphins. Receptors are located at presynaptic and postsynaptic nociceptive afferent nerves. Afferent stimulation results in the release of substance P, glutamate, and calcitonin gene-related peptide. Glutamate acts on AMPA receptors, substance P on neurokinin receptors. The activation of non-NMDA receptors appears to play a role in the development of abnormal responses to chronic pain and the altered response to stimuli. Because of these distinctions it is recommended that pain be describes in terms of its physiologic as well as pathophysiologic responses [7].

Neuropathic pain can be centrally or peripherally generated. It is usually defined as pain persisting at least 3 months. Centrally generated pain may be the result of deafferentation or sympathetic stimulation, the kind of pain arising from phantom limb pain, stroke, or spinal cord injuries. Peripheral pain may occur along the distribution of many peripheral nerves or can be associated with a known peripheral nerve injury from trauma or disease such as you would see in herpetic neuralgia. Neuropathic pain is often described as burning, tingling, or lancinating. Pain can also have associated symptoms related to the affected nerves. Also, neuropathic pain may persist even though there is absence of ongoing disease. It is important to understand these associations to not only aid in diagnostic evaluation, but to effect treatment of the cause of the pain and the pain itself.

The chronic nature of neuropathic pain is a pathophysiologic response to disease or injury. Unlike nociceptive pain, neuropathic pain is not initiated through activation of nociceptors, but is related to reduced inhibition, and thus is not always responsive to narcotics. The development of neuropathic pain continues to be an area of study. There is evidence to suggest that sensitization and cellular hyperexcitability or "wind-up" of nociceptive stimuli contributes to the development of neuropathic pain. This carries import to the practitioner. Preemptive use of narcotics may help to prevent sensitization and development of allodynia from a painful event or surgery. The use of local anesthetics, narotics, and nonsteroidal anti-inflammatory drugs (NSAIDS) have reports of decreasing the need for postprocedure pain medication, and may benefit patients in preventing chronic pain [7].

Pharmaceutical preparations used to treat pain are many. There are three groups of drugs commonly used to treat pain. (1) Nonopioids that includes Acetaminophen and NSAIDS, (2) opioids that include those that are mu agonists and the agonists-antagonists, and (3) adjuvant drugs that includes antidepressants, anesthetics, anticonvulsants, muscle relaxants, alpha-adrenergic agonists, NMDA blockers, neuroleptics, and corticosteroids. Some of these have side effects, dose–tolerance effects, routes of administration considerations, and onset of analgesia and analgesic ceilings to be aware of. These medications offer relief for many, but not all. Those patients looking for additional relief may turn to complementary and alternative medicine for relief.

Complementary alternative medicine

Complementary and alternative medicine is defined as "those medical systems, professions, practices, interventions, modalities, therapies, applications, theories, or claims that are currently not a part of the dominant or conventional medical system" [8]. Many of these therapies may indirectly target neuromodulators and be beneficial as adjunctive treatments for pain.

CAM encompasses nonconventional approaches to healing, beyond traditional medicine. The National Center for Complementary and Alternative Medicine (NCCAM) is a component of the National Institute of Health, and is the Federal government's proponent agency for scientific research on complementary and alternative health practices [9]. Many areas of research are now underway to examine efficacy and therapeutic benefit of some these nontraditional approaches to care. Understanding CAM and integrating its effective therapies add a multidisciplinary approach to care that meet the patients cultural and belief systems.

Patients turn to CAM for a many reasons. Many of the therapies are popular because they place an emphasis on harmony and balance of the mind, body, spirit, and external environment. Patients who choose alternative therapies are not necessarily dissatisfied with conventional medicine; rather, they may want more control and involvement in their care [10]. Many patients seen in the emergency department may be using one or more of these CAM therapies as part of their health practices. It is important to have an understanding of these therapies, the potential benefits, limitations, and potential side effects while caring for your patients.

Complementary and alternative medicine are two different approaches: complementary medicine is any form of therapy used in combination with other alternative treatments or standard/conventional medicine. Complementary therapy usually serves to relieve symptoms and improve quality of life. It is often used to control side effects of conventional therapy.

The theoretical basis for many alternative therapies is derived from Eastern culture, tradition, and philosophy. Some practices are accepted into traditional care without much forethought or hesitation; others are scrutinized for lack of evidenced-based studies proving efficacy. For some of these therapies the benefit is derived from "hypothetical" modulation or reduction in afferent nociceptive input to higher brain centers or a theoretical release of natural endorphins [10].

Six general categories of alternative and complementary therapies have been outlined by NCCAM. These are: mind–body interventions, diet lifestyle modification, herbal remedies, manual healing, bioelectromagnetics (BEM), and pharmacologic–biologic treatments [9]. Some of the therapies included are familiar, and have gained mainstream acceptance. Diet and lifestyle modification are considered important in Healthy People 2010 guidelines. Transcutaneous electrical nerve stimulators (TENS) and acupuncture are well-known therapies. Hypnosis, biofeedback, and relaxation techniques are considered mind–body interventions and have been incorporated in psychiatric practice by many. Vitamin therapy has known preventive benefits for prevention and treatment of illness since the discovery of scurvy by early mariners, in the prevention of neural tube defects in prenatal care, and may play a role in heart disease. There are other additional therapies that exist that are cultural practices used by patients.

Traditional alternative medicine

Traditional alternative medicine has been practiced worldwide for centuries and includes acupuncture, Ayurveda, and Naturopathy, Chinese/Oriental medicine. Understanding the uses and limitations will help navigate through the waters of CAM.

Mind/body treatment approaches

Many types of mind/body treatment approaches are used to reduce pain. Precise mechanisms for pain reduction using these practices are not completely understood, but they may involve the activities of neurotransmitters, serotonin, and catecholamines that influence the mind's perception of pain. Hypnosis, biofeedback, and relaxation techniques, such as meditation and autogenic training, are the primary forms. In some cases, these methods have been found to be both beneficial and economical. Of all the alternative therapies used for pain relief, three techniques are the most widely accepted and are taught in medical schools, and these are available at many hospitals and outpatient clinics.

Numerous research studies support the benefits of mind/body treatment approaches. In 1995, a 35-member National Institute of Health panel was convened to determine the value of specific mind/body techniques for treating pain [11]. In particular, the panel found biofeedback to be effective in the treatment of tension headaches and other types of chronic pain, and hypnosis to be useful in adjunctive treatments for cancer pain, irritable bowel syndrome, temporomandibular joint syndrome, tension headaches, and chronic inflammatory disorders.

Systematic reviews of the literature indicate that mind/body interventions can be effective for health conditions that are caused or made worse by stress [12]. Relaxation techniques can be helpful for pain control [13]; and relaxation and visualization techniques may also be of benefit [14]. These simple techniques can be easily taught in the office or at the bedside, or used during diagnostic procedures in the emergency department, and may provide the pain relief, as well as an enhanced sense of self-efficacy in the setting of chronic pain. Patients using relaxation techniques for pain report improved sense of well-being and score higher on quality-of-life scales after receiving instruction in meditation, affirmation, imagery, and ritual [15].

A cost-effectiveness study in 1991 determined that cancer patients who participated in psychotherapy and relaxation therapies cut their costs and experienced pain reduction and decreased clinic visits by 36% when compared with patients not using these combined techniques [16]. Pediatric patients, and older patients, particularly with some cognitive impairment, may respond better to passive distractions for pain relief than active mind/body therapies, such as an engaging movie or familiar music. But generally, all forms of mind/body do have some benefit in attenuating pain [17].

Massage, body work, and postural therapies

Massage is found to be helpful both physically and emotionally. The rubbing not only soothes sore muscles but the mind as well. A review of six studies in 2004, evaluating massage and chiropractic, failed to demonstrate convincing evidence for prolonged pain relief [18]. Patients do report subjective benefit and relief from massage. The reason for the discrepancy may be emotional benefit. Massaging muscles and soft tissue stimulates nerves, increases blood flow, and relieves stress in the muscles. A number of different types of massage exist today:

- Swedish Massage: this massage technique involves the use of long, smooth strokes, strokes that knead and compress, deep circular movements, vibration, and tapping.

- Oriental Massage: this technique is very gentle and relaxes a person.
- Shiatsu: this Japanese form of massaging is actually a form of acupressure, exerting massaging pressure on certain key points of the body.
- Thai Massage: this massage technique also involves the use of Yoga and certain Chinese traditional medicine methods.

A small study done in 1989 by researchers in Norway measured concentration of plasma beta-endorphins after massage and found that levels increased 16% and remained elevated for approximately 1 hour [19]. This may lend support for the theories that postulate that massage helps control pain by increasing pain-reducing neurochemicals such as endorphins and serotonin in the brain and spinal cord. Variations of Swedish, deep-tissue, sports, and neuromuscular methods are frequently used.

Patients may also explore other types of massage or body work. Generally, body work is nonaerobic movement with controlled breathing that can be practiced to reduce stress and anxiety. Postural body work therapies teach patients how to realign their bodies, improve posture and movement, and reduce structural stress. Only a few controlled studies have been done on these techniques, and most of the reported benefits are subjective. There is moderate evidence of efficacy for mind–body therapies in the areas of hypertension and arthritis; however, more research is needed to determine the benefits in treating chronic back pain, sports injury-related pain, headaches, and joint pain [20].

Tai Chi, an ancient form of martial art based on Taoism, a Chinese belief system, is one form of body work. The practice of Tai Chi includes slow, graceful movements and rhythmic breathing. It is reported to have a beneficial role in pain reduction in patients with arthritis [21]. It is also reported to:

- decrease blood pressure,
- increase stamina, muscle tone, and flexibility,
- improve posture, balance, muscle mass, and strength in older people.

Yoga is an ancient posturing and breathing technique from India. Yoga means "union." Yoga also uses slow movement, in addition to meditation and breathing exercises to reach a state of relaxation. Two limited studies of yoga of patients with osetoarthritis and carpal tunnel syndrome showed improvement in pain relief with the use of yoga. Yoga uses stretching and improves strength, so it theoretically should be beneficial for additional musculoskeletal problems [22]. Yoga is also reported to help:

- reduce stress
- reduce pain associated with some chronic illnesses
- eliminate headaches and insomnia.
- improve stamina for some athletes
- enhance quality of life for some cancer patients.

Chinese medicine

Traditional Chinese medicine is based upon descriptive metaphors for human bioenergetic properties that do not translate well or directly into the English terms used for them. Chinese medicine's basic concept is that a vital force of life surges through the body (also called Qi). Any imbalance to this life force can cause disease and illness. According to traditional Chinese medicine, pain is due to a conflict between blood and Qi, which in turn, results in stagnancy. Relieving this stagnancy, balancing the energy, nourishing the blood, and building up deficient blood are all ways that Chinese medicine treats pain. Traditional Chinese doctors use acupuncture techniques to correct the flow of Qi. They use herbal medicines to reestablish balanced Qi, blood, and moisture in organ networks, to avert excess wind, heat, cold, dryness, and dampness. Perhaps the most well-known Chinese therapy is acupuncture.

Acupuncture is the practice of puncturing the skin with needles at certain anatomic points in the body to relieve specific symptoms associated with many diseases. The anatomic points (acupuncture points) are thought to have certain electrical properties, which affect chemical neurotransmitters in the body.

Acupuncture is one of the oldest, most commonly used medical practices in the world. Originated in China more than 2500 years ago, acupuncture gained attention in this country in the 1970s, when China and the United States opened relations. The practice has been growing in popularity since. Studies support the use of acupuncture for the treatment of acute and chronic types of pain, including osteoarthritis, back pain, dysmenorrhea, and migraines [23]. In an effort to determine precisely how acupuncture works, researchers have isolated changes in the immune, neurochemical, and hormone functions, as well as in pain pathways following acupuncture treatment, but the exact mechanisms of action from a Western perspective remain elusive. Acupuncture may act as a pain preventative, theoretically, by acting on the sympathetic nervous system.

Acupuncture theories today are based on extensive laboratory research, and have become widely known and accepted. In addition, controlled studies have shown evidence of the effectiveness of acupuncture for certain conditions. Approximately 10,000 certified acupuncturists practice in the United States today. Not all certified acupuncturists are physicians, but currently, increasing numbers of certified acupuncturists are US physicians who have incorporated acupuncture into their medical practices.

Acupuncture has been shown to benefit cancer patients who are receiving a stable dose of analgesic. Patients reporting pain scores using a visual analog pain scale had observed reduction in pain intensity from auricular acupuncture [24]. Acupuncture has been shown to be effective in the treatment of facial, dental, and labor pain, knee osteoarthritis, and fibromyalgia [25–28]. Just like many therapies used, acupuncture has had mixed reviews on the treatment of back pain, head ache, and neck pain [29–31].

Chinese herbs

Chinese herbs for pain treatment often have analgesic properties, some of which are extremely potent. In China, as here, herbal medicines are typically taken as teas, capsules, tablets, or extracts. But depending upon the type and severity of the pain, some preparations in China are given in hospitals intravenously or subcutaneously.

Corydalis yanhusuo, or corydalis tuber, is an example of a potent Chinese herb used for neuralgia, painful menstruation, and gastrointestinal spasm. Corydalis contains numerous potent alkaloids that inhibit activity in the brain stem associated with pain perception, and it has sedating properties: the powdered drug has a potency 1% that of opium. One of the predominant alkaloids responsible for these effects is tetrahydropalmatine, which has been isolated and tested on mice to determine its tranquilizing effects. It appears to inhibit postsynaptic dopaminergic receptors and simultaneously to increase the availability of zy-aminobutyricacid receptors. These actions both reduce pain and relieve anxiety. Another corydalis alkaloid, dihydrocorydaline, was used in a clinical study to determine its effects in the treatment of dysmenorrhea. Dihydrocorydaline (50 mg) taken three times a day reduced menstrual pain in 32 of the 44 patients, to varying degrees. Exhaustion, headaches, and decreased menstrual flow were typical side effects [32].

Ayurveda

Ayurveda is a natural system of medicine that originated in India more than 3000 years ago. Ayurveda translates to "knowledge of life." Based on the idea that disease is due to an imbalance or stress in the individual's consciousness, Ayurveda encourages certain lifestyle interventions and natural therapies to regain a balance between the body, mind, and the environment.

Ayurveda treatment begins with an internal purification process, followed by a special diet, herbal remedies, massage therapy, yoga, and meditation. Studies have shown reductions in blood pressure, cholesterol, and reaction to stress in people who practiced Ayurvedic methods.

In India, Ayurveda is considered a form of medical care, equal to conventional Western and homeopathic medicine. Practitioners of Ayurveda in India undergo state-recognized, institutionalized training. However, Ayurvedic practitioners are not licensed in the United States.

Ayurveda can have positive effects when used as an alternative therapy in combination with standard/conventional medical care.

Ayurveda attributes pain syndromes to imbalances and stagnation in constitutional types, known as doshas. The three doshas are vata, kapha, and pitta. The location and type of pain are believed to be dependent on which of three constitutional types is aggravated or stagnant, which in turn, determines the treatment. Often, such treatment is herbal as well as dietary, and involves giving patient's botanical substances or foods that either stimulate or soothe the constitutional imbalance. These preparations are characterized as sweet, sour, salty, bitter, astringent, or pungent, and are often combinations of these types.

For example, vata, which is normally dry, cold, and light in quality, is balanced with substances that are wet, warm, and dark. In Ayurvedic practice, such substances are usually sweet. But in the case of obstructive vata, sweet substances are thought likely to exacerbate blockage, so these patients are given pungent herbs and foods to stimulate the movement of vata.

Triphala and trikatu are two Ayurvedic herbal standards that may be recommended by a practitioner to relieve blockages that cause pain. Trikatu is a blend of black pepper, ginger, and Indian pepper. The Indian pepper used in trikatu (long pepper; pippali) contains elements similar to capsaicin in cayenne pepper. It is used as a topical painkiller for arthritic conditions, and is thought to stimulate and then inhibit pain by destroying substance P. Constituents in ginger can block the cyclooxygenase pathway, preventing the formation of inflammatory prostaglandins [33]. One study done at the Miami Veterans Administration Medical Center and University of Miami found that highly concentrated extract of two ginger species had a beneficial effect on osteoarthritis of the knee [34].

Homeopathy

> "Like cures like. Any substance which can produce a totality of symptoms in a healthy human being can cure that totality of symptoms in a sick human being." — Samuel Hahneman (father of Homeopathic medicine).

The idea behind homeopathy is that if a large dosage of a certain substance produces certain symptoms, a small dosage of the same substance may cause the opposite effect. In other words, if a person suffers from throbbing headaches, he/she might be treated with a very diluted dosage of belladonna, a poisonous herb that causes throbbing headaches in high doses.

Classic homeopathy depends on the assessment of a patient's specific clinical pattern, and relies on individualized treatment strategy. Evidence for applications of homeopathic remedies exists for dental pain, sports injury, and some types of arthritis. Homeopathic remedies for pain may be taken either internally or externally. Homeopathic arnica ointment, for example, has long been recommended for sports-related injuries, such as sprains, with subjective benefit [35].

A double-blind, placebo-controlled crossover trial demonstrated that homeopathic Rhus toxicodendron reduced tender points by 25% in patients with fibromyalgia following 4 weeks of treatment [36]. However, another study of homeopathy and rheumatoid arthritis was negative for effect [37]. Like many treatments and therapies more study needs to be done to determine efficacy in measurable studies versus subjective reports.

Osteopathy and chiropractic

With use of manual manipulation of the spine, chiropractors believe they can improve a person's health without surgery or medication. They believe most illnesses are due to blockages along the nerve bundles in the spinal cord. Spinal manipulation as now performed has extraordinary heterogeneity, making it impossible to form sweeping conclusions about its efficacy [38]. A wide range of techniques is used, varying from extremely gentle contacts or mobilizations to very forceful manipulations. The most common and most studied form is referred to as high-velocity low-amplitude mobilization, where the slack is taken out of a spinal joint and a very rapid short thrust is applied to gap the joint. An audible click is often heard. These manipulations, using either osteopathic or chiropractic techniques, show considerable effectiveness for the treatment of various types of back pain. Research found that chiropractic is beneficial for acute back pain, but that the evidence to support its use in chronic back pain is insufficient [39].

The Agency for Health Care Policy and Research, a federal research and information agency organized in 1989, released its guidelines for the treatment of acute low back pain. The guidelines recommend spinal manipulation, either osteopathic or chiropractic, above more typical forms of physical therapy (including traction, diathermy, TENS, and ultrasound). Osteopathic and chiropractic treatments were found to have benefits that were equal to or superior to placebo. Although the specific physiologic effects of spinal manipulation are largely unknown, the The Agency for Health Care Policy and Research guidelines acknowledge that the methods used often meet with positive results [39].

Several positive meta-analyses and systematic reviews have been done on chiropractic manipulative therapy, but the final evidence of its efficacy remains dependent to some degree on the relative quality of the studies done [40–42]. Spinal manipulation remains immensely popular for back pain, and safety of the procedure is quite good [43].

Osteopathic treatment of acute low back pain has been supported by some positive findings in randomized controlled trials, although most recent studies tend to show little effect [44]. Due to its universal popularity, chiropractic care is sometimes considered the first line of alternative therapy for various types of pain, including fibromyalgia and neck and back pain. Many medical practitioners are now willing to send spinal pain patients for a trial of spinal manipulative therapy, although most would limit the trial to no more than six to eight treatments before wanting to reassess the patient.

Nutritional and botanical dietary supplements

Calcium and magnesium are the two minerals most often recommended for supplementation in the treatment of pain syndromes. Calcium is recommended for conditions such as osteoarthritis, or more as a preventative or corrective supplement in treatment of osteoporosis than as a painkiller. Usual daily dosage is 1000 mg to 1500 mg [45].

Magnesium, a mineral required for musculoskeletal maintenance and health, is used as a tocolytic, and has long been valued in treating migraines. Because it relaxes skeletal and smooth muscles after they contract, magnesium is considered a relaxation-promoting mineral. The recommended daily allowance for magnesium is 320 mg per day for nonpregnant and lactating women, 360 mg per day for pregnant women, and 420 mg per day for men 31 years and older. Dosages up to 1000 mg magnesium a day appear to be safe in healthy women with no significant medical problems.

Current trends in supplemental treatment of pain conditions also include use of essential fatty acids—particularly gamma-linolenic acid (omega-6) and fish-derived eicosapentaenoic acid (omega-3)—and glucosamine sulfate. Essential fatty acids are the starting point from which the body makes both prostaglandins and leukotrienes. Omega-6 fatty acids convert to one- or two-series prostaglandins and to the substances similar to prostaglandin called leukotrienes. The one-series prostaglandins are considered beneficial. They appear to inhibit inflammation, lower cholesterol, and reduce blood pressure. However, the two-series prostaglandins, along with the leukotrienes, are associated with pain and inflammation. The reduction or alteration by essential fatty acids intake may help with the inflammation and pain resulting from the series-2 prostaglandin endpoints [46].

Omega-3 fatty acids, found in marine animal fats and some vegetable oils, are converted to three-series prostaglandins (generally anti-inflammatory in effect) and to a less noxious form of leukotriene. The combination of omega-3 and omega-6 oils may be especially beneficial, as the presence of omega-3 fatty acids tends to prevent the omega-6 oils from being converted to less favorable endpoints.

Fish oil and flax seed oil both provide omega-3 fatty acids. Fish oil is beneficial in the treatment of arthritis [47–49]. The benefits of flax seed oil are less clear because there are more interactions with other vegetable oils.

Glucosamine-sulfate has been shown to be more effective in reducing osteoarthritic pain than NSAIDs, shark cartilage, chondroitin sulfate, or placebo; some investigators feel glucosamine may have disease-modifying properties in osteoarthritis and actually slow the deterioration of joints characteristic of this condition [50,51]. Glucosamine typically takes 4 to

6 weeks to take effect [52]. At doses of 500 mg three times a day, glucosamine-sulfate is considered safe, although mild stomach discomfort and elevation of blood pressure due to salt content is sometimes reported.

Botanical medicine

Pain-reducing botanicals are typically spoken of in terms of their mechanisms of action or in terms of the actions in the same manner as pharmaceutical drugs. Phytochemists (plant chemists) are just beginning to develop an understanding of the mechanisms of action of the many botanical substances in use.

Long et al have reviewed herbal medicines for osteoarthritis, Ernst and Chrubasik have reviewed anti-inflammatory herbs, and Almeid and colleagues have summarized botanical products that have centrally acting analgesic properties [53–55]. Literally hundreds of plants have been found to have antinociceptive and anti-inflammatory properties, including those traditionally thought of for other medicinal purposes [56]. It remains to be seen which plant products will be born out for safety, efficacy, and tolerability in human clinical trials.

Devil's Claw has been studied, and is reported to benefit patients with knee, hip, and back pain with few adverse reactions [57–59]. White willow bark has been studied for pain relief with some success. This plant is a source of salicylate, and as such has the potential to initiate an anaphylactic response in patients with aspirin allergy [60]. Other painkilling herbs include cayenne, which can be taken either internally or rubbed onto painful arthritic joints, the active ingredient being capsaicin [61]. Ginko Biloba, an extract formula that is also gaining popularity as a possible deterrent to Alzheimer's disease and other types of dementia, has also been used for pain relief. One recent trial showed that a proprietary herbal formula, Reumalex, helped reduce chronic arthritis pain [62]. Ginko Biloba extracts have been proven to reduce leg pain associated with intermittent claudication [63]. The mechanism of action of Ginko Biloba is through inhibition of glycine and antagonism of GABA in neurologic tissue. In patients with seizures, this may lower their seizure threshold and precipitate seizures in an otherwise well-controlled epileptic [64,65]. It is these kinds of actions and interactions practitioners must be mindful in when having discussions with patients.

In general, herbal treatments for pain are used topically or internally. One useful topical agent, cajeput oil, is usually administered in combination with other oils, such as peppermint, clove, menthol, eucalyptus, St. John's wort, cayenne, or arnica oil. Cajeput has been shown to relieve musculoskeletal pain, headache, hemorrhoid pain, neuralgia, rheumatic pain, and pain resulting from sports injuries.

With multiple drug prescriptions the provider is always mindful of interactions. The same holds true for patients taking multiple herbal treatments for their self-diagnosed or naturopathically managed conditions. St. John's wort is well known to induce Cytochrome P-450, and now evidence exists that it induces both CYP3A4-catalyzed sulfoxidation and CYP2C19-dependent hydroxylation. For patients treating their depression and pain with these multiple herbal preparations that have gastroesophageal reflux disease and take omeprazole, they may be making their gastroesophageal reflux disease worse. By inducing both CYP3A4 and CYP2C19, plasma concentrations of omeprazole decrease placing them at risk of recurrence of their erosive esophagitis. Clinically relevant interactions with other drugs may occur and must be taken into account when St. John's wort is being taken because metabolism through the CYP3A4 substrates represent at least 50% of all marketed medications [65].

Bioelectromagnetics and magnetic therapy

Electromagnetic (EM) therapy is based on the belief that an imbalance of the EM frequencies or fields of energy can cause illness. By applying electrical energy to the body, the imbalance can be corrected. Many electrical devices and nonelectrical magnetic appliances are available, and are used to treat a variety of symptoms. However, the US Food and Drug Administration do not approve most.

The theory behind BEM is that nonionizing EM fields, in the extremely low-frequency range, may benefit certain conditions, due to EM changes to ligand–receptor interactions at the cell membrane [66,67]. The effects of BEM are thought to result from a change in membrane transport and gene expression. BEM may one day prove to be the effectual factor in therapies that use energetic healing techniques, such as therapeutic touch.

Techniques of nonionizing BEM are either thermal (producing heat in biologic tissue) or nonthermal. Thermal methods are used with laser and radiofrequency (RF) surgery, RF diathermy, and RF hyperthermy. However, the nonthermal applications are more prevalent in alternative medicine. Microwave resonance therapy (MRT) is a method of nonthermal nonionizing BEM used extensively in Russia. MRT incorporates low-intensity sinusoidal microwave radiation, and has had favorable results in treating many conditions, including arthritis, pain, and hypertension. Often, MRT is applied to acupuncture points.

Transcranial EM stimulation of the prefrontal cortex has been shown in multiple studies to have an effect on pain, but this is probably not an alternative or complementary technique [68].

Stationary magnets have been studied for pain of many different body areas, with varying reports of benefit. A summary of success from a number of different studies has been reported in the treatment of knee pain, chronic pelvic pain, postpolio pain, and carpal tunnel pain [69–73]. Little to no benefit was found in treating wrist pain, fibromyalgia, and low back pain, and no benefit in treating heel pain associated with plantar fascitis [74–77].

EM stimulation has been shown to help with knee pain [78,79]. Small studies have been done evaluating therapy on diabetic neuropathy with promising results; however, additional testing and study are needed [80]. Trock and Vallbona have reviewed literature that examined either magnet therapy or pulsed EM fields (PEMF). Trock found that PEMF was a benefit to the growth of bone and cartilage in vitro, and had potential application as an arthritis treatment. PEMF stimulation is already a proven remedy for delayed fractures, with potential clinical application for osteoarthritis, osteonecrosis of bone, osteoporosis, and wound healing. Magnet therapy has had mixed reviews and mostly anecdotal benefits [81,82]. Suffice it to say that the jury is still out on the efficacy of magnetic fields for pain, although generally PEMF seem to be more supported by the literature than are static magnetic fields.

Complementary therapies in palliative care

Attention to palliation in the setting of terminal illness has only recently come to the conventional medical community from its origins in the mid-20th century in England. Although hospice services are widely available, most US hospitals still do not have a palliative care service, including many of the oldest and most prestigious medical institutions. Efforts to remedy this are currently underway in many medical centers.

Palliative care is, by definition, multidisciplinary. The emphasis in palliative care on the social, spiritual, and psychologic needs of the patient is inherently a "holistic" approach. Integration of complementary therapies for pain and other symptoms is a natural extension of this multidisciplinary foundation, both in the hospice setting as well as the hospital units. Although it is clearly not possible to do everything for every patient, select complementary therapies may be helpful to patients approaching the end of life. Conventional nursing, pastoral care, and psychologic services may be appropriately augmented by mind/body therapies, massage, aromatherapy, acupuncture, yoga, or other techniques.

Shumay and colleagues [83] have studied the existing use of CAM techniques in the cancer population, finding more use among women, better educated, Caucasian, and having more severity of symptoms, particularly nausea and vomiting. Pan and colleagues [84] have reviewed 21 studies of CAM therapies, and concluded that although there is still a paucity of data, some CAM therapies are probably useful for the terminally ill. DiGianni and colleagues [85] have studied women with breast cancer and concluded that little evidence exists to support CAM use beyond psychosocial interventions. Power and colleagues [86] have studied the used of CAM therapies in the HIV population.

Although the evidence base may not currently be strong to justify the use of complementary therapies with the terminally ill, many patients do try to request these approaches, and some seem to find benefit from them. The concern exists that patients may delay seeking traditional treatment for cancer and use experimental CAM as initial therapy [87]. From a research viewpoint, that which is unproven is not disproved, but should be used as adjunct to known therapies. One or more of the CAM therapies may be of benefit in the palliative care setting, despite the lack of solid evidence at this time.

Cultural practices not abuse

A number of practices in Southeast Asia Folk medicine practices such as cupping, coining, and moxibustion run counter to accepted norms and are often misinterpreted as physical abuse. These practices may leave marks or discoloration on the skin, and at first glance may appear to be bruises. Coining (cao gio) and cupping (giac) are oriental folk medicine practices, which seem to have surfaced in the country during the Viet Nam era. Coining involves rubbing the skin with a coin producing a welt, while cupping uses a suction device or a piece of cotton soaked in rubbing alcohol is ignited and placed in the cup which is then held horizontally and placed over the skin, extinguishing the flame. This creates heat within the cup. Often leaving a circular area of discoloration. Both coining and cupping bring the "bad wind" to the surface where it can escape and restore balance, and therefore health, to the body. It is generally used for the treatment of minor illnesses, such as colds and fevers. Unfortunately, both produce marks easily interpreted as physical abuse.

Summary

One primary reason patients go to emergency departments is for pain relief. Understanding the physiologic dynamics of pain, pharmacologic methods for treatment of pain, as well CAM therapies used in treatment of pain is important to all providers in emergency care. Asking patients about self-care and treatments used outside of the emergency department is an important part of the patient history. Complementary and alternative therapies are very popular for painful conditions despite the lack of strong research supporting some of their use. Even though evidenced-based studies that are double blinded and show a high degree of interrater observer reliability do not exist, patients will likely continue to seek out CAM therapies as a means of self-treatment and a way to maintain additional life control. Regardless of absolute validity of a therapy for some patients, it is the bottom line: "it seems to help my pain." Pain management distills down to a very simple endpoint, patient relief, and comfort. Sham or science, if the patient feels better, feels comforted, feels less stressed, and more functional in life and their practices pose no health risk, then supporting their CAM therapy creates a true wholistic partnership in their health care.

CAM should be relatively inexpensive and extremely safe. Such is not always the case, as some patients have discovered with the use of botanicals. It becomes an imperative that all providers be aware of CAM therapies and informed about potential interactions and side effects when helping patients manage pain and explore adding CAM strategies for pain relief. The use of regulated breathing, meditation, guided imagery, or a massage for a pain sufferer are simple but potentially beneficial inexpensive aids to care that can be easily employed in the emergency department. Some CAM therapies covered here, while not easily practiced in the emergency department, exist as possibilities for exploration of patients after they leave, and may offer an improved sense of well-being and empowerment in the face of suffering and despair.

The foundations of good nutrition, exercise, stress reduction, and reengagement in life can contribute much to restoring the quality of life to a pain patient. Adding nondrug therapies of physical therapy, cognitive-behavioral therapy, TENS, hypnosis, biofeedback, psychoanalysis, and others can complete the conventional picture. Adding in simple mind/body therapies, touch therapies, acupuncture, or others may be appropriate in select cases, and depending on the circumstances, may effect and enhance a conventional pain management program. Armed with an understanging of pain dynamics and treatments, practitioners can better meet patient needs, avoid serious side effects, and improve care when addressing pain management in the emergency department.

References

[1] Ducharme J, Barber C. A prospective blinded study on emergency pain assessment and therapy. J Emerg Med 1995;13:571–5 [Library Holdings Bibliographic Links].

[2] Lewis LM, Lasater LC, Brooks CB. Are emergency physicians too stingy with analgesics? South Med J 1994;87:7–9 [Library Holdings Bibliographic Links].

[3] Johnston CC, Gagnon AJ, Fullerton L, et al. One-week survey of pain intensity on admission to and discharge from the emergency department: a pilot study. J Emerg Med 1998;16(3): 377–82.

[4] Ducharme J. Acute pain and pain control: state of the art. Ann Emerg Med 2000;35(6): 592–603.

[5] Schnitzer TJ. Non-NSAID pharmacologic treatment options for the management of chronic pain. Am J Med 1998;105:45S–52S.

[6] Gureje O, Von Korff M, Simon GE, Gater R. Persistent pain and well-being: a World Health Organization study in primary care. JAMA 1998;280:147–51.

[7] Siddall PJ, Cousins MJ. Spinal pain mechanisms. Spine 1997;22(1):98–104.

[8] Alternative Medicine. Expanding medical horizons: a report to the National Institutes of Health of alternative medical systems and practices in the United States. Washington: US Government Printing Office; 1994 [Publication No. 017-040-00053770].

[9] National Center for Complementary and Alternative Medicine. http:// nccam.nih.gov.

[10] Gentz BA. Alternative therapies for the management of pain in labor and delivery. Clin Obstet Gynecol 2001;44(4):704–32.

[11] Integration of Behavioral and Relaxation Approaches into the Treatment of Chronic Pain and Insomnia. NIH Technol Assess Statement; 1995. p. 1–34.

[12] Jacobs GD. Clinical applications of the relaxation response and mind-body interventions. J Altern Comp Med 2001;7(Suppl 1):S93–101.
[13] Cole BH, Brunk Q. Holistic interventions for acute pain episodes: an integrative review. J Holistic Nurs 1999;17(4):384–96.
[14] Hoffart MB, Keene EP. The benefits of visualization. Am J Nurs 1998;98(12):44–7.
[15] Targ EF, Levine EG. The efficacy of a mind-body-spirit group for women with breast cancer: a randomized controlled trial. Gen Hosp Psychiatry 2002;24(4):238–48.
[16] Caudill M, Schnable R, Zuttermeister P, et al. Decreased clinic use by chronic pain patients: response to behavioral medicine intervention. Clin J Pain 1991;7(4):305–10.
[17] Fernandez E, Turk DC. The utility of cognitive coping strategies for altering pain perception: a meta-analysis. Pain 1989;38(2):123–35.
[18] Ernst E. Manual therapies for pain control: chiropractic and massage. Clin J Pain 2004; 20(1):8–12.
[19] Kaada B, Torsteinbo O. Increase of plasma beta-endorphins in connective tissue massage. Gen Pharmacol 1989;20(4):487–9.
[20] Astin JA, Shapiro SL, Eisenberg DM, et al. Mind–body medicine: state of the science, implications for practice. J Am Board Fam Pract 2003;16(2):131–47.
[21] Song R, Lee EO, Lam P, et al. Effects of tai chi exercise on pain, balance, muscle strength, and perceived difficulties in physical functioning in older women with osteoarthritis: a randomized clinical trial. J Rheumatol 2003;30(9):2039–44.
[22] Garfinkel M, Schumacher HR Jr. Yoga. Rheum Dis Clin North Am 2000;26(1):125–32.
[23] Kaptchuk TJ. Acupuncture: theory, efficacy, and practice. Ann Intern Med 2002;136(5): 374–83.
[24] Alimi D, Rubino C, Pichard-Leandri E, et al. Analgesic effect of auricular acupuncture for cancer pain: a randomized, blinded, controlled trial. J Clin Oncol 2003;21(22): 4120–6.
[25] Ernst E, Pittler MH. The effectiveness of acupuncture in treating acute dental pain: a systematic review. Br Dent J 1998;184(9):443–7.
[26] Ezzo J, Hadhazy V, Birch S, et al. Acupuncture for osteoarthritis of the knee: a systematic review. Arthritis Rheum 2001;44(4):819–25.
[27] Berman BM, Ezzo J, Hadhazy V, et al. Is acupuncture effective in the treatment of fibromyalgia? J Fam Pract 1999;48(3):213–8.
[28] Skilnand E, Fossen D, Heiberg E. Acupuncture in the management of pain in labor. Acta Obstet Gynecol Scand 2002;81(10):943–8.
[29] Ernst E, White AR, Wider B. Acupuncture for back pain: meta-analysis of randomised controlled trials and an update with data from the most recent studies. Schmerz 2002;16(2): 129–39 [in German].
[30] Leibing E, Leonhardt U, Koster G, et al. Acupuncture treatment of chronic low-back pain—a randomized, blinded, placebo-controlled trial with 9-month follow-up. Pain 2002; 96(1–2):189–96.
[31] White AR, Ernst E. A systematic review of randomized controlled trials of acupuncture for neck pain. Rheumatology (Oxford) 1999;38(2):143–7.
[32] Arnold MD, Thornbrough LM. Treatment of musculoskeletal pain with traditional Chinese herbal medicine. Phys Med Rehabil Clin North Am 1999;10(3):663–71.
[33] Suekawa M, Ishige A, Yuasa K, et al. Pharmacological studies on ginger 1. Pharmacological actions of pungent constituents, [6]-gingerol and [6]-shogaol. Pharmacobiodynamics 1984; 7:836–48.
[34] Altman RD, Marcussen KC. Effects of a ginger extract on knee pain in patients with osteoarthritis. Arthritis Rheum 2001;44(11):2531–8.
[35] Knuesel O, Weber M, Suter A. Arnica montana gel in osteoarthritis of the knee: an open, multicenter clinical trial. Adv Ther 2002;19(5):209–18.
[36] Fisher PA, Greenwood A, Huskisson EC, et al. Effect of homeopathic treatment on fibrosis f(primary fibromyalgia). BMJ 1989;299(6695):365–6.

[37] Fisher P, Scott DL. A randomized controlled trial of homeopathy in rheumatoid arthritis. Rheumatology (Oxford) 2001 Sep;40(9):1052–5.
[38] Gatterman MI, Cooperstein R, Lantz C, et al. Rating specific chiropractic technique procedures for common low back conditions. J Manipulative Physiol Ther 2001;24(7): 449–56.
[39] Bigos SJ, Bowyer OR, Braen GR, et al. Acute low back problems in adults. Clinical practice guideline No. 14. Rockville, MD: Agency for Health Care Policy and Research, Public Health Service, US Department of Health and Human Services; 1994 [AHCPR Publication No. 95–0642].
[40] Bronfort G. Spinal manipulation: current state of research and its indications. Neurol Clin 1999;17(1):91–111.
[41] Koes BW, Assendelft WJ, van der Heijden GJ, et al. Spinal manipulation for low back pain. An updated systematic review of randomized clinical trials. Spine 1996;21(24):2860–71 [discussion 2872–3].
[42] van Tulder MW, Koes BW, Bouter LM. Conservative treatment of acute and chronic nonspecific low back pain. A systematic review of randomized controlled trials of the most common interventions. Spine 1997;22(18):2128–56.
[43] Haldeman S. Neurological effects of the adjustment. J Manipulative Physiol Ther 2000; 23(2):112–4.
[44] Andersson GB, Lucente T, Davis AM, et al. A comparison of osteopathic spinal manipulation with standard care for patients with low back pain. N Engl J Med 1999;314: 1426–31.
[45] NIH Consensus Conference. Optimal calcium intake. NIH Consensus Development Panel on Optimal Calcium Intake. JAMA 1994;272:1942–8.
[46] McCarthy GM, Kenny D. Dietary fish oil and rheumatic diseases. Semin Arthritis Rheum 1992;21(6):368–75.
[47] Gibson RA. The effect of diets containing fish and fish oils on disease risk factors in humans. Aust N Z J Med 1988;18(5):713–22.
[48] Cathcart ES, Gonnerman WA. Fish oil fatty acids and experimental arthritis. Rheum Dis Clin North Am 1991;17(2):235–42.
[49] Henderson CJ, Panush RS. Diets, dietary supplements, and nutritional therapies in rheumatic diseases. Rheum Dis Clin North Am 1999;25(4):937.
[50] Pavelka K, Gatterova J, Olejarova M, et al. Glucosamine sulfate use and delay of progression of knee Osteoarthritis—a 3-year, randomized, placebo-controlled, double-blind study. Arch Intern Med 2002;162(18):2113–23.
[51] McAlindon TE, LaValley MP, Gulin JP, et al. Glucosamine and chondroitin for treatment of osteoarthritis—a systematic quality assessment and meta-analysis. JAMA 2000;283(11): 1469–75.
[52] Matheson AJ, Perry CM. Glucosamine: a review of its use in the management of osteoarthritis. Drugs Aging 2003;20(14):1041–60.
[53] Long L, Soeken K, Ernst E. Herbal medicines for the treatment of osteoarthritis: a systematic review. Rheumatology 2001;40(7):779–93.
[54] Ernst E, Chrubasik S. Phyto-anti-inflammatories—a systematic review of randomized, placebo-controlled, double-blind trials. Rheum Dis Clin North Am 2000;26(1):13.
[55] Almeid RN, Navarro DS, Barbosa-Filho JM. Plants with central analgesic activity. Phytomedicine 2001;8(4):310–22.
[56] Kim SJ, Kim MS. Inhibitory effects of cimicifugae rhizoma extracts on histamine, bradykinin and COX-2 mediated inflammatory actions. Phytother Res 2000;14(8):596–600.
[57] Chrubasik S, Thanner J, Kunzel O, et al. Comparison of outcome measures during treatment with the proprietary Harpagophytum extract doloteffin in patients with pain in the lower back, knee or hip. Phytomedicine 2002;9(3):181–94.
[58] Laudahn D, Walper A. Efficacy and tolerance of Harpagophytum extract LI 174 in patients with chronic non-radicular back pain. Phytother Res 2001;15(7):621–4.

[59] Schmid B, Ludtke R, Selbmann HK, et al. Efficacy and tolerability of a standardized willow bark extract in patients with osteoarthritis: randomized placebo-controlled, double blind clinical trial. Phytother Res 2001;15(4):344–50.
[60] Boullata JI, McDonnell PJ, Oliva CD. Anaphylactic reaction to a dietary supplement containing willow bark. Ann Pharmacother 2003;37(6):832–5.
[61] Nah JJ, Hahn JH, Chung S, et al. Effect of ginsenosides, active components of ginseng, on capsaicin-induced pain-related behavior. Neuropharmacology 2000;39(11):2180–4.
[62] Mills SY, Jacoby RK, Chacksfield M, et al. Effect of a proprietary herbal medicine on the relief of chronic arthritic pain: a double-blind study. Br J Rheum 1996;35(9):874–8.
[63] Pittler MH, Ernst E. Ginkgo biloba extract for the treatment of intermittent claudication: a meta-analysis of randomized trials. Am J Med 2000;108(4):276–81.
[64] Lidija I, Tristan T, Sands J, et al. Terpene trilactones from Ginkgo biloba are antagonists of cortical glycine and GABA(A) receptors. J Biol Chem 2003;278(49):49279–85 [Epub 2003 Sep 22].
[65] Markowitz JS, Donovan JL, DeVane CL, et al. Effect of St John's wort on drug metabolism by induction of cytochrome P450 3A4 enzyme. JAMA 2003;290(11):1519–20.
[66] Rubik B, Becker R, Fowler R, et al. Bioelectromagnetics: applications in medicine. In: Alternative medicine: expanding medical horizons. A report to the National Institutes of Health on alternative medical systems and practices in the United States. Workshop on Alternative Medicine, Chantilly, VA; 1994.
[67] Rubik B. Bioelectromagnetics & the future of medicine. Adm Radiol J 1997;16(8):38–46.
[68] Lefaucheur JP, Drouot X, Keravel Y, et al. Pain relief induced by repetitive transcranial magnetic stimulation of precentral cortex. Neuroreport 2001;12(13):2963–5.
[69] Hinman MR, Ford J, Heyl H. Effects of static magnets on chronic knee pain and physical function: a double-blind study. Altern Ther Health Med 2002;8(4):50–5.
[70] Segal NA, Toda Y, Huston J, et al. Two configurations of static magnetic fields for treating rheumatoid arthritis of the knee: a double-blind clinical trial. Arch Phys Med Rehabil 2001; 82(10):1453–60.
[71] Brown CS, Ling FW, Wan JY, et al. Efficacy of static magnetic field therapy in chronic pelvic pain: a double-blind pilot study. Am J Obstet Gyncol 2002;187(6):1581–7.
[72] Vallbona C, Hazlewood CF, Jurida G. Response of pain to static magnetic fields in postpolio patients: a double-blind pilot study. Arch Phys Med Rehabil 1997;78(11):1200–3.
[73] Weintraub MI, Cole SP. Neuromagnetic treatment of pain in refractory carpal tunnel syndrome: an electrophysiological and placebo analysis. J Back Musculoskel 2000;15(2–3): 77–81.
[74] Carter R, Aspy CB, Mold J. The effectiveness of magnet therapy for treatment of wrist pain attributed to carpal tunnel syndrome. J Fam Pract 2002;51(1):38–40.
[75] Alfano AP, Taylor AG, Foresman PA, et al. Static magnetic fields for treatment of fibromyalgia: a randomized controlled trial. J Altern Complement Med 2001;7(1):53–64.
[76] Collacott EA, Zimmerman JT, White DW, et al. Bipolar permanent magnets for the treatment of chronic low back pain: a pilot study. JAMA 2000;283(10):1322–5.
[77] Winemiller MH, Billow RG, Laskowski ER, et al. Effect of magnetic vs sham-magnetic insoles on plantar heel pain: a randomized controlled trial. JAMA 2004;291(1):43–4.
[78] Jacobson JI, Gorman R, Yamanashi WS, et al. Low-amplitude, extremely low frequency magnetic fields for the treatment of osteoarthritic knees: a double-blind clinical study. Altern Ther Health Med 2001;7(5):54–64 [66–9].
[79] Pipitone N, Scott DL. Magnetic pulse treatment for knee osteoarthritis: a randomised, double-blind, placebo-controlled study. Curr Med Res Opin 2001;17(3):190–6.
[80] Weintraub MI, Cole SP. Pulsed magnetic field therapy in refractory neuropathic pain secondary to peripheral neuropathy: electrodiagnostic parameters pilot study. Neurorehabil Neural Repair 2004;18(1):42–6.
[81] Trock DH. Electromagnetic fields and magnets. Investigational treatment for musculoskeletal disorders. Rheum Dis Clin North Am 2000;26(1):51–62.

[82] Vallbona C, Richards T. Evolution of magnetic therapy from alternative to traditional medicine. Phys Med Rehabil Clin North Am 1999;10(3):729–54.
[83] Shumay DM, Maskarinec G, Gotay CC, et al. Determinants of the degree of complementary and alternative medicine use among patients with cancer. J Altern Complem Med 2002;8(5): 661–71.
[84] Pan CX, Morrison RS, Ness J, et al. Complementary and alternative medicine in the management of pain, dyspnea, and nausea and vomiting near the end of life: a systematic review. J Pain Sympt Manage 2000;20(5):374–87.
[85] DiGianni LM, Garber JE, Winer EP. Complementary and alternative medicine use among women with breast cancer. J Clin Oncol 2002;20(18):34S–8S.
[86] Power R, Gore-Felton C, Vosvick M, et al. HIV: effectiveness of complementary and alternative medicine. Prim Care 2002;29(2):361.
[87] Malik IA, Gopalan S. Use of CAM results in delay in seeking medical advice for breast cancer. Eur J Epidemiol 2003;18(8):817–22.

ELSEVIER
SAUNDERS

Emerg Med Clin N Am 23 (2005) 551–572

EMERGENCY
MEDICINE
CLINICS OF
NORTH AMERICA

Procedural Sedation and Analgesia in the Emergency Department: What Are the Risks?

Michael A. Miller, MD[a,*], Phillip Levy, MD[b], Manish M. Patel, MD, MSc[c]

[a]*Department of Emergency Medicine, Darnall Army Community Hospital, 36000 Darnall Loop, Box 32, Ft. Hood, TX 76544, USA*

[b]*Department of Emergency Medicine, Wayne State University, Detroit Receving Hospital, 4201 St. Antoine 6G. Detroit, MI 48202, USA*

[c]*Emory University School of Medicine, Department of Emergency Medicine, 1365 Clifton Road, Suite B6200 Atlanta, GA 30322, USA*

Practicing emergency medicine physicians routinely administer agents to provide sedation and pain control. An experiment, in effect, is conducted each time this is done; in this experiment we ask, "what are the risks and benefits of achieving our endpoint of this experiment." To best answer this question, the emergency physician must be aware of the risks involved with the procedure as well as the side effects and toxicity associated with the agents used for sedation and pain control. This article will describe the major adverse events the clinician will likely encounter in the emergency department (ED) when conducting procedural sedation and pain control, and will discuss factors that contribute to untoward events.

Epidemiology of procedural sedation and analgesic adverse events

There are many difficulties in determining the prevalence or incidence of adverse events related to procedural sedation and analgesia (PSA) in the ED. There is no uniform definition of an "adverse event." Adverse events following PSA reported in the literature include hypoxia, apnea, stridor, laryngospasm, bronchospasm, cardiovascular instability, paradoxic reactions, emergence reactions, emesis, and aspiration [1]. Prolonged sedation

* Corresponding author.
E-mail address: Michael.miller3@amedd.army.mil (M.A. Miller).

doi:10.1016/j.emc.2004.12.016

emed.theclinics.com

may also be considered an adverse event. In addition, delayed side effects after a patient is discharged to home may also be of significance and may often be overlooked [2]. Malviya et al [2] found that motor imbalance, agitation, and restlessness were not uncommon findings at home in children who were sedated for a diagnostic procedure. Adverse events are also likely to vary with the type of facility where PSA is used, the specialty of the physician administering PSA, patient age and comorbidity, level of patient monitoring, and patient assessment before PSA. One recent pediatric study identified that adverse events after PSA were more likely in nonhospital-based facilities with inadequate or inconsistent monitoring, inadequate presedation medical evaluation, medication errors, and lack of an independent observer [3]. Despite these apparent differences in patient population, hospital facilities, and specialty practicing PSA, the incidence of major adverse events such as respiratory compromise, hypotension, laryngospasm, or dysrhythmias has been reported to be less than 1% in most studies [1]. Incidence of minor events with mild or minimal clinical impact (eg, nausea, pruritis, transient hypoxia) tends to vary depending on the study and the drugs used in the study population. With respect to minor adverse events, a risk–benefit analysis that focuses on whether patients would accept a small risk of suffering an adverse event, given that their pain was adequately managed, might be necessary.

The authors' opinion is that adverse events related to PSA are likely to occur despite the best of scenarios. However, this incidence is likely to be low if proper precautionary measures are taken as outlined by standardized guidelines such as the American College of Emergency Physicians (ACEP) Clinical Policy for PSA in the ED [1]. Inadequate use of sedation and analgesia resulting in a high failure rate (eg, >20%) will result in significant patient dissatisfaction and reduction in patient's quality of life. Arguably, there might be a slight reduction in the overall incidence of adverse events if a higher PSA failure rate is accepted to be the norm. However, a higher incidence of PSA failure with only a marginal reduction in adverse events is unlikely to be desirable by the patient. A more cogent approach might be to provide adequate sedation with appropriate presedation evaluation, monitoring, and preparation for treatment of any potential complication. Given the advanced training of the emergency physician in airway management, vascular access, resuscitation, and pharmacology (of PSA and PSA reversal drugs), the incidence of adverse events are not likely to be higher when an adequate amount, type, and combination of PSA drugs are used with the goal of lower failure rate in mind. The armamentarium of PSA agents available to clinicians today makes the scenario of increased patient satisfaction without increased adverse events possible by allowing for avoidance of agents with unpredictable and life-threatening side effects [4].

Pena et al [5] found the adverse event rate PSA was 2.3% in an urban pediatric ED, although none required intubation or admission. There were no deaths. There were no differences in complications between the various drugs used for sedation, gender, or age groups. Similar studies also suggest that in the right setting (monitoring, physicians with advanced training in resuscitation, vascular access, and pharmacology), complications of PSA in the pediatric ED population are low and manageable [3,6,7].

Patient factors that contribute to adverse events

Patient factors may influence the pharmacologic response to a number of the medications used for PSA. For instance, infants and the elderly have an increased sensitivity to most drugs, necessitating dosing adjustments [8,9]. A careful history, including drug and food allergies, can reveal conditions that may promote susceptibility to an adverse event. The presence of certain underlying medical conditions may direct the choice of agents. Excessive respiratory depression may result from administration of benzodiazepines and barbiturates in patients with chronic obstructive pulmonary disease [10]. Cirrhosis can cause a prolonged duration of action with barbiturates and hepatically metabolized benzodiazepines [11]. An allergy to soybeans or eggs is a contraindication to propofol, because of the composition of its diluent [12]. Seizure disorders may be exacerbated by methohexital [13]. Barbiturates induce porphyrin synthesis and cannot be given to patients with acute intermittent porphyria or porphyria variegata [14]. Ketamine should be avoided in cases where an intracranial mass of bleed is suspected because it increases intracranial pressure through cerebral vasodilatation [15]. The existence of significant comorbidities such as severe coronary artery disease or congestive heart failure may preclude the ED performance of PSA altogether. Therefore, a careful preprocedural history in conjunction with the necessary knowledge of drug–disease–state interaction will allow prevention of many of the predictable adverse occurrences.

A general physical examination should be performed on all patients, with a focused assessment of the airway. Anatomic variants such as mandibular hypoplasia, micrognathia, and macroglossia are important to recognize. Difficulty with bag–valve–mask ventilation can be expected when the patient is >55 years of age, edentulous, bearded, obese, or has a history of snoring [16]. Evaluating an airway for potential intubation difficulty requires a more in-depth approach. The Mallampati classification (see Fig. 1) is commonly used in anesthesiology, and higher classes (≥III) are predictive of difficult vocal cord visualization on direct laryngoscopy [17,18]. Other associated variables include an inability to open the mouth >4 cm, a thyromental distance <6 cm, limitations of neck movement, difficulty protruding the lower jaw, or a history of difficult intubation [19].

Although it is prudent to consider certain factors (see Table 1) that increase the risk of pulmonary aspiration, excessive concern is largely unfounded. There are no cases reports of aspiration related to ED

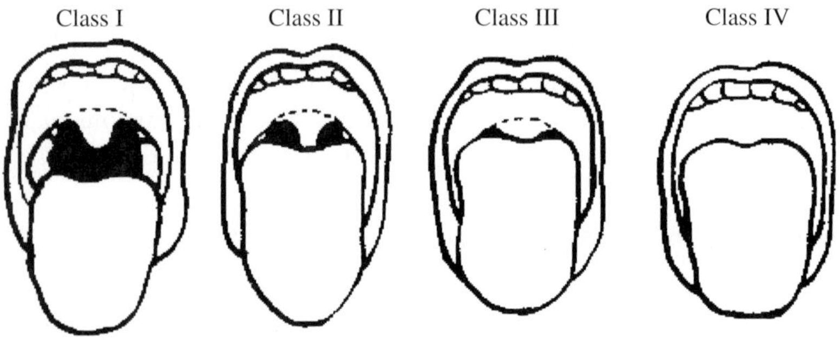

Fig. 1. The Mallampati (modified) classification. (*Data from* Samsoon GL, Young JR. Difficult trachea intubation: a retrospective study. Anesthesia 1987;42:487–90.) Evaluation is performed by inspecting the oropharynx of an upright patient, whose mouth is maximally opened and tongue protruded to the fullest. Increasing obscuration of the uvula and soft palate by the base of the tongue correlates with a higher degree of direct laryngoscopy difficulties.

procedural sedation or analgesia, and the overall incidence from pooled general anesthesia data is low; approximately 1:3420, with an associated mortality rate of 1:125,109. The majority of these aspirations were presumed to have occurred during the process of intubation or extubation; a situation unlikely to arise during ED sedation or analgesia [20]. A significantly lower rate of aspiration (1:8300) has been noted in nonintubated obstetric patients sedated during labor and delivery [21,22]. Given the similar unpredictable and emergent manner with which these patients present, this may represent a truer estimation of the actual ED incidence. Although children have been reported to be more susceptible to aspiration [23], data are conflicting, with aspiration rates ranging from 1:978 to 1:10,060. When data are combined from the largest analyses, the incidence is approximately 1:3708, suggesting

Table 1
Possible risk factors associated with aspiration

Gastric factors
Delayed gastric emptying
Gastroesophageal reflux
Hiatal hernia
Bowel obstruction/ileus
Higher ASA physical status classification
Emergency surgery
Difficulty establishing definitive airway
Head injury with elevated intracranial pressure
Extremes of age

Data from Green SM, Krauss B. Pulmonary aspiration risk during Emergency Department procedural sedation—an examination of the role of fasting and sedation depth. 2002;9:35–42, Engelhardt T, Webster NR. Pulmonary aspiration of gastric contents in anaesthesia. Br J Anaesth 1999;83:453–60.

Table 2
ASA physical status classification

Class	Description	Sedation risk
I	Normal, healthy	Minimal
II	Mild systemic disease without functional limitations	Low
III	Severe systemic disease with functional limitations	Intermediate
IV	Severe systemic disease, which is a constant threat to life	High
V	Moribund patient who may not survive without the procedure	Extremely high

no increase in risk [24–27]. Due to an absence of evidence to support any positive effect on outcomes, the routine administration of antacids, histamine-2 blockers, or proton pump inhibitor in an effort to diminish gastric acidity is no longer recommended [20,23]. The concept of extended preprocedural fasting continues to be endorsed, although multiple studies have shown that administration of clear liquids up to 2 hours before elective surgery results in no increase in gastric volume or acidity and no excess risk for the development of aspiration [20,23]. Agarwal et al recently reported the results of a large (1014 patients) pediatric ED cohort study evaluating the effect of fasting on the development of adverse sedation events [28]. Although the majority (56%) were not "adequately fasted," there were no episodes of aspiration. Additionally, there was no difference in the rate of adverse events between the nonfasted group (6.9%) and the fasted group (8.1%), leading the authors to conclude that the occurrence of adverse events has no association with preprocedural fasting status [28]. The ACEP guidelines for fasting specifically state that "Recent food intake is not a contraindication for administering procedural sedation and analgesia, but should be considered in choosing the depth and target level of sedation" [1]. The American Society of Anesthesiologists (ASA), however, based on consensus opinion with little supporting evidence, continues to recommend a 2-hour fasting period for clear liquids and a 6-hour fasting period for solids and other fluids [29].

Inadequate patient assessment has been shown to be a contributing factor to adverse sedation events [3]. A physical status classification system was developed by the ASA (see Table 2) to assist in determining the negative impact of increasingly poorer health. An ASA physical status of III or greater has been shown to be an independent risk factor for the development of complications with general anesthesia, and has been associated with a higher proportion of sedation-related adverse events in the pediatric population [30–32]. The ASA classification is highly subjective, however, and prone to poor interrater reliability, which diminishes its predictive value [33]. Although the ASA recommends use of this classification system by all nonanesthesiologists performing PSA [34], data regarding the applicability in the ED setting are lacking, and there is no formal support for its routine use by the major academic emergency medicine organizations.

Drug-dosing errors

The greatest proportion of adverse events occurring during the delivery of health care are related to the ordering and administering of medications [35]. The immense implications were highlighted in the 1999 report from the Institute of Medicine, which attributed 7000 deaths each year to medication errors [36]. Approximately 6.5 adverse drug events are thought to occur for every 100 hospital admissions, and in those affected, adverse drug events may be responsible for a near doubling of hospital length of stay. It has been estimated that between 28% and 50% of these are preventable [37,38]. The ED is a setting highly vulnerable to medication errors. Lesar et al [39] found a prescribing error rate of 5.5 per 1000 ED medication orders written. Medications with narrow thresholds of safety, such as some agents used for PSA agents, are particularly susceptible to the effects of error.

Incorrect dosage calculation is one of the leading causes of prescribing error, with an incidence reportedly as high as 15% [37,40]. Nelson et al [41] performed an assessment of EM residents' knowledge of drug dose calculations and found a high rate of inadequacy. After a brief educational intervention, improvements were noted, and it was concluded that targeted education would be beneficial for this group. Ten-fold dosing is a particularly common error in the pediatric ED, and was found to be the predominant cause of ketamine overdose in one series [42,43]. This type of error results from errant decimal point placement or the writing of orders in volume (mL/kg) rather than actual dose (mg/kg) for an agent that has dilute and concentrated preparations available [44]. Dosing errors can result in insufficient medication delivery as well as excess. In an analysis of over 1000 pediatric sedation procedures, Malviya et al [31] found inadequate sedation to be the most common adverse event, noted in 13.2% of patients. Risk factors associated with inadequate ED dosing of sedatives and analgesics include pediatric age and ethnic minority background [45,46]. Administration of the wrong drug may be responsible for 4% to 5% of total medication error cases [39]. Misidentification due to look-alike packaging or sound-alike naming is the primary mechanism by which this occurs [47,48]. Illegible written orders may also contribute. As a group, incorrect dosing is likely the most easily recognized and correctable cause of adverse drug events.

Another source of error of particular concern is the failure to recognize potential drug interactions. In a group of 199 ED patients, Herr et al [49] found that one out of every eight was exposed to a potential adverse drug interaction. Specific interactions relevant to the practice of PSA include: the synergism between fentanyl and midazolam, which may result in enhanced respiratory depressant effects [50], the prolonged duration of action when inhibitors of cytochrome P 450 3A4 such as cimetidine, erythromycin, and ketoconazole are given to patients receiving hepatically metabolized drugs like midazolam [51], and the precipitation of the serotonin syndrome when meperidine is administered to a patient on a monoamine oxidase inhibitor

[52]. The probability of an interaction increases significantly with the combination of several medications. Cote et al [53] found that the use of three or more agents was a significant risk factor for the development of adverse sedation events [53]. Recognition of the potential toxicity of common "lytic cocktails" such as DPT, which includes meperidine (Demerol), promethazine (Phenergan), and chlorpromazine (Thorazine), has prompted recommendations for their removal from hospital formularies [53–55]. If multiple drugs are to be administered, the doses used in combination should be lower than when given individually. A cogent approach to combining agents is a must for minimizing and reducing adverse PSA events.

Minimizing medication errors has been recognized as an important goal for the emergency medicine community [41,56]. Aside from the human cost, prevention of a single adverse drug event may save as much as $4685 in hospital charges [57]. Smaller interventions in the ED such as the use of order checkback techniques and removal of similar looking or sounding medications may enhance teamwork and diminish error due to miscommunication [48]. Larger system-based reorganization may be required to significantly impact hospital medication error rates. Implementation of computerized order entry systems has been shown to decrease adverse drug events by 55% [58]. Automated drug delivery systems like the Pyxis (Pyxis Corporation, San Diego, California) enable more controlled access to medications and allow better inventory control [56]. Twenty-four-hour satellite pharmacies in the ED staffed by pharmacists are particularly effective, offering enhanced drug allergy screening, correct dosing for all medication orders, preparation of intravenous medications, and suggestion of alternative medication options [59].

Adverse effects upon body systems

Cardiovascular

In general, all agents used for PSA typically cause a reduction of sympathetic output from the central nervous system, thereby causing some degree of bradycardia and hypotension [60–62]. This phenomenon is likely to be dose related and when two different classes of agents are combined (eg, benzodiazepines and opiates), as is typical with PSA, there may be a synergistic effect on the reduction of central sympathetic activity [60]. In addition, patients with comorbid conditions (eg, hypovolemia, decreased cardiac reserve) and patients who are on cardiodepressant medications (eg, beta blockers or calcium channel blockers) may be at greater risk for developing hypotension and bradycardia from PSA [63]. However, in most ED-based studies on PSA, clinically relevant hypotension or bradycardia is the exception rather than the rule [1,4], probably due in part to the relatively greater sympathetic tone in ED patients suffering from pain and anxiety.

In addition to reduced sympathetic output, each class of PSA agents has a wide range of effects on the cardiovascular system that might result in adverse effects, such as hypotension or dysrhthmias. Most of these adverse events are more likely to occur in patients with predisposing conditions such as congestive heart failure (CHF), and thus can be anticipated or avoided by choosing agents that might better suit the patient. The clinician today has a wide range of PSA drugs to choose from, thereby avoiding use of drugs with unpredictable adverse events. Drugs with unpredictable side effects will be highlighted and presented only for historic interest.

Barbiturates. Hypotension is the predominant adverse hemodynamic event that might result from use of barbiturates for PSA. The most likely cause of hypotension is venodilation and pooling of blood in the peripheral vascular system [62]. For this reason, caution should be used when using barbiturates in patients with preload-dependent conditions such as CHF, pericardial tamponade, and myocardial ischemia.

Opioids. The primary adverse cardiac event reported with opioids has been rate and rhythm disturbance after use of sufentanil and alfentanil [64,65]. Several case reports of asystole in association with sufentanil and alfentanil have been reported in the anesthesiology literature [64,65]. However, these high-potency opioids are unlikely to be used in the ED setting.

Benzodiazepines. Although benzodiazepines generally have minimal adverse hemodynamic effects, when combined with opiates, the two may have a synergistic effect on reduction of the patient's blood pressure [66]. As with other PSA agents, this effect is more likely to occur in susceptible populations, such as those with ischemic heart disease, and can typically be corrected with fluid resuscitation.

Ketamine. The unique aspect of ketamine is that it may stimulate the cardiovascular system, resulting in tachycardia, hypertension, and increased cardiac output [4]. Because of this increase myocardial work and oxygen consumption, adverse events such as myocardial ischemia might occur in patients with coronary artery disease. However, use of ketamine in adults is not uncommon in anesthesiology, and has even been safely used in patients undergoing coronary artery bypass graft surgery [67]. In the ED, ketamine is most commonly used for pediatric patients, and adverse cardiac events have not been reported.

Etomidate. Transient bradycardia has been rarely reported [68,69]; however, overall, hemodynamic effects with etomidate are unusual, even in patients with ischemic heart disease [70].

Propofol. The most notable adverse cardiac events after use of propofol have included dysrhythmias, heart block, and cardiac arrest, and have typically occurred in conjunction with metabolic acidosis [71,72]. However, these events have all been in critically ill patients (mostly pediatric) receiving high doses of propofol for prolonged periods of time [71]. The most likely hemodynamic consequence with use of propofol in the ED setting is hypotension as a result of venodilation, and a dose-dependent myocardial depression [73]. Propofol-induced hypotension is typically transient and is usually not associated with a reduction in perfusion [72]. Moreover, propofol has a rapid onset of action and a very short duration of action, thereby resulting in rapid resolution of desired and undesired effects after discontinuation of the drug [7].

Chloral hydrate. Historic interest should be the only reason for discussing chloral hydrate. Because of it unpredictable cardiac toxicity, erratic analgesic and amnestic effects, and the availability of better PSA agents, chloral hydrate should not have any role in modern PSA. Many reports of cardiac dysrhythmias and deaths from chloral hydrate toxicity have been reported, mostly after therapeutic dosing errors and intentional drug overdoses [74]. Arrhythmias are dose dependent, and attributed to both chloral hydrate and its active metabolite, trichloroethanol.

Pulmonary

Respiratory depression is the most prominent adverse effect of PSA, and is found to some degree with nearly all agents. Other pulmonary effects such as brochospasm, bronchorrhea, laryngospasm, and muscular rigidity occur more rarely, and in general, are a consequence of specific medications. The occurrence of respiratory depression is usually dose dependent, but can be related to the rate of infusion. For this reason, careful titration and slow administration are recommended [1]. Monitoring for respiratory depression is essential. For this purpose, pulse oximetry is widely employed. Reliant on recognition of hypoxemia (defined as oxygen saturation $<90\%$), pulse oximetry may be less sensitive with concurrent oxygen administration due to delayed onset of desaturation [75]. Detection of rising carbon dioxide levels using end-tidal carbon dioxide ($ETCO_2$) monitoring has been shown to be an effective adjunct. Using validated criteria (an absence of waveform, an $ETCO_2 > 50$ mmHg, or an increase from baseline >10 mmHg), it is possible to identify subclinical respiratory depression [76]. Theoretically, this may be beneficial, especially with medications that decrease hypoxic ventilatory drive, but there is no evidence that this impacts patient outcome [77].

Opiod medications, when used at analgesic doses, have a clear depressant effect on respiratory drive. This appears to be mediated through dose-dependent agonism at the μ_2 opiod receptor in the brain stem, with a resultant decrease in respiratory activity (respiratory rate, minute volume, and tidal volume) as well as a blunting of both hypoxic and hypercarbic ventilatory responses [78–80]. Antitussive effects, noted primarily with codeine and dextromethorphan, may also be moderated by the μ_2 receptor, possibly in conjunction with the 5-HT_{1A} serotonin receptor [81]. For morphine, maximal respiratory depression is seen within 5 to 10 minutes if administered intravenously and within 30 to 90 minutes if given intramuscularly or subcutaneously. The onset of respiratory depression is more rapid with lipid soluble agents (fentanyl and its derivatives), but for all opiods, at equianalgesic doses, the absolute degree is equivalent. Delayed effects on respiration can be seen for up to 4 hours, possibly due to drug redistribution or to enterohepatic circulation [82]. Partial agonist-antagonist opiods such as buprenorphine and nalbuphine are associated with a ceiling effect on respiratory depression, due largely to a predominance of κ rather than μ_2 agonist activity [80]. Opiate-mediated respiratory depression is easily reversible with the administration of antagonists such as naloxone. Conservative intravenous dosing, starting with 0.05 mg, followed subsequently with 0.4 mg, 2 mg, and finally 10 mg as indicated, will reduce the potential for abrupt withdrawal and its accompanying adverse effects [83]. Although a causal relationship between naloxone-precipitated opiate withdrawal and the development of opiod-related noncardiogenic pulmonary edema (now termed acute lung injury) has been noted, no clear corollary exists. Based on animal models, it has been suggested that naloxone may induce acute lung injury by stimulating a massive central nervous system release of catecholamines, with resultant oversensitization of the myocardium [84]. Numerous case reports exist, however, including William Osler's seminal observation in 1880, in which opiod-related acute lung injury developed in the absence of naloxone [85]. There is no single explanation for the etiology of opiate-related acute lung injury, and it may be that naloxone simply reveals underlying pathology. Presumably, it involves an increase in the permeability of the alveolar-capillary membrane, but there is no evidence that opiates directly induce alveolar toxicity [86]. A plausible mechanism proposed by Nelson suggests that edema develops as a result of intraalveolar fluid translocation from excessive negative intrathoracic pressure caused by inspiration against an opiod-induced lax glottis (the Müller maneuver) [87].

Fentanyl is the opiod agent most often selected for procedural sedation. Rapid intravenous injection and doses of in excess of 15 μg/kg have been associated with the development of glottic and chest wall rigidity [88,89]. A similar reaction has been noted with the ultrashort-acting fentanyl derivatives such as alfentanyl, sufentanil, remifentanil, and rapifentanil. Difficulty with respiration and an inability to adequately supplement oxygenation with bag–valve–mask ventilation typically develop. Delayed onset of up to 6 hours has been noted, and is thought to be a result of secondary redistribution from adipose tissue and the gastrointestinal tract [90]. The etiology is uncertain, but may involve effects at the μ receptors in the locus ceruleus, or may be mediated through central α_2-adrenergic receptors [91]. The latter is supported by the observation that pretreatment with dexmedetomidine, a central acting α_2-adrenergic agonist, may prevent the development of rigidity [92]. Rigidity may also be mitigated by pretreatment with midazolam or diazepam [93]. Naloxone can effectively reverse rigidity in the majority of cases, but neuromuscular blocking agents may be required in refractory situations, especially those involving mechanical ventilation [87,89]. At doses commonly used in the ED, however, this occurrence is rare. Chudnofsky et al [89] evaluated the safety of fentanyl in the 841 ED patients. The average dose per patient was 180 μg (range, 25 to 1400 μg), and there were no episodes of chest wall rigidity noted. The incidence of respiratory depression was remarkably low as well; only six (0.7%) patients developed respiratory complications, three of which required transient noninvasive ventilatory support [89]. The respiratory depressant effects of fentanyl are markedly potentiated by concurrent administration of midazolam [94]. Appropriate precautions should be exercised when using this combination, and it is recommended that the fentanyl be given first, with the midazolam dose titrated to the desired effect [1].

Both midazolam and diazepam have been shown to be safe for procedural sedation in the ED, but midazolam is generally preferred due to a faster onset and shorter duration of action [95]. Overall, the incidence of respiratory complications with these agents is low, which may be secondary to a paucity of benzodiazepine receptors in the brain stem [96]. Midazolam has been associated with fatal respiratory depression and apnea, but the majority of cases involved improper monitoring and a failure to recognize the synergistic effect of opioids [97]. It was initially thought that rapid infusion of midazolam might have been a precipitating factor, but the rate of administration has been shown to have no effect on the development of respiratory complications [98]. As a class, benzodiazepines decrease alveolar ventilation and depress the hypoxic ventilatory drive in a dose-dependent manner. Subclinical oxygen desaturation may result from hypoventilation, but clinical hypoxemia is rare, especially with short-acting agents such as midazolam [99]. In instances when respiratory depression does occur with midazolam, the effect is usually brief, with spontaneous resolution or improvement after verbal stimulation and oxygen therapy [94]. Flumazenil can be used to reverse more severe cases of midazolam-induced respiratory depression when the use of this reversal agent is not contraindicated [100].

Midazolam is frequently used with ketamine to prevent emergence reactions. The combination has been associated with varying rates of adverse respiratory events. Slonim et al [101] evaluated the use in 295 pediatric intensive care unit procedures and noted minor respiratory complications in only two cases (0.7%). Parker et al [102] analyzed a larger sample of procedures in general pediatric patients, reporting a similar incidence (1.1%) of transient respiratory depression (desaturation only).

Chudnofsky et al [103], however, studied an adult ED population and found a 6% incidence of respiratory events, with two episodes of apnea requiring bag–valve–mask ventilation. In another ED-based study, Wathen et al [104] compared the effects of ketamine versus ketamine–midazolam coadministration. The combined rate of respiratory complications was 4.5%. There was an equivalent incidence of apneic episodes (0.8% versus 0.7%), but the occurrence of oxygen desaturation increased with the addition of midazolam from 1.6% to 7.3%. Of note, all respiratory events resolved spontaneously, and repositioning or oxygen was the only therapy required. Although not proven, midazolam may suppress ketamine metabolism through competitive inhibition, prolonging the duration of action [105].

Ketamine alone produces a mild, dose-dependent effect on respiration, primarily due to a decrease in the hypercarbic ventilatory response [106]. Even at fully dissociative doses (1.5 mg/kg), ketamine produces no clinically evident respiratory depressant effects, and may slightly increase respiratory rate [107]. Apnea has been reported when only when given by rapid intravenous bolus necessitating slow administration (over 1 minute) [15,107]. Partial airway obstruction from positional malalignment has been seen, and may cause oxygen desaturation. It is easily reversible with repositioning of the head [105]. A bronchodilating effect exists as well, resulting from an inhibition of catecholamine reuptake and direct smooth muscle relaxation [108].

Ketamine is associated with hyperdynamic laryngeal reflexes, which can result in laryngospasm [15,105]. Predisposing risk factors include active upper respiratory infections (especially croup), an age <3 months, and stimulation of the posterior oropharynx. As a result, all are considered contraindications to the use of ketamine [103,105]. Suctioning may also be a precipitant of laryngospasm. Because tracheobronchial secretions and excessive salivation are stimulated by ketamine and may require suction removal, adjunctive treatment with anticholinergic agents such as atropine (0.01 mg/kg, maximum 0.5 mg) is recommended [109]. Glycopyrrolate (0.005 mg/kg, maximum 0.25 mg) is equally efficacious, and produces less tachycardia [110] Laryngospasm is a rare occurrence. In 1022 pediatric ED patients given intramuscular ketamine, Green et al [105] observed an incidence of laryngospasm of only 0.4%. Spontaneous resolution without the need for intubation was noted in all cases. This is consistent with pooled-data analysis that has shown that airway intervention for laryngospasm is infrequent, noted in only 2 of 11,589 (0.017%) reviewed ketamine administrations [111].

Hyperdynamic respiratory reflexes may also be seen with the barbiturates. Zink et al [112] found that coughing or hiccups occurred in 7 of 102 (6.9%) of their patients who were given methohexital. There observed no episodes of laryngospasm or brochospasm. Barbiturates have the potential for induction of severe respiratory depression. Smaller hypnotic doses blunt the hypoxic and hypercarbic stimulation of respiration. Increasingly higher doses produce a deep unconscious state, with a loss of the central neurogenic respiratory drive and protective airway reflexes. Of the short acting barbiturates, methohexital causes less respiratory depression than thiopental [8]. Reports of apnea with methohexital vary with older studies noting rates of 17% to 30% and newer studies finding rates of 2.6% to 10.5% [112,113]. Brief respiratory assistance with a bag–valve–mask may be required in approximately 10% to 20% of patients given methohexital [112]. There are no apparent synergistic respiratory depressant interactions between methohexital and opioids or benzodiazepines [14].

Miner et al [114] performed a recent comparison trial of methohexital versus propofol. Using $ETCO_s$ and pulse oximetry criteria, the authors found a 48.5% rate of respiratory depression overall, with an equivalent occurrence in each group. Apnea was seen in 7.7% of those receiving methohexital and 3.9% of those given propofol [114]. Propofol has undergone several similar trials, with less stringent definitions of respiratory depression. In a pediatric ED study, propofol (11.6%) and midazolam (10.9%) induced a similar degree of hypoxemia without any episodes of significant clinical respiratory depression [115]. In a pediatric intensive care unit study, however, propofol was three times more (10%) likely to induce apnea than ketamine (3%) [116]. Apnea was also noted in 10% of patients (2 of 20) when propofol was added to fentanyl in an ED observational study by Swanson et al [117]. Propofol's respiratory depressant effects are dose-dependent, and mediated in part through a diminution of the hypoxic ventilatory drive. Effects such as brochospasm are not noted to occur with propofol administration, and lower loading (0.8 mg/kg) and infusion doses (30 μg/kg/min) may limit the development of clinically significant respiratory depression without significantly compromising sedation [118].

Based on studies conducted during the performance of cardioversion, etomidate appears to induce a lesser degree of apnea than equipotent dosing of propofol [119]. Comparison information on the incidence of respiratory complications during ED procedural sedation is limited, but suggests that it is equivalent to midazolam [120]. Etomidate is known to produce respiratory depression through a decrease in tidal volume and minute ventilation. A recent ED observational trial of etomidate conducted by Ruth et al [68] noted a relatively low occurrence of respiratory events, with an 8.9% rate of desaturation, none requiring respiratory assistance, and no episodes of apnea. In a similar study by Vinson and Bradbury [69], however, 5 of 150 (3.3%) patients developed apnea, with four requiring brief bag–valve–mask-assisted ventilation, and three of the episodes lasting 30 minutes or longer. All five patients received slightly higher doses and were >55 years of age, leading the authors to conclude that advanced age was a risk factor for the development of respiratory depression with etomidate [69].

Chloral hydrate is used infrequently with the advent of more effective medications. Although thought to be a generally safe agent, recent reports have observed a high rate of adverse events [3]. Malviya et al [31] found that 73% (46 of 63) of patients who experienced a respiratory complication, received chloral hydrate as the sole sedative agent. Chloral hydrate has no effect on the hypercarbic or hypoxic respiratory response, and respiratory rate may slightly increase [121]. There are depressant effects on the genioglossus muscle, which can cause upper airway obstruction [122]. Obstructive sleep apnea syndrome, tonsillar/adenoid hypertrophy, and genetic conditions such as trisomy 21 are associated with a greater risk of developing this complication. Hypoventilation may result from the addition of 30% or 50% nitrous oxide [123]. It is the authors' opinion that the pulmonary and cardiovascular adverse effects of chloral hydrate should preclude its choice as a PSA agent in the ED.

Nitrous oxide alone has limited effects on the respiratory system. It does induce a potent but selective vasodilatory effect on pulmonary vasculature, which can be used therapeutically in newborn pulmonary hypertension [124]. Methemoglobinemia development is a known complication, and significant concentrations should be suspected with a persistent pulse oximetry reading of 85%, despite oxygen therapy. Nitrous oxide is eliminated unchanged by the lungs. Moderate to high concentrations can displace oxygen from the alveoli and result in a diffusional hypoxia. Delayed onset of this effect may be seen due to redistribution kinetics. Dosing adjustments are recommended when used at high altitude to prevent hypoxia [8]. At higher concentrations (>50 ppm) nitrous oxide may cause pulmonary toxicity. This is partially due to the formation of nitrogen dioxide, which is capable of producing ciliary loss and bronchiolar hyperplasia [125].

Gastrointestinal

Although typically minor, gastrointestinal (GI) side effects of PSA will be experienced by a significant minority of patients [126]. Nausea and vomiting are the most common GI adverse events, and the rates vary depending upon the group of agents or combination of agents used [69,126]. Opiods predictably cause nausea and occasional vomiting [127]. Overall the incidence of nausea and vomiting associated with PSA ranges from 4% with etomidate, 6% with ketamine and midazolam, to 28.6% with morphine sulfate [69,126,127]. In addition to the nausea and vomiting that occurs shortly following the procedure, patients may experience nausea and vomiting after discharge. In the pediatric study by Pitetti and colleagues, 9.8% of patients undergoing PSA had minor complications following discharge with vomiting occurring in 76.7% of those patients (7.5% of all patients undergoing PSA) [126]. Patient instruction in this regard may help reduce unnecessary patient concern and ED visits.

Renal and adrenal

Although many medications used for analgesia such as nonsteroidal anti-inflammatory drugs and acetaminophen can affect the kidneys, significant renal injury from isolated PSA is not reported [128]. Even with agents that are well recognized to cause analgesic nephropathy, large overdoses of nonsteroidal anti-inflammatory drugs and acetaminophen do not consistently cause nephrotoxicity, with only 8.9% of severe acetaminophen overdoses having associated renal impairment [129,130]. In the ED, renal function is much more likely to be a concern with regard to which agents undergo renal metabolism than which agent(s) will induce a nephrotoxic effect.

Adrenocortical dysfunction is routinely and predictably induced by the use of Etomidate; however, clinically important suppression is very unusual after a single dose for PSA or rapid-sequence intubation (RSI). In the study by Schenarts, a dose of 0.3 mg/kg used for RSI induced abnormal cosyntropin stimulation tests in 70% of patients. However, the cosyntropin stimulation tests returned to normal in all patients at 12 hours. Normal serum cortisol levels were present throughout this early, post-RSI period, and no significant clinical events related to hypoadrenalism occurred. Although the effect of PSA upon the adrenal axis is quite unlikely to be of significance, it is the authors' opinion that its use for PSA or RSI in the patient with concomitant septic shock may benefit from corticosteroid supplementation, as there may already be a component of adrenocortical dysfunction [131].

Dermatologic, allergic, and neurologic

Dermatologic side effects of PSA may involve Immunoglobulin E (IgE)-mediated effects, direct mast-cell degranulation events, or idiosyncratic, non-IgE–related allergic mechanisms. Although rash during and following sedation varies depending upon the agents used, the incidence is generally between 1% to 2%, with most reactions being mild [126,132]. Opiods are most commonly implicated in rashes that develop in the PSA patient, and these are generally due to direct stimulation of histamine release from cutaneous mast cells, producing a wheal and flare appearance [133]. Most drug-induced urticaria is not IgE mediated; one study reported that only 6% of patients with drug-induced urticaria demonstrated IgE mechanisms [134]. Of course, use of an agent to which the patient has a stated "allergy" must be approached with caution. Serious allergic reactions during PSA have occurred, for example, with the use of propofol in a child with egg and peanut allergy [12]. Opiod-related massive mast-cell degranulation has been implicated as a possible cause of death in some heroin addicts [135].

Short-term neurologic effects during and following PSA are not uncommon, with the most common event being recurrence of the sedated state with concurrent hypoxia [126]. Many highly variable and odd neurologic side effects have been described to include hiccups, myoclonus, diplopia, ataxia, mild to severe recovery agitation, and even clinical B-12 deficiency in the use of nitrous oxide as an anesthetic adjunct [105,111,136].

Assuring that the patient is safe for discharge should be a primary endpoint to any PSA protocol. When neurologic adverse effects do occur, the practioner should ensure that they are sufficiently minor or have resolved before patient discharge.

Summary

The practitioner of emergency medicine is routinely faced with patients in need of emergent procedures and pain control and sedation. Our challenge is to make our patients' experiences as painless and as safe as possible, while maximizing our ability to perform the procedure at hand; this is not always an easy task given the propensity of each human body to react differently to interventions and stimuli. We can best meet this challenge by understanding how our patients and pharmaceutical agents intermingle in the risk–benefit equation we formulate before starting our "experiment." Coupling this information with fundamentally sound patient care and monitoring will mimimize bad experiences with PSA for both the patient and practitioner.

References

[1] Clinical policy for procedural sedation and analgesia in the emergency department. American College of Emergency Physicians. Ann Emerg Med 1998;31:663–77.
[2] Malviya S, Voepel-Lewis T, Prochaska G, et al. Prolonged recovery and delayed side effects of sedation for diagnostic imaging studies in children. Pediatrics 2000;105:E42.
[3] Cote CJ, Notterman DA, Karl HW, et al. Adverse sedation events in pediatrics: a critical incident analysis of contributing factors. Pediatrics 2000;105:805–14.
[4] Blackburn P, Vissers R. Pharmacology of emergency department pain management and conscious sedation. Emerg Med Clin North Am 2000;18:803–27.
[5] Pena BM, Krauss B. Adverse events of procedural sedation and analgesia in a pediatric emergency department. Ann Emerg Med 1999;34:483–91.
[6] Rothermel LK. Newer pharmacologic agents for procedural sedation of children in the emergency department—etomidate and propofol. Curr Opin Pediatr 2003;15:200–3.
[7] Skokan EG, Pribble C, Bassett KE, et al. Use of propofol sedation in a pediatric emergency department: a prospective study. Clin Pediatr (Phila) 2001;40:663–71.
[8] Sacchetti A, Schafermayer R, Gerardi M, et al. Pediatric analgesia and sedation. Ann Emerg Med 1994;23:237–50.
[9] Cepeda MS, Farrar JT, Baumgarten M, et al. Side effects of opioids during short-term administration: effect of age, gender, and race. Clin Pharmacol Ther 2003;74:102–12.
[10] Gross JB, Zebrowski ME, Carel WD, et al. Time course of ventilatory depression after thiopental and midazolam in normal subjects and in patients with chronic obstructive pulmonary disease. Anesthesiology 1983;58:540–4.
[11] Guglielminotti J, Maury E, Alzieu M, et al. Prolonged sedation requiring mechanical ventilation and continuous Flumazenil infusion after routine doses of clorazepam for alcohol withdrawal syndrome. Intensive Care Med 1999;25:1435–6.
[12] Hofer KN, McCarty MW, Buck ML, et al. Possible anaphylaxis after propofol in a child with food allergy. Ann Pharmacother 2003;37:398–401.
[13] Zink BJ, Darfler K, Salluzzo RF, et al. The efficacy and safety of methohexital in the emergency department. Ann Emerg Med 1991;20:1293–8.

[14] Charney DA, Mihic SJ, Harris RA. Hypnotics and sedatives. In: Hardman JG, Limbird LE, editors. Goodman and Gilman's the pharmacologic basis of therapeutics. 10th edition. New York: McGraw-Hill; 2001. p. 399–427.
[15] Green SM. Ketamine sedation for pediatric procedures: part 2, review and implications. Ann Emerg Med 1990;19:1033–46.
[16] Langeron O, Masso E, Huraux C, et al. Prediction of difficult mask ventilation. Anesthesiology 2000;92(5):1229–36.
[17] Samsoon GL, Young JR. Difficult trachea intubation: a retrospective study. Anaesthesia 1987;42:487–90.
[18] Mallampati SR, Gatt SP, Gugino LD. A clinical sign to predict difficult tracheal intubation: a prospective study. Can Anesth Soc J 1985;32:429–34.
[19] El-Ganzouri AR, McCarthy RJ, Tuman KJ. Preoperative airway assessment: predictive value of a multivariate risk index. Anesth Analg 1996;82:1197–204.
[20] Green SM, Krauss B. Pulmonary aspiration risk during Emergency Department procedural sedation—an examination of the role of fasting and sedation depth. Acad Emerg Med 2002;9:35–42.
[21] Krantz ML, Edwarda WL. The incidence of nonfatal aspiration in obstetric patients [letter]. Anesthesiology 1973;39:359.
[22] Soreide E, Bjornestad E, Steen PA. An audit of perioperative aspiration pneumonitis in gynecological and obstetric patients. Acta Anaesthesiol Scand 1996;40:14–9.
[23] Engelhardt T, Webster NR. Pulmonary aspiration of gastric contents in anaesthesia. Br J Anaesth 1999;83:453–60.
[24] Borland LM, Sereika SM, Woefel SK, et al. Pulmonary aspiration in pediatric patients during general anesthesia: incidence and outcome. J Clin Anesth 1998;10:95–102.
[25] Olsson GL, Hallen B, Hambraeus-Jonzon K. Aspiration during anaesthesia; a computer-aided study of 185,358 anaesthetics. Acta Anaesthesiol Scand 1986;30:84–92.
[26] Tiret L, Nivoche Y, Hatton F, et al. Complications related to anaesthesia in infants and children. A prospective survey of 40,240 anaesthetics. Br J Anaesth 1988;61:263–9.
[27] Warner MA, Warner ME, Warner DO, et al. Perioperative pulmonary aspiration in infants and children. Anesthesiology 1999;90:66–71.
[28] Agarwal D, Manzi SD, Gupta R, et al. Preprocedural fasting state and adverse events in children undergoing procedural sedation and analgesia in a pediatric emergency department. Ann Emerg Med 2003;42:636–46.
[29] American Society of Anesthesiologists. Practice guidelines for preoperative fasting and the use of pharmacologic agents to reduce the risk of pulmonary aspiration: application to healthy people undergoing elective procedures. Anesthesiology 1999;90:896–905.
[30] Jastak JT, Peskin RM. Major morbidity or mortality from office anesthetic procedures: a closed-claim analysis of 13 cases. Anesth Prog 1991;38:39–44.
[31] Malviya S, Voepel-Lewis T, Tait A. Adverse events and risk factors associated with the sedation of children by nonanesthesiologists. Anesth Analg 1997;86(6):1207–13.
[32] Malviya S, Voepel-Lewis T, Eldevik OP, et al. Sedation and general anaesthesia in children undergoing MRI and CT: adverse events and outcomes. Br J Anaesth 2000;84:743–8.
[33] Aronson WL, McAuliffe MS, Miller K. Variability in the American Society of Anesthesiologists Physical Status Classification Scale. AANA J 2003;71:265–74.
[34] American Society of Anesthesiologists Task Force on Sedation and Analgesia by Non-Anesthesiologists. Practice guidelines for sedation and analgesia by non-anaesthesiologists. Anesthesiology 1996;84:459–70.
[35] Brennan TA, Leape LL, Laird N, et al. Incidence of adverse events and negligence in hospitalized patients. Results of the Harvard Medical Practice Study I. N Engl J Med 1991; 324:370–6.
[36] Kohn LT, Corrigan JM, Donaldson MS, editors. To err is human: building a safer health system. Report of the Institute of Medicine. Washington (DC): National Academy Press; 1999.

[37] Bates DW, Cullen DJ, Laird N, et al. Incidence of adverse drug events and potential adverse drug events: implications for prevention. JAMA 1995;274:29–34.
[38] Chassen DC, Pestotmik SL, Evans RS, et al. Adverse drug events in hospitalized patients: excess length of stay, extra costs and attributable mortality. JAMA 1997;277: 301–6.
[39] Lesar TS, Lomaestro BM, Pohl H. Medication prescribing errors in a teaching hospital: a 9-year experience. Arch Intern Med 1997;157:1569–76.
[40] Lesar TS, Briceland L, Stein DS. Factors related to errors in medication prescribing. JAMA 1997;277:312–7.
[41] Nelson LS, Gordon PE, Simmons MD, et al. The benefits of houseofficer education on proper medication dose calculation and ordering. Acad Emerg Med 2000;7:1311–6.
[42] Selbst SM, Fein JA, Osterhoudt K, et al. Medication errors in a pediatric emergency department. Pediatr Emerg Care 1999;15:1–4.
[43] Green SM, Clark R, Hostetler MA, et al. Inadvertent ketamine overdose in children: clinical manifestations and outcome. Ann Emerg Med 1999;34:492–7.
[44] Koren G, Haslam RH. Pediatric medication errors: predicting and preventing tenfold disasters. J Clin Pharmacol 1994;34:1043–5.
[45] Hostetler MA, Szilagyi PG, Auinger P. Do children in the emergency department really receive less analgesia and sedation than adults? Acad Emerg Med 2000;7:549.
[46] Todd KH, Samaroo N, Hoffman JR. Ethnicity as a risk factor for emergency department analgesia. JAMA 1993;269:1537–9.
[47] Leape LL, Bates DW, Cullen DJ, et al. Systems analysis of adverse drug events. ADE Prevention Study Group. JAMA 1995;274(1):35–43.
[48] Chisolm CD, Klanduch F. Inadvertent administration of sufentanil instead of fentanyl during sedation/analgesia in a community hospital emergency department: a report of two cases. Acad Emerg Med 2000;7:1282–4.
[49] Herr RD, Caravati EM, Tyler LS, et al. Prospective evaluation of adverse drug interactions in the emergency department. Ann Emerg Med 1992;21:1331–6.
[50] Bailey P, Pace N, Ashburn M, et al. Frequent hypoxemia and apnea after sedation with midazolam and fentanyl. Anesthesiology 1990;73:826–30.
[51] Klotz U, Arvela P, Rosenkranz B. Effect of single doses of cimetidine and ranitidine on the steady-state plasma levels of midazolam. Clin Pharmacol Ther 1985;38:652–5.
[52] Browne B, Linter S. Monoamine oxidase inhibitors and narcotic analgesics: a critical review of the implications for treatment. Br J Psychiatry 1987;151:210–2.
[53] Cote CJ, Karl HW, Notterman DA, et al. Adverse sedation events in pediatrics: analysis of medications used for sedation. Pediatrics 2000;106:633–44.
[54] Stambaugh JE, Wainer IW. Drug interactions. Meperidine and chlorpromazine, a toxic combination. J Clin Pharmacol 1981;21:140–6.
[55] Brown ET, Corbett SW, Green SM. Iatrogenic cardiopulmonary arrest during sedation with meperidine, promethazine and chlorpromazine. Pediatr Emerg Care 2001;17: 351–3.
[56] Schenkel S. Promoting safety and preventing medical error in emergency departments. Acad Emerg Med 2000;7:1204–19.
[57] Bates DW, Spell N, Cullen DJ, et al. The costs of adverse drug events in hospitalized patients. JAMA 1997;277:307–11.
[58] Bates DW, Leape LL, Cullen DJ, et al. Effect of computerized physician order entry and a team intervention on prevention of serious medication errors. JAMA 1998;35:70–3.
[59] Powell MF, Solomon DK, McEachern RA. Twenty-four hour emergency pharmaceutical services. Am J Hosp Pharm 1985;42:831–5.
[60] Flacke JW, Davis LJ, Flacke WE, et al. Effects of fentanyl and diazepam in dogs deprived of autonomic tone. Anesth Analg 1985;64:1053–9.
[61] Lowenstein E, Hallowell P, Levine FH, et al. Cardiovascular response to large doses of intravenous morphine in man. N Engl J Med 1969;281:1389–93.

[62] Skovsted P, Price ML, Price HL. The effects of short-acting barbiturates on arterial pressure, preganglionic sympathetic activity and barostatic reflexes. Anesthesiology 1970; 33:10–8.
[63] Tomicheck RC, Rosow CE, Philbin DM, et al. Diazepam-fentanyl interaction—hemodynamic and hormonal effects in coronary artery surgery. Anesth Analg 1983;62: 881–4.
[64] Sherman EP, Lebowitz PW, Street WC. Bradycardia following sufentanil–succinylcholine. Anesthesiology 1987;66:106.
[65] Rivard JC, Lebowitz PW. Bradycardia after alfentanil–succinylcholine. Anesth Analg 1988;67:907.
[66] Reves JG, Croughwell N. Valium–fentanyl interaction. In: Reves JG, Hall K, editors. Common problems in cardiac anaesthesia. Chicago: Year Book; 1987. p. 356.
[67] Savege TM, Colvin MP, Weaver EJ, et al. A comparison of some cardiorespiratory effects of althesin and ketamine when used for induction of anaesthesia in patients with cardiac disease. Br J Anaesth 1976;48:1071–81.
[68] Ruth WJ, Burton JH, Bock AJ. Intravenous etomidate for procedural sedation in emergency department patients. Acad Emerg Med 2001;8(1):13–8.
[69] Vinson DR, Bradbury DR. Etomidate for procedural sedation in emergency medicine. Ann Emerg Med 2002;39(6):592–8.
[70] Gooding JM, Weng JT, Smith RA, et al. Cardiovascular and pulmonary responses following etomidate induction of anesthesia in patients with demonstrated cardiac disease. Anesth Analg 1979;58:40–1.
[71] Parke TJ, Stevens JE, Rice AS, et al. Metabolic acidosis and fatal myocardial failure after propofol infusion in children: five case reports. BMJ 1992;305:613–6.
[72] Rothermel LK. Newer pharmacologic agents for procedural sedation of children in the emergency department—etomidate and propofol. Curr Opin Pediatr 2003;15:200–3.
[73] Claeys MA, Gepts E, Camu F. Haemodynamic changes during anaesthesia induced and maintained with propofol. Br J Anaesth 1988;60:3–9.
[74] Sing K, Erickson T, Amitai Y, et al. Chloral hydrate toxicity from oral and intravenous administration. J Toxicol Clin Toxicol 1996;34:101–6.
[75] Rubin DM, Eisig S, Freeman K, et al. Effect of supplemental gases on end-tidal CO2 and oxygen saturation in patients undergoing fentanyl and midazolam outpatient sedation. Anesth Prog 1997;44:1–4.
[76] Miner JR, Heegaard W, Plummer D. End-tidal carbon dioxide monitoring during procedural sedation. Acad Emerg Med 2002;9:275–80.
[77] Wright S. Procedural sedation and analgesia in the emergency department: the value of capnography and pulse oximetry. Ann Emerg Med 1992;25:551–5.
[78] Ling GS, Spiegel K, Lockhart SH, et al. Separation of opioid analgesia from respiratory depression: evidence for different receptor mechanisms. J Pharmacol Exp Ther 1985;232: 149–55.
[79] Weil JV, McCullough RE, Kline JS, et al. Diminished ventilatory response to hypoxia and hypercapnia after morphine in normal man. N Engl J Med 1975;292:1103–6.
[80] Shook JE, Watkins WD, Camporesi EM. Differential roles of opioid receptors in respiration, respiratory disease and opiate-induced respiratory depression. Am Rev Respi Dis 1990;142:895–909.
[81] Kamei J. Role of opioidergic and serotonergic mechanisms in cough and antitussives. Pulm Pharmacol 1996;9:349–56.
[82] Gutstein HB, Akil H. Opioid analgesics. In: Hardman JG, Limbird LE, editors. Goodman and Gilman's the pharmacologic basis of therapeutics. 10th edition. New York: McGraw-Hill; 2001. p. 569–619.
[83] Howland MA. Antidotes in depth: opioid antagonists. In: Goldfrank LG, Flomenbaum NE, Lewin NA, Howland MA, Hoffman RS, Nelson LS, editors. Goldfrank's toxicologic emergencies. 7th edition. New York: McGraw-Hill; 2002. p. 924–8.

[84] Mills CA, Flacke JW, Miller JD, et al. Cardiovascular effects of fentanyl reversal by naloxone at varying arterial carbon dioxide tensions in dogs. Anesth Analg 1988;67: 730–6.
[85] Osler W. Oedema of left lung-morphina poisoning. Montreal Gen Hosp Rep 1880;1: 291–3.
[86] Dettmeyer R, Schmidt P, Musshoff F, et al. Pulmonary edema in fatal heroin overdose: immunohistological investigations with IgE, collagen IV and laminin—no increase of defects of alveolar-capillary membranes. Forensic Sci Int 2000;110:87–96.
[87] Nelson LS, Opioids. In: Goldfrank LG, Flomenbaum NE, Lewin NA, Howland MA, Hoffman RS, Nelson LS, editors. Goldfrank's toxicologic emergencies. 7th edition. New York: McGraw-Hill; 2002. p. 910–23.
[88] Rosenberg M. Muscular rigidity with fentanyl; a case report. Anesth Prog 1977;24:50–2.
[89] Chudnofsky CR, Wright SW, Dronen SC, et al. The safety of fentanyl use in the emergency department. Ann Emerg Med 1989;18(6):635–9.
[90] Klausner JM, Caspi J, Lelcuk S, et al. Delayed muscular rigidity and respiratory depression following fentanyl anesthesia. Arch Surg 1988;123:66–7.
[91] Wang SW, Tsou MY, Lee TY, et al. Antagonization of fentanyl-induced muscular rigidity by neurotensin at the locus coeruleus of the rat. Regul Pept 1994;51:33–40.
[92] Weinger MB, Segal IS, Maze M. Dexmedetomidine, acting through central alpha-2 adrenoceptors, prevents opiate-induced muscle rigidity in the rat. Anesthesiology 1989;71: 242–9.
[93] Sanford TJ, Weinger MB, Smith NT, et al. Pretreatment with sedative-hypnotics, but not nondepolarizing muscle relaxants, attenuates alfentanil-induced muscle rigidity. J Clin Anesth 1994;6:473–80.
[94] Bailey PL, Pace NL, Ashburn MA, et al. Frequent hypoxemia and apnea after sedation with midazolam and fentanyl. Anesthesiology 1990;73:826–30.
[95] Wright SW, Chudnofsky CR, Dronen SC, et al. Comparison of midazolam and diazepam for conscious sedation in the emergency department. Ann Emerg Med 1993;22:201–5.
[96] Study RE, Barker JL. Cellular mechanisms of benzodiazepine actions. JAMA 1982;247: 2147–51.
[97] Classen DC, Pestonik SL, Evans RS, et al. Intensive surveillance of midazolam use in hospitalized patients and the occurrence of cardiopulmonary arrest. Pharmacotherapy 1992;12:213–6.
[98] Alexander CM, Teller LE, Gross JB. Slow injection does not prevent midazolam-induced ventilatory depression. Anesth Anal 1992;74:260–4.
[99] Nordt SP, Clark RF. Midazolam: a review of therapeutic uses and toxicity. J Emerg Med 1997;15:357–65.
[100] Blouin RT, Conard PF, Perreault S, et al. The effect of flumazenil on midazolam-induced depression of the ventilatory response to hypoxia during isohypercarbia. Anesthesiology 1993;78:635–41.
[101] Slonim AD, Oginbene FP. Sedation for pediatric procedures, using ketamine and midazolam, in a primarily adult intensive care unit; a retrospective evaluation. Crit Care Med 1998;26:1900–4.
[102] Parker RI, Mahan RA, Giugliano D, et al. Efficacy and safety of intravenous midazolam and ketamine as sedation for therapeutic and diagnostic procedures in children. Pediatrics 1997;99:427–31.
[103] Chudnofsky CR, Weber JE, Stoyanoff PJ, et al. A combination of midazolam and ketamine for procedural sedation and analgesia in adult emergency department patients. Acad Emerg Med 2000;7:228–35.
[104] Wathen JE, Robcak MG, Mackenzie T, et al. Does midazolam alter the clinical effects of intravenous ketamine sedation in children? A randomized, double-blind, controlled emergency department trial. Ann Emerg Med 2000;35:229–38.

[105] Green SM, Rothrock SG, Lynch EL, et al. Intramuscular ketamine for pediatric sedation in the emergency department: safety profile in 1022 cases. Ann Emerg Med 1998;31: 688–97.
[106] Hamza J, Ecoffey C, Gross JB. Ventilatory response to CO2 following intravenous ketamine in children. Anesthesiology 1989;70:422–5.
[107] Kim G, Green SM, Denmark TK, et al. Ventilatory response during dissociative sedation in children—a pilot study. Acad Emerg Med 2003;10:140–5.
[108] Hirshman Cam Downes H, Farbood A, Bergman NA. Ketamine block of bronchospasm in experimental canine asthma. Br J Anaesth 1979;51:713–8.
[109] Morgensen F, Muller D, Valentin N. Glycopyrrolate during ketamine and diazepam anesthesia: a double blind comparison with atropine. Acta Anesthesiol Scand 1986;30: 332–6.
[110] Toft P, Romer UD. Glycopyrrolate compared with atropine in association with ketamine anaesthesia. Acta Anesthesiol Scand 1987;31:438–40.
[111] Green SM. Ketamine sedation for pediatric procedures: part 1, a prospective series. Ann Emerg Med 1990;19:1024–32.
[112] Zink BJ, Darfler K, Salluzzo RF, et al. The efficacy and safety of methohexital in the emergency department. Ann Emerg Med 1991;20:1293–8.
[113] Lerman B, Yoshida D, Levitt MA. A prospective evaluation of the safety and efficacy of methohexital in the emergency department. Am J Emerg Med 1996;14:351–4.
[114] Miner JR, Biros M, Kreig S, et al. Randomized clinical trial of propofol versus methohexital for procedural sedation during fracture and dislocation reduction in the emergency department. Acad Emerg Med 2003;10:931–7.
[115] Havel CJ, Strait RT, Hennes H. A clinical trial of propofol vs midazolam for procedural sedation in a pediatric emergency department. Acad Emerg Med 1999;6:989–97.
[116] Vardi A, Salem Y, Padeh S, et al. Is propofol safe for procedural sedation in children? A prospective evaluation of propofol versus ketamine in pediatric critical care. Crit Care Med 2002;30:1231–6.
[117] Swanson ER, Seaberg DC, Mathias S. The use of propofol for sedation in the emergency department. Acad Emerg Med 1996;3:234–8.
[118] Yoon HD, Yoon ES, Dhong ES, et al. Low-dose propofol infusion for sedation during local anesthesia. Plast Reconstr Surg 2002;109:956–63.
[119] Hullander RM, Leivers D, Wingler K. A comparison of propofol and etomidate for cardioversion. Anesth Analg 1993;77:690–4.
[120] Burton JH, Bock AJ, Strout TD, et al. Etomidate and midazolam for reduction of anterior shoulder dislocation: a randomized, controlled trial. Ann Emerg Med 2002;40:496–504.
[121] Hunt CE, Hazinski TA, Gora P. Experimental effects of chloral hydrate on ventilatory response to hypoxia and hypercarbia. Pediatr Res 1982;16:79–81.
[122] Hershenson M, Brouillette RJ, Olsen E, et al. The effect of chloral hydrate of genioglossus and diaphragmatic activity. Periatr Res 1984;18:516–9.
[123] Litman RS, Kottra JA, Verga KA, et al. Chloral hydrate sedation: the additive sedative and respiratory depressant effects of nitrous oxide. Anesth Analg 1998;86:724–8.
[124] Kinsella JP, Truog WE, Walsh WF, et al. Randomized, multicenter trial of inhaled nitric oxide and high frequency oscillatory ventilation in severe, persistent pulmonary hypertension of the newborn. J Pediatr 1997;131:55–62.
[125] Steudel W, Hurford WE, Zapol WM. Inhaled NO: basic biology and clinical applications. Anesthesiology 1999;91:1090–121.
[126] Pitetti RD, Singh S, Pierce MC. Safe and efficacious use of procedural sedation and analgesia by nonanesthesiologists in a pediatric emergency department. Arch Pediatr Adolesc Med 2003;157(11):1090–6.
[127] Chew ST, Ip-Yam PC, Kong CF, et al. Recovery following tonsillectomy a comparison between tramadol and morphine for analgesia. Singapore Med J 2003;44(6):296–8.

[128] Bach PH, Nguyen TK. Renal papillary necrosis—40 years and on. Toxicol Pathol 1998;26(1):73–91.
[129] Hall AH, Smolinske SC, Stover B. Ibuprofen overdose in adults. J Toxicol Clin Toxicol 1992;30(1):23–37.
[130] Boutis K, Shannon M. Nephrotoxicity after acute sever acetaminophen poisoning in adolescents. J Toxicol Clin Toxicol 2001;39(5):441–5.
[131] Cooper MS, Stewart PM. Corticosteroid insufficiency in acutely ill patients. N Engl J Med 2003;348(8):727–34.
[132] Slonim AD, Ognibene FP. Sedation for pediatric procedures, using ketamine and midazolam, in a primarily adult intensive care unit: a retrospective evaluation. Crit Care Med 1998;26(11):1900–4.
[133] Levy JH, Brister NW, Shearin A, et al. Wheal and flare responses to opiods in humans. Anesthesiology 1989;70(5):756–60.
[134] Cousin F, Catelain A, Phillips K, et al. Immediate hypersensitivity is rarely implicated in drug induced uticaria. Ann Dermatol Venereol 2003;130(3):321–4.
[135] Edston E, van Hage-Hamsten M. Anaphylactoid shock—a common cause of death in heroin addicts? Allergy 1997;52(9):950.
[136] Felmet K, Robins B, Tilford D, et al. Acute neurologic decompensation in an infant with cobalamin deficiency exposed to nitrous oxide. J Pediatr 2000;137(3):427–8.

ELSEVIER
SAUNDERS

EMERGENCY MEDICINE CLINICS OF NORTH AMERICA

Emerg Med Clin N Am 23 (2005) 573–584

Legal Issues in Pain Management: Striking the Balance

Linda L. Lawrence, MD, FACEP

4301 Jones Bridge Road, Bethesda, MD 20814, USA

Pain is a symptom, but can often be the presenting chief complaint for many patients in the emergency department. Although the disease or condition causing the pain may not be within the realm of the emergency physician to definitively manage or even in some cases diagnose, there still remains an expectation to treat the symptom. In recent years, due to changes in accreditation standards, many have come to argue that pain has become the fifth vital sign, and new expectations have been created for health care providers [1].

Physicians have an ethical obligation to treat patient's pain and suffering as outlined in the Hippocratic Oath, American Medical Association Code of Medical Ethics, and more specifically, for emergency physicians in the American College of Emergency Physicians (ACEP) Code of Ethics [2,3]. In the ACEP Code of Ethics, the principle of beneficence would suggest the responsibility for physicians to "respond quickly to acute illnesses and injuries to prevent or minimize pain and suffering" [2]. In addition, the ACEP policy statement, Ethical Issues for Resuscitation, outlines physician responsibility to provide appropriate comfort measures to the dying patient when resuscitation is not indicated [4].

However, despite the above obligations, several studies still cite physician's continued failure to appropriately treat pain [5–7]. Inadequate pain management is becoming recognized as a serious public health concern [8]. Undertreatment of pain has been well documented in a diversity of patient populations [9–11], with the greatest frequency being noted in patients with chemical dependency [12], a group of patients frequently encountered in some emergency departments.

Disclaimer: The opinions or assertions contained herein are the private ones of the author and are not to be construed as official or reflecting the views of the Department of Defense, Department of the Air Force, or the Uniformed Services University of the Health Sciences.

E-mail address: llawrence@usuhs.mil (L.L. Lawrence).

doi:10.1016/j.emc.2004.12.018 **emed.theclinics.com**

In an earlier article, Changing Attitudes about Pain and Pain Control in Emergency Medicine, Drs. Fosnocht, Swanson, and Barton discuss the problem of oligoanalgesia and some of the barriers to effective pain treatment. In this article I will expand on what some consider one of the major reasons for undertreatment of pain: the external threat of legal action or other sanctioning by a licensing board against a physician [13].

Consistently, physician fear of investigation or sanction by federal, state, or local regulatory agencies to include medical licensing boards remains a common reason for the inadequate or inappropriate treatment of patients with chronic pain [14,15]. There has been a national and international plea in the past decade to address the mounting problem of inadequate pain treatment. Organizations who have recognized the impact of regulatory barriers and drug abuse control policies on pain management have included the World Health Organization, International Narcotics Control Board, Institute of Medicine, and National Institutes of Health, to name a few [15]. During the past several years significant actions have occurred among the licensing and regulatory community in an attempt to reduce this fear and promote legitimate medical use of controlled substances while striking a balance with efforts to curb the diversion of controlled substances for illegitimate use. The following discussion will explore this transformation and the impact it has had on clinical practice.

In addition to the regulatory movement to promote a more aggressive approach to the treatment of all types of pain, especially intractable pain, the change in standards of care have opened the door for increased liability issues, especially in the realm of undertreatment of pain. It can be argued that failure to properly manage pain may also be professional negligence [13,16]. Although the number of court cases citing physicians for breach of care related to undermedicating for pain or other failures to manage patient's pain remains rare [13], the threat of malpractice suit for under-treatment of pain is on the rise, and can pose increased liability issues for emergency physicians. As the medical practice of pain management is more clearly defined by state policies and regulations, clinical practice guidelines, and accreditation requirements, the number of lawsuits is expected to rise. This article will discuss potential liability issues associated with undertreatment of pain management.

Definitions

To engage in a discussion about legal aspects of pain management certain definitions should be clearly understood. As a refresher, the following definitions as they pertain to pain management are provided for review. These definitions have been adopted with slight modification and addition from the University of Wisconsin Pain & Policy Studies Group (PPSG) Glossary of Terms and other sources [17]. The PPSG provides an excellent resource for easy Internet access to a wide range of policies, guidelines, articles, and other activities related to pain management.

Acute pain—normal predicted physiologic response to adverse stimuli associated with surgery, injury, or illness. Typically it is time limited and responds to opioids and other treatment modalities [14].

Addiction—sociologic term for compulsive drug use, psychologic dependence, and continued use despite harm. Physical dependence and tolerance are not sufficient in defining addiction.

Chronic pain—persistent pain state associated with a long-term incurable or intractable medical condition or disease [14].

Guideline—official policy statement that does NOT have force of law.

Law—broad term that refers to rules of conduct subject to legal force. Law can include treaties, constitutional provisions, decisions of the court, statutes, and regulations, and can be at the international, federal, state, or local levels.

Narcotic—legal, not scientific, term for some of the drugs controlled under the US Controlled Substances Act (CSA). Includes opioids, marijuana, cocaine.

Opioid—scientific term for both natural and synthetic drugs with pharmacologic effects mediated by specific receptors in nervous system. Also applies to agonists and antagonists with morphine-like activity.

Physical dependence—physical adaptation of body to presence of chronic opiod therapy that is characterized by signs of withdrawal when the opioid is stopped or an antagonist is administered. This is expected with chronic use and is not synonymous with addiction.

Pseudoaddiction—*d*rug-seeking behavior pattern in pain patients resulting from inadequate pain management. Often this is mistaken for addiction [14].

Regulation—official rule or order issued from agencies of the executive branch of government. Regulations have the force of law, and are intended to implement a specific statute. Typically related to the conduct of those regulated by the agency.

Statute—law created by a federal, state, county, or city legislative body.

Tolerance—physical adaptation of the body to a drug resulting in need to increase the dose to achieve same medical effect or a reduced effect is noticed when the dose remains constant.

Barriers in federal policy and state policy

The Food and Drug Administration, pursuant to the Food, Drug and Cosmetic Act of 1962, initially approve all medications for marketing and medical use. The Food, Drug and Cosmetic Act does not place any limitations on physicians as to the dosage of a medication or prescribing of controlled substances to patients with addictive disease. However, because of the potential for abuse, the CSA adopted by Congress in 1970 further regulates controlled substances [18]. This statute requires all individuals and businesses involved in the manufacturing, prescribing, distribution, and dispensing of controlled substances to be registered to ensure control and availability. The CSA is not to interfere in legitimate medical practice while controlling the abuse and diversion of controlled substances [8]. The Drug Enforcement Administration (DEA) enforces the provisions of the CSA and is responsible to enact programs to reduce the availability of illicit drugs and diversion of controlled substances [19]. Despite the fact that the CSA does not interfere with legitimate medical practice, it has been argued that the fear of investigation and loss of DEA license often hinders physicians from appropriately prescribing pain medications to patients [20]. Yet in actuality, the states, not the federal government, hold the authority to regulate medical practice.

Numerous state policies exist regarding the use of controlled substances, and initially, many of these failed to recognize the medical value of controlled substances [8]. State policy has been cited as being so restrictive that it places barriers to the appropriate prescribing of pain medications for any patient, not just those with chemical dependency [21–23]. Policy language has included the characterization of opioids as a medical treatment of last resort, or suggests medical use of opioids is not within the legitimate scope of medical practice. Some state regulatory requirements limit prescribing based on quantity or duration or require informed consent in every case [24]. States have required special licenses and the use of special government-issued forms when prescribing controlled substances. These are among the several reasons why physicians have become reluctant to use opioids even when medically indicated.

In addition, it has been noted in studies that members of state medical boards lack proper legal understanding of legitimate opioid use in medical practice [22]. In 1991, a total of 627 medical board members were surveyed on their opinion of the legality of prescribing opioids for chronic pain patients with and without cancer. Although 75% of respondents felt prescribing opioids for chronic cancer pain was a legal and acceptable medical practice, only 12% agreed when the pain was from a nonmalignant source [24]. When the patient had a history of drug abuse an even greater percentage of board members felt prescribing of opioids was illegal.

Initiatives to reduce regulatory barriers

Impact of the Mayday Project

One of the most pivotal activities in changing the regulatory environment and reducing the real and perceived barriers imposed by the legal system on effective pain management has been through the work of the Mayday Project. The Mayday Project is operated by the American Society of Law,

Medicine, and Ethics (ASLME), and began in 1995, due to the generous financial support obtained from the Mayday Fund and the Emily Davie and Joseph S. Kornfeld Foundation [25]. Working with health care providers, state policy makers, attorneys, pharmacists, nurses, health care administrators, and patient advocates the project has supported scholarship through research, national meetings, and other functions, resulting in a wealth of knowledge and subsequent policies promoting a shift in both the medical and legal communities.

An area of strong emphasis in the Mayday Project has been the focus on standards, policies, and practices relating to medical licensure and discipline, resulting in a significant change of public policy. In 1996, the ASLME under the Mayday Project held a national meeting with leadership from the groups identified above. One of the critical concepts that evolved from this meeting and the research published afterward in the ASLME journal was the recognition that standards used by medical boards failed to recognize best practices in pain management, and in addition, the medical board review process had a negative impact on care [26]. From this concept through the Project on Legal Constraints on Access to Effective Pain relief came the Pain Relief Act, which is a model statute governing pain relief for state legislators to enact [27].

The Pain Relief Act provided protection to health care providers involved in the prescribing of controlled substances for chronic pain patients. The proposed statute was broader than existing state pain statutes in several respects. First, the act covered not only physicians but all health care providers involved in the treatment of pain to even include pharmacists and nurses [26,27]. Second, the Act required state medical boards to use expert clinical testimony when attempting to prove a physician did not adhere to clinical practice standards [26,27]. Finally, it specifically addressed the treatment of intractable pain and the protection applied to the treatment of chemically dependent patients [26,27]. The Act strongly promoted the use of clinical practice guidelines as the accepted standard of care. It is important to note the intent was not to require compliance with the guidelines but instead had the guidelines serve more as a shield from disciplinary or criminal actions. For example, if a physician followed a professionally recognized clinical practice guideline supporting the use of larger doses of opioids for treatment of cancer pain, then the physician would be protected from disciplinary actions. However, it was not the intent to prosecute departure from the guidelines for those who choose less aggressive treatment plans [28].

When the Act was first published only 10 states had statutes that addressed treatment of intractable pain, and only six of these offered some protection from unwarranted disciplinary action [20]. Since 1996, when the Act was first proposed, the number of states with legislation addressing concerns associated with the treatment of intractable pain has more than doubled to at least 26 states [26]. Almost all of these provide physicians with some degree of legal immunity from disciplinary action when in compliance with state medical board identified written guidelines.

Model guidelines from Federation of State Medical Boards

Almost simultaneous to the development of the Pain Relief Act, the Federation of State Medical Boards (FSMB) met to review standards used by medical boards when reviewing physician prescribing practices. In 1997, the FSMB, in response to the escalating demand for improved patient rights to adequate treatment of pain, initiated a project to develop model guidelines for use by state medical boards and other health care regulatory boards to promote the appropriate use of controlled substances [14]. The goals of the project were to define uniform standards for use by boards in evaluating cases involving controlled substances that would protect the public from substandard use of controlled substances while simultaneously promoting improved public access to appropriate and effective pain relief [29]. An important tactic in the approach was to promote nonlegislative avenues for improving regulation of physician prescribing of controlled substances and avoiding addition of unnecessary requirements through legislative actions that may hinder provider prescribing. Thus, by advocating a pain management policy approach it was hoped that legislative intervention would be curtailed.

Collaborating groups for the development of the FSMB's *Model Guidelines for the Use of Controlled Substances for the Treatment of Pain* included ASLME, the American Pain Society, the American Academy of Pain Medicine, The PPSG, pharmaceutical companies, and state medical boards [29]. In 1998, the FSMB's House of Delegates adopted the *Model Guidelines*, and since then, it has been widely distributed to state medical boards, medical professional organizations, health care regulatory boards, patient advocacy groups, and other regulatory agencies with the intent to foster development of guidelines to promote legitimate prescribing of controlled substances by providers.

The *Model Guidelines* advocates for use of clinical practice guidelines to promote a sound approach to the management of pain. It acknowledges that proper pain management will often require the use of controlled substances, and cases should be evaluated on an individual basis with medical assessment and treatment outcome setting the standard when evaluating physician conduct rather than the quantity or chronicity of prescribing. Appropriate documentation in medical records of patient assessment, treatment plan, informed consent, periodic review, and consultation when necessary are essential to the success of this model. Similar to the Pain Relief Act, the *Model Guidelines* also recognized the need for physicians to use controlled substances when treating chemically dependent patients with intractable pain. In addition, physicians must adhere to applicable state and federal regulations for prescribing, dispensing, or administering controlled substances.

By establishing these guidelines when evaluating use of controlled substances by physicians the FSMB hoped to alleviate physician fear of disciplinary action, thus promoting appropriate pain management while still maintaining a boundary of professional practice that prevents diversion of drugs for illegitimate use. The National Association of State Controlled Substances Authorities endorsed the *Model Guidelines* in 1999 as a reasonable set of principles to guide health care professionals, regulators, and law enforcement [30]. The Annual Review of State Pain Policies, in 2000, attributed the significant increase in state policies in 1999 to the publication of *Model Guidelines* [31]. Fifteen states were noted to have adopted in full or in part the *Model Guidelines*.

Drug enforcement agency actions

In 2001, the DEA for the first time ever joined 21 health care organizations including the American Medical Association in issuing a joint consensus statement aimed at maintaining the balance between patient care and diversion prevention [32]. The collaboration resulted out of increased attention to abuse of OxyContin and other opioids and concern for generating a sense of fear reducing the legitimate use of opioids in pain management [33]. This statement publicly acknowledged that the undertreatment of pain was a serious problem, and patients were entitled to effective pain therapy that often included opioid analgesics. Although discussing the seriousness of drug abuse, the statement noted that focusing on the abuse potential of a drug could result in the medication being avoided when medically indicated [32]. In addition, the DEA developed an educational brochure to assist providers in identifying the potential for patient drug abuse yet still encourage appropriate medical use of opioids [34].

State pain policies and regulations—where are we today?

The previously mentioned actions have been instrumental in creating almost a decade of change in state pain policy. For this discussion the term "state pain policy" refers to statutes, regulations, and medical board guidelines and policy statements affecting the professional practice of pain management and use of controlled substances [31]. The central principle of balance is a term used to depict the dual obligation of governments to ensure medical availability of controlled substances while simultaneously implementing a system that prevents drug abuse, trafficking, and diversion [15].

According to the PPSG, efforts over the past several years have resulted in positive changes as well as additional unintended restrictions [15]. The PPSG, with funding from the Robert Wood Johnson Foundation, evaluated state pain policies as of March 2003 and in September 2003 and published *Achieving Balance in State Pain Policy: A Progress Report Card* [15]. The report grades the language in state pain policy that governs the medical use of opioid analgesia on whether it enhances or impedes pain management. The intent is for this report to be used as a tool to achieve more positive and consistent state pain policy while not disturbing the principle of balance within the system between control of illegitimate use with maintenance of drug availability for legitimate medical use.

In their evaluation of state pain policy the PPSG developed 17 criteria based on the central principle of balance. The grades are based on the principle of balance, with higher grades being awarded to those states that achieve this balance while effectively promoting opioid use for pain management. In summary, 39% of states scored a grade of better than C, 35% a grade of C and 25% below a grade of C [15]. No state scored an A or F. Compared with a similar review 3 years earlier, 14 states exhibited positive policy changes. The report identified three major sources of change in state pain policy: (1) adoption of palliative care or end-of-life care policies, (2) removal of single or multiple copy prescription programs, (3) removal of ambiguous or restrictive language in policies [15].

Media coverage

It is without question that pain management has been an important topic in the medical community in the past several years with enhanced research, publication of guidelines, and educational mandates [35]. One would postulate a similar increase in media coverage involving pain issues. In 2002, the MayDay Fund commissioned an analysis to examine trends in major newspaper and news magazine coverage from 1997 to 2001. During the 4-year period in 11 major newspapers and two major news magazines a total of 922 articles were published. There was a sharp increase from 1997 to 1999, followed by an unexplained precipitous drop after 1999 [36]. More recently, articles on political and legal issues appear to include stories written about lawsuits on the undertreatment of pain [35]. It is important for physicians to recognize the impact of media on the public and their medical care expectations.

Liability concerns

With increased media attention, Joint Commission on Accreditation of Health Care Organizations pain standards and regulatory changes can be expected as professional and public awareness increases; so will patient expectations for improved pain management. Failure for a physician to appropriately treat a patient's pain may be considered medical malpractice

[37,38]. In 1990, a North Carolina negligence lawsuit, *James v. Hillhaven Corp* [39], a health care provider for the first time was held liable for failure to appropriately treat a dying patient's pain. Another case, *State v. McAfee* [40], also demonstrated a responsibility for providers to incorporate pain management in medical care plans. Although this case focused on a patient's right to refuse unwanted medical care, it implied that providers must remain responsible for providing measures to ensure patient comfort. Thus, it is important for physicians to understand the elements of medical malpractice and potential liability issues associated with pain management.

The plaintiff, when alleging professional negligence, must prove four elements. First, the provider must have a duty to treat the patient. This is easily met in emergency medicine, as we must medically assess and stabilize all patients who come through our doors. Second, the provider must breach this duty by failing to provide treatment that meets accepted reasonable standards. Third, the breach in duty is the principal cause of injury to the patient. Fourth, that the patient has suffered from a compensable injury.

Although proving negligent pain management can be challenging for a plaintiff, it is important to recognize that it is plausible, and some postulate that it may become more prevalent in the future. A physician is not held to a standard of perfection nor would they be expected to completely resolve patient's pain. However, it can be argued that physicians are expected to provide treatment commensurate with standard of care for our practice environment. The development and proliferation of clinical practice guidelines by professional medical organizations has pushed medical practice to national standards [38]. Clinical practice guidelines are becoming more evidence-based, and although these are recommendations for care, the more scientifically based the easier it becomes for plaintiffs to argue these as standard of care and harder for the defendant to dispute.

A search on the National Guidelines Clearinghouse (www.guideline.gov/search) in December 2003, using pain management elicited 238 related guidelines. Limiting the search to key words of "acute pain management" located 143 matches. Seven current ACEP clinical guidelines mention pain management in particular situations. Coupled with the preponderance of clinical guidelines is the easy availability of guidelines and medical information through the Internet. Ignorance of guidelines will become a difficult defense, as a plaintiff attorney readily displays in the courtroom the results of a computer search and their relative ease of access [38]. Also, scientific knowledge continues to rapidly grow surrounding effective pain management therapies and disputing the commonly held urban myths previously discussed that result in undertreatment of pain. The judicial system, through a variety of cases to include malpractice, workers compensation, and medical discipline, has respected aggressive opioid use by physicians, thus promoting a standard that increasingly expects proper pain management [38]. Medical opinion now strongly supports the use of opioids for chronic intractable pain and, as discussed previously, many state statutes and medical licensing board guidelines endorse the use of opioids for chronic pain. Therefore, even though the threat of a malpractice suit for undertreatment of pain remains relatively low, it can be agued that a standard of care promotes appropriate pain management.

The challenge to plaintiffs in proving negligence from undertreatment of pain will lie in proving some tangible injury resulted from breach of duty. Before an award for pain and suffering damages can be granted, proximate cause must be demonstrated. In mismanagement of pain cases the provider is not necessarily responsible for the patient's condition causing the pain, but instead, the pain is a symptom of underlying disease and possibly something terminal. Therefore, pain becomes the only component of the damages. Medical literature has supported that pain alone can be physically and emotionally damaging. Untreated pain can "rewire" neurologic pathways, promoting persistent or worsening pain. Chronic pain patients loose their ability to function, and thus can have loss of wages and other concrete damages.

Untreated pain can result in emotional distress for not only the patient but arguably even the family member. In *Oswald v. Legrand*, a married couple successfully sued for mental injury as a result of series of obstetric events citing negligent infliction of emotional distress under egregious circumstances compounded by the "crass insensitivity" of the medical staff [41]. It can be argued that the doctrine of negligent infliction of emotional distress can be applied to cases of poor management of intractable pain.

It is speculated that the courts will engage in judicial standard-setting by recognizing current pain management guidelines as the standard of care for treatment of chronic, intractable pain, thus curbing the customary practice of undertreatment of pain through threat of malpractice litigation. As emergency physicians it is essential to recognize both our ethical and legal obligation to adequately treat patient suffering, and appreciate the regulatory changes that provide greater protections to us when operating by acceptable medical standards.

Summary

The momentum over the past several years resulting in positive change to state pain policy is encouraging, especially as the medical community meets greater expectations from patients for appropriate pain management. As the trend for increased medical use of opioid medications continue it is important that medical professionals continue to work with government officials to ensure efforts to curb drug abuse do not impede patient access to pain management. Essential to maintaining that balance is an expansion of scholarly work supporting the medical use of opioids and promotion of research through educational activities. In 2004, the Mayday Project at ASLME will host a national conference, with an emphasis on pain management in the emergency department [26]. The previous noted success of Mayday Project activities should give all of us hope that through scholarly activity further guidance will be provided in finding that critical balance between effective pain management and drug diversion.

References

[1] JCAHO. Standards, intents, examples and scoring questions for pain assessment and management—comprehensive accreditation manual for hospitals. Oakbrook Terrace (IL): JCAHO Department of Standards; 1999. p. 1–11.
[2] American College of Emergency Physicians Policy Statement #400188: code of ethics for emergency physicians. Dallas (TX). Reaffirmed 2001. Available at: http://www.acep.org. Accessed Nov 2003.
[3] American Medical Association. Council on Ethical and Judicial Affairs: code of medical ethics. Chicago: American Medical Association; 1996.
[4] American College of Emergency Physicians Policy Statement #400133: ethical issues for resuscitation. Dallas (TX). Reaffirmed 2001. Available at: http://www.acep.org. Accessed Nov 2003.
[5] Fosnocht DE, Swanson ER, Bossart P. Patient expectations for pain medication delivery. Am J Emerg Med 2001;19(5):399–402.
[6] Petrack EM, Christopher NC, Kriwinsky J. Pain management in the emergency department: patterns of analgesic utilization. Pediatrics 1997;99(5):711–4.
[7] Todd KH, Samaroo N, Hoffman JR. Ethnicity as a risk factor for inadequate emergency department analgesia. JAMA 1993;269:1537–9.
[8] Gilson AM, Joranson DE. US policies relevant to the prescribing of opioid analgesics for the treatment of pain in patients with addictive disease. Clin J Pain 2002;18:S91–8.
[9] Todd KH, Deaton C, D'Adamo AP, et al. Ethnicity and analgesic practice. Ann Emerg Med 2000;35(1):11–6.
[10] Breitbart W, Rosenfeld BD, Passik SD, et al. The undertreatment of pain in ambulatory AIDS patients. Pain 1996;65(2–3):243–9.
[11] Bonham VL. Race, ethnicity and pain treatment: striving to understand the causes and solutions to the disparities in pain treatment. J Law Med Ethics 2001;29:52–68.
[12] Portenoy R, Dole V, Joseph H, et al. Pain Management and chemical dependency: evolving perspectives. JAMA 1997;278:592–3.
[13] Furrow BR. Pain management and liability issues. Hemato/Oncol Clin N Am 2002;16(6): 1483–94.
[14] Federation of State Medical Boards of the United States. Model guidelines for the use of controlled substances for the treatment of pain. Euless (TX): Federation of State Medical Boards; 1998. Available at: http://www.fsmb.org. Accessed Nov 2003.
[15] Pain & Policy Studies Group. Achieving balance in state pain policy: a progress report card. Madison (WI): University of Wisconsin Comprehensive Cancer Center; 2003.
[16] Cherny NI, Catane R. Professional negligence in the management of cancer pain: a case for urgent reforms. Cancer 1995;76(11):2181–5.
[17] University of Wisconsin Pain & Policy Studies Group. Glossary of terms. Available at: http://www.medsch.wisc.edu/painpolicy/glossary.htm. Accessed Nov 2003.
[18] Controlled Substances Act. Pub. L. 91–513, title II, Sec. 301, Oct 27, 1970, 84 Stat. 1253. Available at Drug Enforcement Administration Website http://www.usdoj.gov/dea/pubs/csa.html. Accessed Dec 2003.
[19] Mission Statement DEA. Drug Enforcement Administration; US Department of Justice. Available at Drug Enforcement Administration website http://www.usdoj.gov/dea/agency/mission.htm. Accessed Dec 2003.

[20] Hyman C. Pain Management and Disciplinary Action: how medical boards can remove barriers to effective treatment. J Law Med Ethics 1996;24(4):338–43.
[21] Joranson DE, Gilson AM, Ryan KM, et al. Achieving balance in federal and state pain policy: a guide to evaluation. Madison (WI): The Pain & Policy Studies Group, University of Wisconsin Comprehensive Cancer center; 2000.
[22] Joranson DE, Cleeland CS, Weissman DE, et al. Opioids for chronic cancer and non-cancer pain: a survey of state medical boards. Fed Bull 1992;79(4):15–49.
[23] Joranson DE, Gilson AM. State intractable pain policy: current status. APS Bull 1997;7(2): 7–9.
[24] Joranson DE, Gilson AM. Controlled substances, medical practice and the law. In: Schwartz HI, editor. Psychiatric practice under fire: the influence of government, the media and special interests on somatic therapies. Washington (DC): American Psychiatric Press Inc.; 1994. p. 173–94.
[25] Lo B, Rothnberg KH, Vasko M. Appropriate management of pain: addressing the clinical, legal, and regulatory barriers. J Law Med Ethics 1996;24(4):285–6.
[26] Johnson S. Providing relief to those in pain: a retrospective on the scholarship and impact of the Mayday Project. J Law Med Ethics 2003;31:15–20.
[27] Project on Legal Constraints to Effective Pain Relief. The Pain Relief Act. J Law Med Ethics 1996;24(4):317–8.
[28] Johnson S. Disciplinary actions and pain relief: analysis of the pain relief act. J Law Med Ethics 1996;24(4):319–27.
[29] Federation of State Medical Boards. Position of the Federation of State Medical Boards in support of adoption of pain management guidelines. Euless (TX): Federation of State Medical Boards; 1998. Available at: http://www.medsch.wisc.edu/painpolicy/domestic/FSMBwp.htm. Accessed Nov 2003.
[30] National Association of State Controlled Substances Authorities. Resolution 99-01 adopted 1999. Couer d' Alene (ID). Available at: www.medsch.wisc.edu/painpolicy/domestic/nascsa.htm. Accessed Dec 2003.
[31] Joranson DE, Maurer MA, Gilson AM, et al. Annual review of state pain policies, 2000. Madison (WI): Pain & Policy Studies Group University of Wisconsin Comprehensive Cancer Center; 2001.
[32] Joint Statement from 21 Health Organizations and the Drug Enforcement Administration. Promoting pain relief and preventing abuse of pain medications: a critical balancing act. Drug Enforcement Administration: US Department of Justice; Washington (DC): 2001.
[33] Media Advisory. DEA to join pain advocates in issuing statement on prescription pain medications. Available at: http://www.medsch.wisc.edu/painpolicy/consensus2.pdf. Accessed Dec 2003.
[34] Drug Enforcement Administration. Don't be scammed by a drug abuser. An informational brochure by the Drug Enforcement Administration. US Department of Justice: Washington (DC): 1999.
[35] Gallagher RM. Physician variability in pain management: are the JCAHO standards enough? Pain Med 2003;4(1):1–3.
[36] Mayday Fund. Analysis of media coverage involving pain issues. Jun 02. Available at: http://www.painandhealth.org/media-pain/media-report.html. Accessed Nov 2003.
[37] Shapiro RS. Health care providers' liability exposure for inappropriate pain management. J Law Med Ethics 1996;24(4):360–4.
[38] Furrow BR. Pain management and provider liability: No more excuses. J Law Med Ethics 2001;29:28–51.
[39] *Estate of Henry James v. Hillhave Corp.* Super. Ct. Div. 89CVS64, Hertford County (NC) (Nov. 20, 1990).
[40] *State v. McAfee*, 259 Ga. 579, 385 S.E.2d 651 (1989).
[41] *Oswald v. Legrand* 453 N.W.2d 634 (Iowa 1990).

ELSEVIER
SAUNDERS

Emerg Med Clin N Am 23 (2005) 585–601

EMERGENCY MEDICINE CLINICS OF NORTH AMERICA

Pain Management in the Wilderness and Operational Setting

Ian S. Wedmore, MD, FACEP[a,*], Troy Johnson, MD[b], Jim Czarnik, MD[c], Steve Hendrix, CRNA[d]

[a]*University of Washington School of Medicine, Madigan Army Medical Center, Ft. Lewis, WA 98431, USA*
[b]*University of Health Sciences, Washington, DC, USA*
[c]*WOMAC Medical Center, Ft. Bragg, NC, USA*
[d]*Eisenhower Army Medical Center, Ft. Gordon, GA, USA*

The wilderness and operational setting places unique constraints on one's ability to treat pain. In this article we will discuss methods for treating pain both in the wilderness and operational setting. By operational we mean the austere deployed military setting, to include both noncombat and combat operations. The authors combined experience with wartime trauma pain management consists of experience in Operation "Just Cause" (Panama Invasion), Operation "Desert Storm" (the Persian Gulf War), Operation "Uphold democracy" (Haiti liberation), Operation "Enduring Freedom" (Afghanistan conflict), and Operation "Iraqi Freedom" (OIF) (Iraq conflict).

Because of the austerity of care for patients in these settings, there is limited evidence based information for "ideal" pain control. We will present what little literature is available as well as providing much information on what is done, what seems to work, and some novel ideas in the area. Much of what will be described will include actual patient care cases. It is hoped this article will provide some basic pain management principles for those who practice in the austere environment.

The information in this article represents only the views and experiences of the authors. It does not represent the official policies of the Department of Defense, the US Army, or any subordinate commands of either.

* Corresponding author.

E-mail address: wedmorei@msn.com (I.S. Wedmore).

doi:10.1016/j.emc.2004.12.017 ***emed.theclinics.com***

Overview

The wilderness and operational setting provides unique challenges for pain assessment and management. The diversity and quantity of pain control medication is limited by the quantity and type of medication one can carry with them into the austere setting. The type of medication may further be limited by the lack of or difficulty in obtaining intravenous (IV) access. This is often due to the difficulty in carrying heavy, bulky IV supplies. In the operational setting there is often difficulty in obtaining IV placement due to a given tactical situation, that is, doing so in a moving tactical vehicle or while under enemy fire. The inability to use IV medications therefore often limits the choice of pain medication that may be used. Consideration must also be given to cases where one must treat multiple casualties at one time, and how to best safely manage pain with limited resources.

The patient in the austere setting may also be required to assist with or actively be involved in his evacuation, limiting the type of medication that can be administered to something nonsedating. In the operational setting a wounded individual may still be required to defend himself and his comrades, also limiting the type of pain control he receives. Other factors of concern include the hydration status of a patient, individuals in the wilderness or military operations tending to be at least minimally dehydrated on a frequent basis. Environmental considerations also become paramount, not only for the patient but for the storage of the medications; for example, any medication requiring refrigeration is poorly suited for austere use. These multiple factors often decide what medications will be ideal for a given situation.

The ideal pain medication for wilderness and operational use would be:

- Light
- Compact
- Can be carried and stored without concern for environment or temperature
- Have a very high therapeutic index particularly with regard to ensuring that airway reflexes are protected
- Not require an IV or other equipment to administer
- Can be used regardless of a patients level of stability

Although no pain control agents perfectly meet these criteria, we will discuss those most commonly used with some of their specific considerations for austere use.

Nonsteroidal anti-inflammatory drugs

Nonsteroidal anti-inflammatory drugs (NSAIDS) have long been the mainstay for oral treatment of mild to moderate pain in the austere setting. So much so that in the operational setting Ibuprofen is colloquially known as "Ranger Candy." NSAIDS have been shown to be both effective for moderate pain control as well as to reduce the dosage of narcotics required for adequate pain control [1], thus reducing the risk of oversedation of patients in the austere setting. Ketorolac has often been the military intramuscular (IM) choice of moderate or greater pain control. Ketorolac has variously been shown to have analgesic properties equal to everything from acetaminophen to standard doses of narcotic agents depending on the disease process being treated [2]. Despite its having been shown to have this variable analgesic effect, it is often used as a first-line IM agent. Oral NSAIDs as well as acetaminophen have remained the most commonly used oral medications in the austere environment; they have been covered in detail elsewhere, so we will only discuss their side effects and its influence on austere use.

Three problems with NSAIDs that cause concern with their use in the austere environment are: (1) increased incidence of gastrointestinal distress and bleeding [3,4], (2) the possible risk of inducing renal failure in those already somewhat dehydrated [5,6], and (3) inhibition of effective clot formation due to NSAID "poisoning" of platelet function [7].

These side effect profiles have led to consideration, particularly in the operational setting, of the use of selective cyclooxygenase-2 (COX2) inhibitors. The COX2s do have a lower incidence of gastrointestinal side effects [8]. The risk of inducing renal failure, however, is no different between regular NSAIDs and COX2 [9,10]. There is, furthermore, no difference in pain control between the two classes [11]. Of greater concern, particularly in the tactical environment, is the effect of NSAIDS on platelet function and bleeding time. The COX2s do have an advantage here in they do not appear to effect platelet function and bleeding time [12,13]. Because of this, the Committee on Tactical Combat Casualty Care consensus panel recommended the use of COX2 inhibitors as the NSAID of choice for combat operations [14].

Some military units have, in fact, developed "wound packs," which are to be taken in the event that a soldier receives a penetrating extremity wound of any type. The packs contain acetaminophen, a COX2, and a fluroquinolone. Immediately upon wounding the individual will open the pack and take these medications. The addition of acetaminophen to an NSAID has been felt to increase the degree of pain relief while not increasing sedation (Fig. 1).

Anecdotal experience in OIF showed this to be very effective in treating pain from minor penetrating soft tissue injuries (fragment wounds, an so on), although the numbers involved have thus far been small.

The risk of renal injury remains a consideration with NSAID use in the austere environment. Fortunately, the risk of this in healthy individuals is extremely small, the incidence of hospitalization for acute renal failure being 0.6 per 100,000 person years of NSAID use in individuals younger than 64 [5]. Theoretically, one would expect the incidence to be higher in individuals

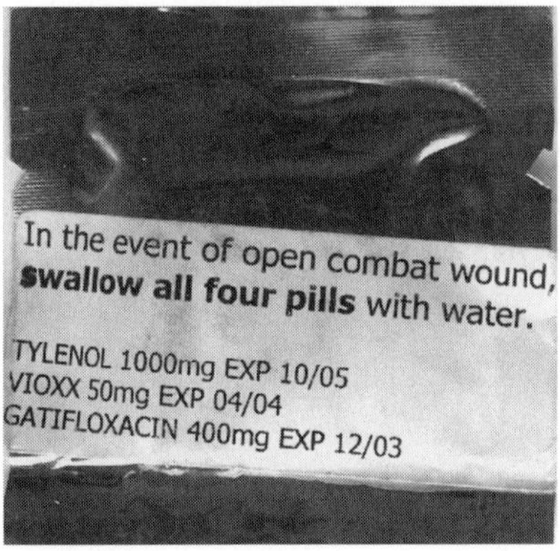

Fig. 1. Wound Pack utilized in OIF (Courtesy of Troy Johnson, MD, Washington, DC.)

with mild dehydration, as is often seen in the wilderness and combat environment. There is, however, no good data on the effect of mild dehydration on the incidence of NSAID-induced renal failure. If we assume that the increased risk of renal failure is probably similar to that seen in older individuals (> 65 years old) who often have impaired renal function due to age, medication use and other factors including volume depletion that decrease renal blood flow, then the risk from NSAID use causing renal failure incidence increases to 4.6 per 100,000 person years [5]. An increased risk to be considered, although again not a high risk.

Oral and IM NSAIDs are the most common types used; however, other forms of NSAIDs have some utility in the austere environment. Topical NSAIDS have some excellent utility in specific situations. They have been shown to be very effective for reducing pain associated with corneal abrasions [15], with a number of them approved for ophthalmologic use [16]. An ibuprofen gel for use in acute soft tissue injuries has also been found to be as effective as oral ibuprofen with obviously less gastrointestinal upset [17].

Opiates

Opiate analgesia is by far the most effective pain management drug class for severe pain. Frequently encountered situations involving injuries in the austere environment will often require opiate medication for adequate pain management. Morphine has been the standard IV opiate analgesic for operational use [18], its familiar dosing and side effect profile being the primary reason to recommend it. Opioids can be given via the oral, IM, and IV routes. IV has been the route of choice due to variable absorption and "first-pass effect" seen with oral and IM dosing methods. The IV method of delivery, however, may be difficult in the combat setting; the medical experience in the Falklands conflict found the use of IV narcotics to be impractical [19]. Specifics of opiates have been covered in depth elsewhere, so we will not repeat them here. There have been, however, some recent innovations in the use of oral opiates in the tactical setting. Oral opiates are commonly used for pain control, but up until recently oral opiate analgesia have been slow in onset and difficult to titrate to effect without having significant side effects or prolonged absorption profiles. Before OIF, several physicians in the Special Operations community addressed this problem.

Several choices were available; none were perfect. Our ideal opiate analgesic agent would have to be given orally, potentially self-administrable, have a significant safety profile, low side effect profile, and be rapid in onset. Pill-form opiate medications such as oral morphine were of limited use secondary to the prolonged time of onset and limitations in dosages. Liquid agents were limited by the significant first-pass effect of opiate metabolism and the administration and packaging in the field environment. The recent release of an oral preparation of fentanyl citrate under the trade name of Actiq appeared to fit our requirements. Actiq (Oral Transmucosal Fentanyl Citrate, OTFC) is a crystalline form of fentanyl citrate incorporated into a sweetened white lemon-flavored lozenge on a plastic handle (Fig. 2).

Fentanyl citrate is a highly lipophilic synthetic phenylpiperidine derivative that is approximately 80 to 100 times more potent than morphine, and selectively binds to the mu-1 and mu-2 receptors. OTFC is intended to be administered orally over 15 minutes, and reaches maximal serum levels after 10 to 20 minutes following administration. It undergoes metabolism in the liver and intestinal mucosa by the cytochrome P450 3A4 isozyme to an inactive metabolite, norfentanyl. The mechanism of action is both transmusocal and gastrointestinal. OTFC is rapidly absorbed through the oral mucosa, and has an onset of action of 5 to 10 minutes. Only 25% of the total dose is absorbed in this way. The rest of the medication is swallowed and absorbed through the intestinal mucosa. There is a significant first-pass metabolism with the only one third of the swallowed dose reaching the systemic circulation (25% of the total). This gives a total functional absorbed dose of 50% of the administered preparation. The mucosal-absorbed medication accounts for its rapid onset, while the swallowed preparation accounts for the duration effect. The terminal half-life is 6 to 7 hours, and serum concentration increases in a dose-dependent manner. The side effect profile also appears to follow a dose-dependent graph, with the

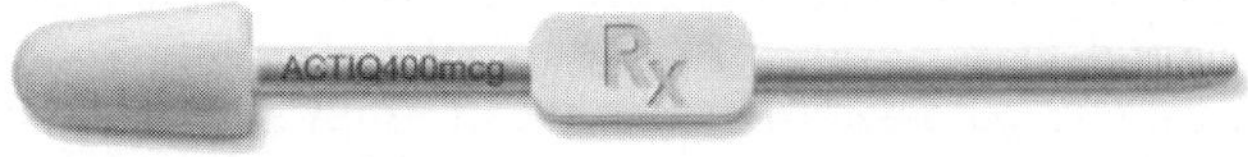

Fig. 2. Actiq Fentanyl Lozenges. (Courtesy of Troy Johnson, MD, Washington DC.)

most severe side effect, respiratory depression, starting to occur at serum levels of 2 ng/mL. This serum level is reached by using dosages greater than 800 μg [20].

Oral fentanyl citrate is Federal Drug Administration-approved as two preparations, oralet and actiq. Oralet is no long available on the market due to financial reasons. The current Federal Drug Administration approval for Actiq is for opiate-dependent pain in cancer patients that have breakthrough pain. There are several studies documenting its efficacy in this area [21–24]. Several studies using Oralet have also documented its efficacy in the hospital setting with children [25–28]. There is also one study documenting its effectiveness for the use of acute pain in the emergency department setting [29]. In a yet unpublished observational study documenting its use by Special Operations Forces in OIF, it again proved to be a safe and effective analgesic agent (Johnson T, personal communication, pending publication). The packaging held up well to significant wear and tear, and the preparation tolerated a variety of temperatures. Common side effects seen in most studies are pruritis (50–60%), vomiting (40%), and transient oxygen desaturation below 94% (0–24%). Severe side effects can include respiratory depression, bradycardia, and chest wall rigidity, but these have not been seen with standard dosing [30]. The absorption profile can also be altered by swallowing the preparation, which will delay the maximal concentration 20 to 30 minutes [30]. However, the significant first-pass metabolism will lower the serum concentration to 25% of the total swallowed dose. OTFC has been shown to have a morphine equivalency of 8 to 14:1 [31].

Overall, OTFC appears to be ideal for administering safe rapid-onset oral opiate analgesia in the prehospital austere setting.

This was used very effectively during an episode in OIF. Nine patients required care for extremity fractures simultaneously. Due to the tactical situation the placement of IVs was, at best, difficult. Of the nine patients, seven had significant fractures and all had significant pain. All were given OTFC with 90% plus reduction in pain within 15 minutes. Several fell asleep but maintained airway reflexesand oxygen saturation. Two, however, fell asleep with the "lollipop stick" hanging out of their mouth. Because of this it is recommended that the OTFC be taped to the patient's finger while they use it to prevent inadvertent choking on the same if they became somulent. Two developed nausea and one had one episode of emesis. All did well with effective pain relief during transport to definitive care.

Another opiate form recommended for austere use includes intranasal butorphanol (Stadol NS). Nasal butorphanol has been shown to be effective for postoperative pain with an onset of approximately 15 minutes [32,33]. It has also been used in the third world as a method of providing postoperative analgesia without the need for IV access [34]. The authors have no experience with this medication, although it shows promise as another method of providing rapid onset pain relief in the austere environment.

Ketamine

Ketamine, a dissociative anesthetic agent, has been used extensively as an anesthetic agent for traumatic war wounds [35,36]. Ketamine fits many of the criteria for an ideal pain control agent: it provides effective analgesia, it provides amnesia to pain and events, and the patient's airway reflexes remain intact despite dissociation. Airway reflexes are protected to the point where patients maintain oxygen saturations even while spontaneously breathing air during austere surgery [37]. Ketamine is also cardiovascularly stable, and it has both a rapid onset as well as being both relatively short acting and titrateable [38].

Ketamine has been found to be a very effective pain control method for both painful procedures, that is, in burn care [39], as well as for treating pain not otherwise well controlled by other means, that is, in refractory cancer pain [40]. It has been used as a narcotic "sparing agent" to effectively treat postoperative pain [41]. Ketamine has also been used independently as an infusion to treat postoperative pain [42]. Ketamine has also been used preoperatively as an infusion for analgesia of war-wounded individuals awaiting treatment for wounds incurred in fighting along the Thai–Cambodian border. In this situation, ketamine infusion significantly reduced pain, particularly with landmine injuries [43], and was the drug of choice for pain control in hemodynamically compromised individuals.

The doses used for analgesia are less than the typical procedural "conscious sedation doses." Recommended dose ranges are 0.44 to 1.0 mg/kg IM or 0.2 to 0.5 mg/kg IV [44,45]. The authors typically start with 0.1 mg/kg IV and titrate to effect.

In OIF, a patient with a traumatic knee fracture/dislocation was in significant pain despite IV morphine. The injury was unstable, but fortunately, the popliteal artery appeared intact. To control pain for placement of the injury in a splint as well as for transport, 0.1 mg/kg IV of ketamine was given. The patient's pain was effectively controlled, allowing stabilization of the injury and transport of the patient to definitive care.

In an incident related by a NATO physician several years earlier, ketamine was also effectively used. A patient with an ankle fracture/dislocation during a parachute training event suffered a fracture/dislocation of the ankle. The physician gave 1 mg/kg of IM ketamine, and was both able to reduce the injury as well as control pain for the patient without the need for an IV.

Author Czarnik had a similar experience with ketamine use in the emergency department. A 27-year-old male sustained an open fracture of the third to fifth metatarsals secondary to a motorcycle accident. He had no other injury and 8/10 pain. A single dose of IV ketamine at 0.5 mg/kg brought on marked pain relief, reducing the pain to 1/10. The patient remained coherent and cooperative throughout.

Because of its limited side effect profile ketamine has been suggested as an easy and effective method of pain control in mass casualty/disaster situations [46,47], the idea being that it can be used quickly on multiple individuals as a single IM injection. Ketamine has furthermore been used as an agent for intravenous anesthesia in very austere surgery. In one study it was used in Somalia and Uganda to perform a number of significant surgeries with spontaneous ventilation and no monitoring equipment [48]. It has likewise been used in diverse warfare conditions from combat injuries in the Falklands to the Thai border to conflict in Afghanistan [19]. Ketamine is not, however, without side effects, although true toxicity is extremely rare [49].

The major side effects of ketamine include "bad dreams" as well as more severe emergence phenomena. Although the "bad dreams" are not so problematic, a patient suffering emergence with access to loaded weapons in a combat zone could be a significant potential problem. The incidence of these side effects does appear to be somewhat dose related [50], with less delirium noted with typical "pain" doses. The concomitant use of benzodiazepines with the ketamine has been shown to reduce psychotomimetic side effects [51–53]. This combination, however, increases the incidence of cardiovascular and respiratory side effects, and is therefore not routinely recommended for austere use, although in the Uganda study the combination was used with little problem [48]. Falkland War experience also showed there to be no problems with emergence when diazepam was coadministered [54]. It has also been shown that the isomer makeup of ketamine determines both its potency and incidence of psychogenic side effects [55]. The typical ketamine used today is a racemic mixture of d and l forms. The d form has been shown to be more potent, and also to have less psychotomimetic side effects [55,56]. Work is being done to use the d-isomer as a pain control medication.

Ketamine is most commonly given IM or IV; however, it is also available in oral, sublingual, rectal, and nasal preparations. Oral tablets appear to have approximately 20% bioavailability. Rectal and sublingual preparations appear to be 30%, and intranasal at least 45% [57]. Intranasal ketamine is being studied for use as an intranasal pain control agent in the operational setting. When using the d-isomer, intranasal ketamine may hold promise as an effective analgesic without the requirement of an IV and with a decreased incidence of psychotomimetic side effects.

Regional anesthesia

The most often discussed and written [58] about method of wilderness [59] and operational pain control is the use of regional anesthesia, which offers many advantages for the austere environment [18]. Although the following section is written primarily from an operational standpoint, regional anesthesia works equally well in the wilderness setting.

Wounds received during military conflicts present as challenges that require medical providers to possess a mastery of manifold anesthesia management techniques to deliver optimum care. The mechanism of injury, desires of the patient, and the skills of the practitioner dictate the type of regional anesthesia administered for any military wound. This section will briefly review the physiologic variables, technical highlights, and austere environment considerations for the administration of regional anesthesia to the trauma patient. In addition, common potential complicating factors present in the trauma patient will be discussed. The regional anesthetics discussed below were used whenever time allowed. For example, numerous amputations were performed on Iraqi soldiers during the Persian Gulf War using regional anesthesia and supplemental ketamine.

Regional anesthesia has been administered in one form or another during all major conflicts involving the United States over the last 100 years [60]. It has even been used as the sole method of anesthesia for cranial surgery [61]! Its use has been limited due to sterile environment considerations and the anesthesia provider's regional anesthesia comfort level. Despite this, it has been recommended as a pain control technique of choice in mass casualty situations as it "provides complete and instantaneous pain relief...and provides an economy in personnel, time and money" [62]. There have been no studies that demonstrate a higher risk of infection with regional anesthetics administered outside of the operating room setting. The level of regional anesthesia experience among anesthesia providers varies greatly due to varying levels of emphasis demonstrated in the different training programs in the United States. This lack of training and familiarity with the involved techniques will likely present the greatest deterrent to use of regional anesthesia for austere pain control.

Regional blocks most frequently used in the austere setting include femoral blocks, ankle blocks, axillary blocks, wrist blocks, facial blocks, and digital blocks. Blocks that have been used by the authors in the field environment include all of these.

The majority of these blocks have been covered elsewhere in this text. We will, therefore, only discuss the techniques for those blocks not previously covered or where the authors have a slightly different approach. Many blocks can be performed in a variety of ways, all of which are acceptable, and dependent solely on the preference of the practitioner.

The femoral nerve block is relatively simple to administer and provides reliable anesthesia. In the hospital setting the common indications for use of femoral nerve block include knee arthroscopy, patella tendon repair, repair of patella fracture, and skin grafting from the anterior aspect of the thigh. The femoral-sciatic block, in particular, has been shown to be effective in reducing postoperative pain after outpatient knee surgery [63].

The femoral nerve originates from the L2 to L4 lumbar roots, and it descends between the psoas major and iliac muscles. In the inguinal region, the nerve is positioned anterior to the iliopsoas muscle (medial to the femoral artery) and inferior to the inguinal ligament. It innervates the muscles of the anterior thigh (quadriceps and sartorius muscles), and supplies articular branches to the hip and knee joints. Sensory branches innervate the skin of the medial thigh, medial part of the lower leg, and the medial part of the foot. With certain injuries, this regional anesthetic may mask the onset of compartment syndrome in the affected extremity; this must be considered if the femoral block is used.

The landmarks for the femoral nerve are inferior to the femoral crease. The insertion point is immediately lateral to the pulse of the femoral artery. The mnemonic NAVES is used to remember the relationship between the femoral nerve and the femoral artery. Structures are ordered lateral to medial: nerve, artery, vein, empty space, lymphatics, pubic symphysis.

To place this block, position the patient in the supine position with a fully extended lower extremity. This block may be accomplished with an iodine-based antiseptic solution and a 22-gauge 2-inch needle in addition to local anesthetic. Successful placement of the block can be performed by eliciting a paresthesia with a needle in the sensory/motor distribution of the femoral nerve. Light sedation of the patient is acceptable, but the use of the paresthesia technique requires an awake and responsive patient.

The landmark region is prepped and draped sterilely. Cutaneous anesthesia at the point of needle insertion may be obtained with a skin wheel of local anesthetic. A 2-inch 22-gauge (B bevel/dull point) needle is introduced through the skin at a 45-degree angle directed cephalad and medially toward the umbilicus. An evoked response of the rectus femoris is sought as the needle is carefully advanced. Movement of the patella indicates stimulation of the femoral nerve. If this motion is not found, the needle is brought back to the skin and redirected in a more lateral or medial direction. Once the desired nerve response is elicited, aspirate and inject the local anesthetic (0.5% bupivacaine) in 5-mL increments. A total of 30 mL of local anesthetic is usually injected [64].

In Operation Just Cause, a soldier had sustained an open tib/fib fracture from the airborne insertion. A femoral nerve block was placed, with immediate pain relief lasting several hours until the soldier could be taken to the operating room.

In Operation Desert Storm, an enemy combatant had his foot blown off in combat. A femoral nerve block allowed amputation of the remaining affected limb without pain.

Ankle blocks and brachial plexus blocks may be used to provide surgical anesthesia or pain control. The ankle block is described as the impulse blockade of the five nerves that provide motor and sensory innervation to the foot. These nerves include the superficial peroneal, deep peroneal, saphenous, sural, and tibial nerves. Procedures that lend themselves to use of an ankle block include foot debridement, amputations of toes, or short-term pain relief. Anesthesia of the medial foot requires blockade of the superficial, deep peroneal, saphenous, and tibial nerves. Surgery of the lateral aspect of the foot requires blockade of all but the saphenous nerve. The ankle block has been covered elsewhere in this text.

In Operation Desert Storm, an enemy combatant had suffered a gunshot wound to the foot. An ankle block was placed for wound debridement. The procedure as well as subsequent transport of the soldier was done without pain.

Brachial plexus anesthesia will provide excellent anesthesia to the forearm and hand. An axillary block is the most commonly performed variety of brachial plexus anesthesia. The landmarks are easy to identify, and it is associated with fewer complications than other approaches to the brachial plexus. The axillary block does not provide reliable anesthesia above the elbow.

Insert an IV in the opposite arm. With the patient lying supine the arm is abducted to about 90 degrees, externally rotated, and flexed at the elbow. Prepare the axilla using a skin sterilizing solution. Palpate the axillary artery and place a finger on its as high in the axilla as possible. Cutaneous anesthesia at the point of needle insertion may be obtained with a skin wheal of local anesthetic. Slowly advance the 2-inch 22-gauge (B bevel/dull point) needle perpendicular to the skin through the weal toward the artery. A "pop" may be felt as the needle enters the nerve sheath. Correct placement in the sheath is confirmed if the needle gently pulsates, indicating close proximity to the artery or if the patient complains of pararesthesia in nerve distribution areas. Aspirate to exclude intravascular placement of the needle and then inject the local anesthetic in 5-mL intervals. During injection aspirate again to ensure the needle has not changed position and entered a vessel. Injection is easier if an extension set (K-52 tubing) between the syringe and the needle is used. This allows the syringe to be changed without moving the needle. Some anesthesia providers elect to place a plastic cannula in the sheath for further injections. The volume of the local anesthetic injected is between 30 to 40 mL. If an arterial puncture occurs, slowly advance the needle until blood cannot be aspirated (thus indicating needle position in the nerve sheath posterior to the axillary artery) and then slowly inject 5-mL increments while watching for local anesthetic toxicity [65].

In Operation Just Cause, a soldier shot through the hand was given an axillary block. This allowed debridement of the wound as well as pain control for transport back to the United States.

Intercostal (Rib) blocks have been shown to be effective in providing immediate, sedation free pain relief in thoracic trauma, thereby reducing respiratory splinting and the pulmonary complications, which are resultant thereof [66]. Intercostal blocks have been previously covered elsewhere in this volume.

Perhaps the easiest of all blocks, the digital block, has been covered elsewhere in this text, but it is probably the most frequently used by all levels of health care providers.

The authors have used digital blocks on occasions too numerous to individually mention, both in the wilderness and combat zone settings, for injuries to the fingers as well as the toes, all with effective pain relief.

Another simple but effective block that can be used specifically in fracture pain is the hematoma block. This has been shown to be an effective method of providing analgesia for fracture reduction [67,68], and in some cases superior to IV sedation [69]. To perform the hematoma block one first sterilely preps the skin over the fracture site. One then inserts a needle into the hematoma at the fracture site, correct placement is confirmed by aspiration of blood. Local anesthesia (5–15 cc) is then injected into the hematoma. This technique should not be used in open fractures or through a dirty skin site [70].

The length of surgical procedure and duration of desired analgesia dictate the best choice of local anesthetic. Procedures lasting 1 to 1.5 hours lend themselves to the use of 3% chloroprocaine (anesthesia onset within 5–10 minutes) with 1:200,000 epinephrine. Mepivacaine or lidocaine 1.5% with 1:200,000 epinephrine will provide dense anesthesia for surgical procedures lasting 2 to 2.5 hours. Bupivacaine 0.5% with 1:200,000 epinephrine will provide anesthesia for over 4 hours. More dilute concentrations of local anesthetic (0.25% bupivacaine) may be used to provide analgesia.

In all of the blocks discussed one must be aware of the toxic doses and signs and symptoms of LA toxicity. These signs follow a pattern associated with the total dose of absorbed local anesthetic include ringing in the ears, metallic taste in the mouth, numbness of the tongue, blurred vision, drowsiness with impaired mentation, restlessness, and apprehension [71]. With larger doses delirium may progress to overt seizure activity. Asphyxia leading to metabolic and respiratory acidosis with cardiac depression and eventual cardiac arrest may develop if the convulsions are not treated rapidly and adequately. Treatment is aimed at maintaining the airway and suppressing seizures. In general, slow intermittent injection and close observation of patient status will prove to be the best safeguard against local anesthetic toxicity.

The use of regional anesthesia is an effective alternative to the use of general anesthesia for both surgical procedures as well as for effective pain control in an austere environment. With practice, the provider can safely administer local anesthesia for nerve blocks in a very expedient manner. The pain relief obtained and patient satisfaction achieved by the authors has shown that regional blocks with IV sedation are a very adequate technique for health care providers. The greatest limitation to use of these techniques is a lack of familiarity and experience with them by medical providers. The authors therefore recommend their increased use in training programs to overcome this shortfall.

Nonpharmacologic pain control

In addition to pharmacologic pain control, several other techniques have been described and used for austere environments. These include the physical pain relief modalities of splinting, compression, cold and heat therapy, as well as the complimentary medical technique of acupuncture [72].

Splinting is a well-known and used technique, which provides pain control by preventing further injury and nerve stimulation by inhibiting movement of injured extremities. It will not be covered, as there is only reason to recommend its continued use and no recommendations against, based on practical experience as well as literature review.

Compression anesthesia tends to be an inadvertent result of wrapping an injured limb either for splinting or hemostasis of bleeding. This typically occurs as an ace wrap is placed over a gauze hemostatic dressing. The resultant compression may also compress the involved peripheral nerves leading to distal anesthesia [73]. Placing a proximal compression bandage on a limb proximal to the injury can likewise induce this.

The authors do not recommend this technique, but if it is used, one must be extremely careful to ensure the paresthesia is not a sign of compartment syndrome.

Cryoanalgesia or application of cold to decrease pain has been used for soft tissue injuries for centuries. This may be done with ice packs, snow, cold water compresses, or commercial cold packs. The standard recommendation is to place a towel or other barrier between the skin and cold pack and apply it for 15 to 20 minutes every few hours [74]. Care must be taken to not cause cold injury to the underlying tissues. Cold application has been shown to have variable efficacy, from no effect [75] to effective in decreasing pain, depending on how it is applied as well as what the treatment is for [76]. If one is careful to avoid cold injury to the tissue, however, there is little downside, and this adjunctive technique is recommended. Heat therapy has not been shown to be particularly effective for acute pain control, and is therefore not recommended.

Acupuncture is another complimentary medicine technique that has been suggested for use in austere pain management [72]. Developed in austere settings thousands of years ago in Asia, acupuncture has been found to be of benefit in certain conditions [77]. It has also shown promise in use in the wilderness setting [78,79]. The supplies themselves are lightweight and compact. Unfortunately, acupuncture requires lengthy prior training. Given the positive recommendations of the National Institutes of Health Consensus Panel on Acupuncture it seems that this is a modality of potential adjunctive use for pain control in the hands of a properly skilled provider.

The austere wilderness and operational setting puts increased strain on injured individuals and those attempting to asses and treat the pain of the injured. We have attempted to cover some of the unique aspects of pain control in these settings. It is hoped this information will both aid the provider going into the austere environment as well as initiate further discussion and research in this area.

References

[1] Garibaldi JA, Elder MF. Evaluation of ketorolac with varying amounts of codeine for postoperative extraction pain control. Int J Oral Maxillofac Surg 2002;31(3):276–80.
[2] Gillis JC, Brogden RN. Ketorolac. A reappraisal of its pharmacodynamic and pharmickinetic properties and therapeutic use in pain management. Drugs 1997;53(1):139–88.
[3] Lewis SC, Langman MJ, Lapoetl JR, et al. Dose–response relationships between individual nonaspirin nonsteroidal anti-inflammatory drugs (NANSAIDs) and serious upper gastrointestinal bleeding: a meta-analysis based on individual patient data. Br J Clin Pharmacol 2002;54(3):320–6.
[4] Adamopoulos A, Efstathiou S, Tsioulos D, et al. Acute upper gastrointestinal bleeding: comparison between recent users and nonusers of nonsteroidal anti-inflammatory drugs. Endoscopy 2003;35(4):327–32.
[5] Gutthan P, Perez GS, Garcia RL, et al. Nonsteroidal anti-inflammatory drugs and the risk of hospitalization for acute renal failure. Arch Intern Med 1996;156:2433–9.
[6] Epstein M. Non-steroidal anti-inflammatory drugs and the continuum of renal dysfunction. J Hypertens 2002;20(Suppl 6):S17–23.
[7] Buttar N, Wang K. The "aspirin" of the new millennium: cyclooxygenase-2 inhibitors. Mayo Clin Proc 2000;75:1027–38.
[8] Hawkey CJ, Laine L, Simon T, et al. Incidence of gastroduodenal ulcers in patients with rheumatoid arthritis after 12 weeks of rofecxib, naproxen or placebo: a multicentre, randomized, double blind study. Gut 2003;52(6):820–6.
[9] Giovanni G, Giovanni P. Do non-steroidal anti-inflammatory drugs and COX-2 selective inhibitors have different renal effects? J Nephrol 2002;15(5):480–8.
[10] Papaioannides D, Bouropoulos C, Sinapides D, et al. Acute renal dysfunction associated with selective COX-2 inhibitor therapy. Intern Urol Nephr 2001;33(4):609–11.
[11] Katz N. Coxibs: evolving role in pain management. Semin Arthritis Rheum 2002;32(3 Suppl 1):15–24.
[12] Chavez NL, DeKorte CJ. Valdecoxib:a review. Clin Ther 2003;25(3):817–51.
[13] McCrory C, Lindahl SGE. Cyclooxygenase inhibition for postoperative analgesia. Anesth Analg 2002;95:169–76.
[14] The Committee on Tactical Combat Casualty Care. Tactical combat casualty care. In: The prehospital trauma life support anual. 5th edition. The Committee on Tactical Combat Casualty Care. St. Louis (MO): Mosby; 2003.
[15] Weaver CS, Terrell KM. Evidence based emergency medicine. Update: do ophthalmic nonsteroidal anti-inflammatory drugs reduce the pain associated with simple corneal abrasion without delaying healing? Ann Emerg Med 2003;41(1):134–40.
[16] Schalnus R. Topical nonsteroidal anti-inflammatory therapy in ophthalmology. Opthalmologica 2003;217(2):89–98.
[17] Whitefield M, O'Kane CJ, Anderson S. Comparative efficacy of a proprietary topical ibuprofen gel and oral ibuprofen in acute soft tissue injuries: a randomized, double blind study. J Clin Pharmacol Ther 2002;27(6):409–17.
[18] Anesthesia and analgesia. In: Emergency war surgery Nato handbook. 2nd revision. US Government Printing Office, Washington DC, 1988.
[19] Jowitt MD, Knight RJ. Anaesthesia during the Falklands campaign the land battles. Anaesthesia 1983;38(8):776–83.

[20] The FDA Center of Drug Evaluation and Research. Application Number NDA 20747. Oct 1998.
[21] O'Mahony S. Multidisciplinary care of the terminally ill patient. Surg Clin North Am 2000; 80(2):729–45.
[22] Carver AC. Symptom assessment and management. Neurol Clin 2001;19(4):921–47.
[23] Li JM. Pain management in the hospitalized patient. Med Clin North Am 2002;86(4): 771–95.
[24] Coluzzi PH. Breakthrough cancer pain: a randomized trial comparing oral transmucosal fentanyl citrate (OTFC) and morphine sulfate immediate release (MSIR). Pain 2001;91(1–2): 123–30.
[25] Proudfoot J. Analgesia, anesthesia, and conscious sedation. Emerg Med Clin North Am 1995;13:357–79.
[26] Sacchetti A, Schafermeyer R, Gerardi M, et al. Pediatric analgesia and sedation. Ann Emerg Med 1994;23:237–50.
[27] Ashburn MA, Streisand JB, Tarver SD, et al. Oral transmucosal fentanyl citrate for premedication in pediatric outpatients. Can J Anesth 1990;37:857–66.
[28] Schutzman SA, Burg J, Liebelt E, et al. Oral transmucosal fentanyl citrate for premedication of children undergoing laceration repair. Ann Emerg Med 1994;24:1059–64.
[29] Lind GH, Marcus MA, Mears SL, et al. Oral transmucosal fentanyl citrate for analgesia and sedation in the emergency department. Ann Emerg Med 1991;20:1117–20.
[30] Wheeler M. Uptake pharmacokinetics of the Fentanyl Oralet in children scheduled for central venous access removal: implications for the timing of initiating painful procedures. Paediatr Anaesth 2002;12(7):594–9.
[31] Lichtor JL, Sevaning FB, Joshi GP, et al. The realative potency of oral transmucosal fentanyl citrate compared with intravenous morphine in the treatment of moderate to severe postoperative pain. Anesth Analg 1999;89(3):732–42.
[32] Desjardins PJ, Norris LH, Cooper SA, et al. Analgesic efficacy of intranasal butorphanol (Stadol NS) in the treatment of pain after dental impaction surgery. J Oral Maxillofac Surg 2000;58(10 Suppl. 2):19–26.
[33] Bennie RE, et al. Transnasal butorphanol is effective for postoperative pain relief in children undergoing myringotomy. Anesthesiology 1998;89(2):385–90.
[34] Tobias JD, Rasmussen GE. Transnasal butorphanol for postoperative analgesia following paediatric surgery in a third world country. Paediatr Anaesth 1995;5(1):63–6.
[35] Levin JM, Bornstein LA. The treatment of burns in the recent Middle East conflict. Plast Reconstr Surg 1974;54(4):432–6.
[36] Bion JF. Infusion analgesia for acute war injuries: a comparison of pentazocine and ketamine. Anaesthesia 1984;39:560–4.
[37] Pesonen P. Pulse oximitry during ketamine anaesthesia in war conditions. Can J Anaesth 1991;38(5):592–4.
[38] Cohen ML, Chan SL, Way WL, et al. Distribution in the brain and metabolism of Ketamine in the rat after intravenous administration. Anesthesiology 1973;39:370–6.
[39] Pal Sk, Cortiella J, Herndon D. Adjunctive methods of pain control in burns. Burns 1997; 23(5):404–12.
[40] McQueen AL, Baroletti SA. Adjuvant Ketamine analgesia for the management of cancer pain. Ann Pharmacother 2002;36(10):1614–9.
[41] Javery KB, et al. Comparison of morphine and morphine with Ketamine for postoperative analgesia. Can J Anaesth 1996;43(3):212–5.
[42] Stehle R. Anesthesiological care in a field hospital in Thailand with special regard to ketamine. Anaesthesist 1983;32(3):130–3.
[43] Bion JF. Infusion analgesia for acute war injuries: a comparison of pentazocine and ketamine. Anaesthesia 1984;39:560–4.
[44] Bennet RC, Stewart RD. Ketamine. In: Paris PM, Stewart RD, editors. Pain management in emergency medicine. Norwalk (CT): Appleton & Lange; 1988. p. 295–310.

[45] Sadove MS, Shulman M, Hatano S, et al. Analgesic effects of ketamine administered in subdissociative doses. Anaesth Analg 1971;50(3):452–7.
[46] Bonica JJ. Pain control in mass casualties. In: Manni C, Magalini SI, editors. Emergency and disaster medicine: proceedings of the Third World Congress in Rome, 1983. Berlin: Springer-Verlag; 1985. p. 151–66.
[47] Dick W, Hirlinger WK, Mehrkens HH. Intramuscular ketamine: an alternative pain treatment for use in disasters? In: Manni C, Magalini SI, editors. Emergency and disaster medicine: proceedings of the Third World Congress in Rome, 1983. Berlin: Springer-Verlag; 1985. p. 167–72.
[48] Bonanno FG. Ketamine in war/tropical surgery (a final tribute to the racemic mixture). Injury 2002;33(4):323–7.
[49] Gren SM, Clark R, Hostetler MA, et al. Inadvertent ketamine overdose in children: clinical manifestations and outcome. Ann Emerg Med 1999;34:492–7.
[50] Liang HS, Liang HG. Minimizing emergence phenomena: subdissociative dosage of ketamine in balanced surgical aesthesia. Anesth Analg 1975;54:312–6.
[51] Beekhuis GJ, Kahn DL, Klegon RB, et al. Anesthesia for facial cosmetic surgery: low dosage ketamine-diazepam anesthesia. Laryngoscope 1978;88:1709–12.
[52] Tucker MR, Hann JR, Phillips CL, et al. Subanesthetic doses of ketamine, diazepam and nitrous oxide for adult outpatient sedation. J Oral Maxillofac Surg 1984;42:668–72.
[53] Cartwright PD, Pingel SM. Midazolam and diazepam in ketamine anesthesia. Anaesthesia 1984;39:439–42.
[54] Bull PT, et al. Anaesthesia during the Falklands campaign, the experience of the Royal Navy. Anaesthesia 1983;38:770–5.
[55] White PF, Ham J, Way WL, et al. Pharmacology of ketamine isomers in surgical patients. Anesthesiology 1980;52:231–9.
[56] White PF, Schuttler J, Shafer A, et al. Comparative pharmacology of the ketamine isomers: studies in volunteers. Br J Anaesth 1985;57:197–203.
[57] Yanagihara Y, Ohtan M, Kariya S, et al. Plasma concentration profiles of ketamine and norketamine after administration of various ketamine preparations to healthy Japanese volunteers. Biopharmaceut Drug Disp 2003;24(1):37–43.
[58] Calkins MD, Kuzma PJ, Larkin TM, et al. Pain management in the special operations environment: regional anesthetics. Mil Med 2001;166:211–6.
[59] Dickison AE. Pain management in the field. In: Wilderness medical society summer conference & annual meeting compendium. Colorado Springs (CO): Wilderness Medical Society; 2001. p. 189–211.
[60] Barton CR, Beeson M. Anesthesia for trauma during wartime. CRNA 1997;8(1):2–12.
[61] Medell RJ, et al. Field block for cranial surgery in World War II. Mil Med 1998;163(2):80–3.
[62] Whiffler K, Leiman BC. The application of regional anesthesia in a disaster situation. S Afr Med J 1983;63:409–10.
[63] Williams BA, Kentor ML, Vogt MT et al. Femoral-sciatic blocks for complex outpatient knee surgery are associated with less postoperative pain before same day discharge: a review of 1,200 consecutive cases from the period 1996–1999: Anesthesiology 2003;98(5):1206–13.
[64] Vloka JD, Hadzic A, Drobnik L, et al. Anatomical landmarks for femoral nerve block: a comparison of four needle insertion sites. Anesth Analg 1999;89:1467–70.
[65] Zenz M. Brachial plexus block—the axillary approach. In: Horester W, et al, editor. Regional anesthesia. 2nd edition. St Louis (MO): Mosby; 1990. p. 66–72.
[66] Desai SM, Bernhard WN, McAlary B. Regional anesthesia: management considerations in the trauma patient. Crit Care Clin 1990;6(1):85–101.
[67] The efficacy and safety of the hematoma block for fracture reduction in closed, isolated fractures. Orthopedics 1997;20(5):423–6.
[68] Alioto RJ, Furia JP, Maruart JD. Hematoma block for ankle fractures: a safe and efficacious technique for manipulations. J Orthop Trauma 1995;9(2):113–6.

[69] Singh GK, et al. Analgesia for reduction of Colles fracture. A comparison of hematoma block and intravenous sedation. J Curr Clin Trials 1992;23 (Online).
[70] Orlinsky M, Dean E. Local and topical anesthesia. In: Roberts JR, Hedges JR, editors. Clinical procedures in emergency medicine. 3rd edition. Philidelphia: WB Saunders; 1998. p. 464–5.
[71] Naguib M, et al. Adverse effects and drug interactions associated with local and regional anesthesia. Drug Saf 1998;18:221–50.
[72] Frank BL. Principles of pain management. In: Auerbach PS, editor. Wilderness medicine. 4th edition. St. Louis (MO): Mosby; 2001. p. 399–412.
[73] Madigan SR, Raj PP. History and current status pain management. In: Raj PP, editor. Practical management of pain. 2nd edition. St. Louis (MO): Mosby; 1992.
[74] Swenson C, Sward L, Karlsson J. Cryotherapy in sports medicine. Scand J Med Sci Sports 1996;6(4):193–200.
[75] Konrath GA, Lock T, Gontz HT, et al. The use of cold therapy after anterior cruciate ligament reconstruction. A prospective, randomized study and literature review. Am J Sports Med 1996;24(5):629–33.
[76] Albrecht S, et al. Cryotherapy as analgesic technique in direct, postoperative treatment following elective joint replacement. Z Orthop Ihre Grenzgeb 1997;135(1):45–51.
[77] NHI Consensus Conference. Acupuncture. JAMA 1998;280(17):1518–24.
[78] Frank BL. Medical acupuncture enhances standard wilderness medical care: a case study from the Inca trail, Machu Picchu, Peru, April 2, 1997. Wild Environ Med 1997;8(3):161–3.
[79] Frank BL. Medical acupuncture and wilderness medicine; an integrated medical model in the third world setting. Med Acupuncture 1996;8:11–4.

EMERGENCY MEDICINE CLINICS OF NORTH AMERICA

Emerg Med Clin N Am 23 (2005) 603–608

Index

Note: Page numbers of article titles are in **boldface** type.

doi:10.1016/S0733-8627(05)00032-5

Changing Your Address?

Make sure your subscription changes too! When you notify us of your new address, you can help make our job easier by including an exact copy of your Clinics label number with your old address (see illustration below.) This number identifies you to our computer system and will speed the processing of your address change. Please be sure this label number accompanies your old address and your corrected address—you can send an old Clinics label with your number on it or just copy it exactly and send it to the address listed below.

We appreciate your help in our attempt to give you continuous coverage. Thank you.

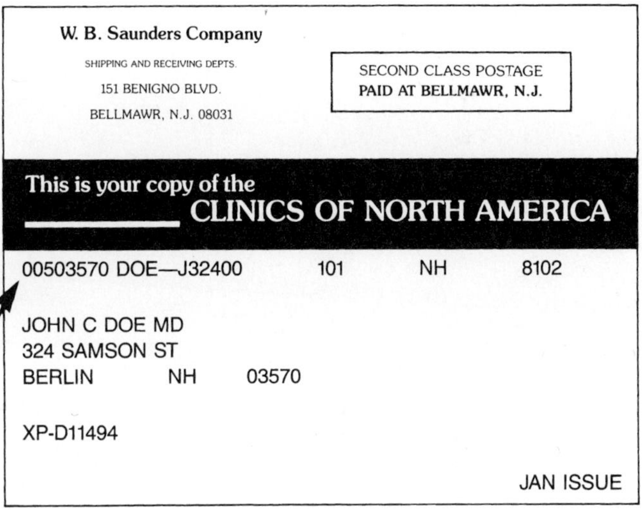

W. B. Saunders Company
SHIPPING AND RECEIVING DEPTS.
151 BENIGNO BLVD.
BELLMAWR, N.J. 08031

SECOND CLASS POSTAGE
PAID AT BELLMAWR, N.J.

This is your copy of the
________ CLINICS OF NORTH AMERICA

00503570 DOE—J32400 101 NH 8102

JOHN C DOE MD
324 SAMSON ST
BERLIN NH 03570

XP-D11494

JAN ISSUE

Your Clinics Label Number

Copy it exactly or send your label along with your address to:
W.B. Saunders Company, Customer Service
Orlando, FL 32887-4800
Call Toll Free 1-800-654-2452

Please allow four to six weeks for delivery of new subscriptions and for processing address changes.

Order your subscription today. Simply complete and detach this card and drop it in the mail to receive the best clinical information in your field.

YES! Please start my subscription to the **CLINICS** checked below with the ❑ first issue of the calendar year or ❑ current issues. If not completely satisfied with my first issue, I may write "cancel" on the invoice and return it within 30 days at no further obligation.

Please Print:

Name ______________________

Address ______________________

City ______________ State ____________ ZIP __________

Method of Payment

❑ Check (payable to **Elsevier**; add the applicable sales tax for your area)

❑ VISA ❑ MasterCard ❑ AmEx ❑ Bill me

Card number ______________ Exp. date __________

Signature ______________________

Staple this to your purchase order to expedite delivery

❑ **Adolescent Medicine Clinics**
- ❑ Individual $95
- ❑ Institutions $133
- ❑ *In-training $48

❑ **Anesthesiology**
- ❑ Individual $175
- ❑ Institutions $270
- ❑ *In-training $88

❑ **Cardiology**
- ❑ Individual $170
- ❑ Institutions $266
- ❑ *In-training $85

❑ **Chest Medicine**
- ❑ Individual $185
- ❑ Institutions $285

❑ **Child and Adolescent Psychiatry**
- ❑ Individual $175
- ❑ Institutions $265
- ❑ *In-training $88

❑ **Critical Care**
- ❑ Individual $165
- ❑ Institutions $266
- ❑ *In-training $83

❑ **Dental**
- ❑ Individual $150
- ❑ Institutions $242

❑ **Emergency Medicine**
- ❑ Individual $170
- ❑ Institutions $263
- ❑ *In-training $85
- ❑ Send CME info

❑ **Facial Plastic Surgery**
- ❑ Individual $199
- ❑ Institutions $300

❑ **Foot and Ankle**
- Individual $160
- Institutions $232

❑ **Gastroenterology**
- ❑ Individual $190
- ❑ Institutions $276

❑ **Gastrointestinal Endoscopy**
- ❑ Individual $190
- ❑ Institutions $276

❑ **Hand**
- ❑ Individual $205
- ❑ Institutions $319

❑ **Heart Failure (NEW in 2005!)**
- ❑ Individual $99
- ❑ Institutions $149
- ❑ *In-training $49

❑ **Hematology/ Oncology**
- ❑ Individual $210
- ❑ Institutions $315

❑ **Immunology & Allergy**
- ❑ Individual $165
- ❑ Institutions $266

❑ **Infectious Disease**
- ❑ Individual $165
- ❑ Institutions $272

❑ **Clinics in Liver Disease**
- ❑ Individual $165
- ❑ Institutions $234

❑ **Medical**
- ❑ Individual $140
- ❑ Institutions $244
- ❑ *In-training $70
- ❑ Send CME info

❑ **MRI**
- ❑ Individual $190
- ❑ Institutions $290
- ❑ *In-training $95
- ❑ Send CME info

❑ **Neuroimaging**
- ❑ Individual $190
- ❑ Institutions $290
- ❑ *In-training $95
- ❑ Send CME inf0

❑ **Neurologic**
- ❑ Individual $175
- ❑ Institutions $275

❑ **Obstetrics & Gynecology**
- ❑ Individual $175
- ❑ Institutions $288

❑ **Occupational and Environmental Medicine**
- ❑ Individual $120
- ❑ Institutions $166
- ❑ *In-training $60

❑ **Ophthalmology**
- ❑ Individual $190
- ❑ Institutions $325

❑ **Oral & Maxillofacial Surgery**
- ❑ Individual $180
- ❑ Institutions $280
- ❑ *In-training $90

❑ **Orthopedic**
- ❑ Individual $180
- ❑ Institutions $295
- ❑ *In-training $90

❑ **Otolaryngologic**
- ❑ Individual $199
- ❑ Institutions $350

❑ **Pediatric**
- ❑ Individual $135
- ❑ Institutions $246
- ❑ *In-training $68
- ❑ Send CME info

❑ **Perinatology**
- ❑ Individual $155
- ❑ Institutions $237
- ❑ *In-training $78
- ❑ Send CME inf0

❑ **Plastic Surgery**
- ❑ Individual $245
- ❑ Institutions $370

❑ **Podiatric Medicine & Surgery**
- ❑ Individual $170
- ❑ Institutions $266

❑ **Primary Care**
- ❑ Individual $135
- ❑ Institutions $223

❑ **Psychiatric**
- ❑ Individual $170
- ❑ Institutions $288

❑ **Radiologic**
- ❑ Individual $220
- ❑ Institutions $331
- ❑ *In-training $110
- ❑ Send CME info

❑ **Sports Medicine**
- ❑ Individual $180
- ❑ Institutions $277

❑ **Surgical**
- ❑ Individual $190
- ❑ Institutions $299
- ❑ *In-training $95

❑ **Thoracic Surgery (formerly Chest Surgery)**
- ❑ Individual $175
- ❑ Institutions $255
- ❑ *In-training $88

❑ **Urologic**
- ❑ Individual $195
- ❑ Institutions $307
- ❑ *In-training $98
- ❑ Send CME info

*To receive in-training rate, orders must be accompanied by the name of affiliated institution, dates of residency and signature of coordinator on institution letterhead. Orders will be billed at the individual rate until proof of resident status is received.